Ethical Issues and Security Monitoring Trends in Global Healthcare:

Technological Advancements

Steven A. Brown
Capella University, USA

Mary Brown
Capella University, USA

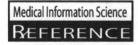

MEDICAL INFORMATION SCIENCE REFERENCE

Hershey · New York

Senior Editorial Director:	Kristin Klinger
Director of Book Publications:	Julia Mosemann
Editorial Director:	Lindsay Johnston
Acquisitions Editor:	Erika Carter
Development Editor:	Joel Gamon
Typesetters:	Michael Brehm and Milan Vracarich, Jr.
Production Coordinator:	Jamie Snavely
Cover Design:	Nick Newcomer

Published in the United States of America by
Medical Information Science Reference (an imprint of IGI Global)
701 E. Chocolate Avenue
Hershey PA 17033
Tel: 717-533-8845
Fax: 717-533-8661
E-mail: cust@igi-global.com
Web site: http://www.igi-global.com/reference

Library of Congress Cataloging-in-Publication Data

Ethical issues and security monitoring trends in global healthcare :
technological advancements / Steven A. Brown and Mary Brown, editors.
       p. cm.
  Summary: "This book identifies practices and strategies being developed
using the new technologies that are available and the impact that these tools
might have on public health and safety practices"-- Provided by publisher.
  Includes bibliographical references and index.
  ISBN 978-1-60960-174-4 (hardcover) -- ISBN 978-1-60960-176-8 (ebook) 1.
Medical care--Technological innovations. 2. Medical technology--Moral and
ethical aspects. 3. Medical care--Safety measures. I. Brown, Steven A.,
1962- II. Brown, Mary, 1955-
  R855.3.E84 2011
  362.1--dc22
                              2010051760

British Cataloguing in Publication Data
A Cataloguing in Publication record for this book is available from the British Library.

Table of Contents

Section 1
Trends in Global Healthcare

Section 2
Security in the Healthcare Industry

Section 3
Ethical Implications of Security Monitoring In in Health Care

Detailed Table of Contents

Section 1
Trends in Global Healthcare

Chapter 1

    Mary Brown, Capella University, USA

Federal incentives and regulations are being offered to healthcare stakeholders in order to accelerate the adoption of electronic health systems and health exchange networks. These technologies will be used to support widespread health outcomes research with the goal of identifying superior outcomes and reducing the cost of healthcare. This chapter looks at the impact these technologies and outcomes research might have on the rationing of healthcare.

Chapter 2

    John Beswetherick, Capella University, USA

The increase in the use of electronic health systems results in the need to consider the impact on privacy. The disabled, as a result of more frequent interactions with the health system tend to generate more sensitive health data more frequently than the average person. This chapter looks at strategies to support the privacy rights of disabled individuals as related to their personally identifiable health information.

Chapter 3

    Terry Dillard, Dillard Systems, LLC

The European "Directive of Data Protection" is the framework for a number of international data privacy laws designed to provide direction to organizations as to how data can and cannot be shared. This chapter explores the details of these laws including the challenges in compliance and enforcement. Available technological solutions are identified as support for addressing some of those challenges.

The healthcare industry has advanced the use of Electronic Health Records making a large amount of health data available via the Internet. There are potential benefits and challenges providers will face when attempting to leverage the Internet to engage in bio-surveillance and other public health monitoring activities. This chapter offers insight into some of the obstacles that have the potential to impede these activities.

The healthcare industry is not unique in looking for methods to save operating expenses. One potential solution being adopted includes the use of self-service kiosks that allow patients to control their own information and to make their own appointments. This chapter describes some of the ways that this technology is being implemented within the healthcare industry.

Scotland is, like the rest of the developed world, moving towards integration of technology into core healthcare processes. This chapter replicates an earlier study to evaluate the readiness of the Scottish health system to adopt these new technologies.

Section 2
Security in the Healthcare Industry

As the healthcare industry moves more rapidly towards adoption of electronic medical records and other forms of electronic decision support systems it becomes more critical that there are effective business continuity and disaster recovery plans in place to ensure continuation of business in the face of a potential event. This chapter identifies some of the potential technologies and strategies that are available to healthcare organizations interested in ensuring they are prepared to handle a loss of access or availability of the data needed to engage in core business processes.

Chapter 8

Vasupradha Vasudevan, Management Sciences and System, USA
H.R. Rao, Management Sciences and System, USA

The move to electronic collection and storage of health data have had an impact on the potential discovery of evidence that happens as part of healthcare litigation. This chapter explores the impact that adoption of new technologies has had on healthcare litigation and on the activities involving e-discovery of evidence useful in litigation.

Chapter 9

Omotunde Adeyemo, TEKsystems, USA

The information security field, particularly in regulated industries including the healthcare industry, is more often considering two factor authentications as the minimum standard for securing sensitive health information. This chapter explores the use of biometrics as an effective solution for meeting the criteria of strong authentication.

Chapter 10

Bandar Alhaqbani, Queensland University of Technology, Australia
Colin J. Fidge, Queensland University of Technology, Australia

Some of the challenges to widespread use and sharing of health data for outcomes research include ensuring the quality and privacy of the data. This chapter proposes a formal methodology for validating the trustworthiness of medical data.

Chapter 11

Dennis Backherms, Capella University, USA

Biometric solutions come in a range of methodologies and approaches. This chapter reviews some of the ways that biometrics can be integrated into a healthcare data security framework, in particular, as a means to combat the potential for using patient data for identity theft which has become a more frequent issue within the industry.

Section 3
Ethical Implications of Security Monitoring In in Health Care

Chapter 12

RFID technologies are finding their way into a variety of healthcare applications. This chapter explores some of these applications of RFID and the ethical implications that are a part of these implementations.

Chapter 13

The healthcare system has been moving at an accelerated pace towards adoption of electronic data collection and storage. An additional component of this shift in practice involves the connectivity of this electronic health data with the Internet. This chapter explores some of the ethical implications of making sensitive health information available via the Internet.

Chapter 14

The field of nursing has been uniquely impacted by the introduction of technology into the healthcare field. This chapter considers some of the ethical issues that nurses are facing from local to national and even international perspectives.

Chapter 15

The history of technology adoption within the healthcare industry has been fractured and has developed within a number of silo systems. This chapter is intended as an analysis and evaluation of the approach that the healthcare industry has so far adopted and includes recommendations for how the industry might change this approach for more effective use of technology to treat patients.

Foreword

In today's global environment, the protection of patient privacy, compliance with regulations, effectiveness and efficiency of collaboration, and ability to control costs are all key necessities for healthcare professionals. Healthcare also continues to be focused on the impact of electronic health records (EHRs), gaining higher utilization rates, and achieving interoperability. The challenge of meeting each of these respective key requirements is concurrently protecting private patient information. In their book, *Ethical Issues and Security Monitoring Trends in Global Healthcare*, Drs. Steven and Mary Brown provide a comprehensive look at ongoing technology advances within the healthcare industry. The comprehensive approach taken in the book provides the reader in-depth insight to the challenges facing the industry with regards to the use and implementation of information technology. Recognizing the challenges are vast, the Drs. Brown provide recommendations and considerations that should be taken into account by all healthcare professionals working to more effectively streamline their operations. This book is a must read for all those interested in understanding the challenges and concerns related to the protection of patient information and the use of technology.

Brett Miller

Preface

The cost of care today has created incentives for many of the stakeholders within the healthcare industry and government health agencies to devote time and resources towards acceleration of technology adoption to help manage those costs. While individual countries approach how to integrate technology into their own particular healthcare system depending on their own cultures and experience, this book demonstrates that regardless, they are all increasingly reliant on the use of technology to create efficiencies in those systems.

The first section of this book is designed to elaborate on some of the new trends within health technologies. The healthcare industry has long operated using paper records along with a combination of silo-based clinical specialization systems. There is a significant push going on in the United States, Europe and in other developing countries. The United Kingdom, in particular, has been one of the leaders of leading technology trends within the healthcare industry.

The first chapter speaks to one of the most comprehensive and far reaching healthcare technology efforts that are currently under way in the United States. This project is an extension of previous efforts by the federal government to accelerate the use of Electronic Health Records (EHR). There has been sufficient progress made towards this adoption that the legislative efforts have shifted focus to the potential uses of this electronic data that is being collected and stored via EHRs. One of the primary uses facilitated through the most recent legislation directed at economic stimulus and health reform includes the creation of the technical, procedural, semantic framework that is necessary to engage in widespread, large scale medical research projects. These medical research projects are expected to identify superior therapies and medications which will be applied to best practice. The assumption is that through creation of a National Health Information Network (NHIN) to allow for easy exchange of large amounts of health data these best practices can be identified and integrated into the system in such a way as to reduce the cost of healthcare delivery. This form of research is known as Comparative Effectiveness Research (CER). One of the biggest potential barriers to the success of the NHIN and CER is the perception that this will result in rationing of healthcare. The proponents of the NHIN and CER are pouring substantial financial incentives into the system to advance their usage, while the opponents of the NHIN and CER are pledging to 'repeal and replace' much of what has been proposed.

The 2nd chapter in the book identifies the impact of technology adoption on the privacy rights of disabled individuals. The author makes a case for the fact that disabled individuals have the potential to be more directly impacted by potential privacy threats of electronic health data. This increase in the potential risk relates to the fact that the disabled are more likely to have private medical issues that could present barriers in insurance and employment. The disabled population is also more likely to be more often seen by more individual providers than their able bodied peers. These more frequent interactions with the healthcare system that generates more sensitive health information puts this population at higher risk of having the information compromised.

The move towards electronic health data collection and storage has motivated stakeholders within the healthcare industry to explore technical controls to assist with the protection of this data. The Hippocratic Database and Active Enforcement are examples of technologies being proposed to accomplish this goal through granular access and audit controls built in to clinical systems. The author outlines how these technologies can be used to support protection of health data and makes a case for how it can also be helpful in meeting more stringent health protection laws that impact the global use and exchange of health data.

The National Health Information Network (NHIN) is one of the most ambitious proposals of how technology can be used to support the healthcare industry among a number of proposals. The preliminary efforts towards creation of the NHIN involve several federal agencies and a small handful of private providers. The intent is to leverage the Internet as the backbone for this network and the existing pilot is intended to prove the viability of this approach. The author identifies a range of potential barriers and challenges that have the potential to impede or prevent these plans from coming to fruition.

One of the objectives behind the promotion of accelerated adoption of technology by governments all over the developed world is the need or desire to reduce the cost of administering healthcare. This author identifies one approach being used in the UK that will reduce the cost of maintaining patient demographic and activity information by providing a kiosk approach that allows patients to do their own data entry into these systems. The various kiosk solutions that are available to fill this role are explored and the benefits and challenges of their use are explored, as well.

The final chapter in this section of the book consists of a study that looks at the readiness of the Scottish health system to leverage the principles and benefits of eHealth solutions. The study is a follow-up of a previous study and is meant to confirm or deny the results of that previous study.

The second section of the book involves a look at the security solutions that are being implemented in the healthcare industry in response to the adoption of changing trends and new technologies.

The move towards electronic health records has created a new and more urgent need for healthcare providers to have and maintain an aggressive and comprehensive disaster recovery and business continuity program. Failure to invest time and resources in hardware, software and data redundancy can be a fatal mistake for healthcare providers who will no longer have a paper record to use as backup. This author explores the important components that are critical to an effective disaster recovery and business continuity plan for those organizations that have made the move to electronic health data collection and storage.

Those information security professionals that work in the finance industry have long been aware of the potential for risks pertaining to discovery of electronic data as part of a criminal or civil lawsuit. As the healthcare industry moves towards electronic data collection and storage the potential for the industry to face some of these same risks increases as well. This author explores some of those unexpected outcomes and offers advice as to how healthcare organizations might mitigate some of those risks.

The healthcare industry has been identified by criminals as high potential for engaging in identify theft. The industry has long collected and used social security numbers as a means to differentiate patients and as a part of their payment process. Much of the risk and activity involving identify theft involves trusted insiders making this particular problem particularly tough for the industry to manage. This author explores the role that biometric controls might play in mitigation of the risk of identity theft by associating this biometric with a transaction.

A large challenge facing those who are working towards widespread, large scale health research projects is having the tools necessary to evaluate the trustworthiness of this data that is coming from a large number of different providers. There are a range of factors that contribute to trustworthiness including accuracy, validity, rigor in collection processes, integrity controls etc. This author considers the factors that contribute to trustworthiness of health data and proposes a model that researchers or others who are interested in secondary use of health data can apply to mitigate some of the risks of using data from multiple sources.

There is a trend in the information security industry towards implementation of two factor authentication as a replacement for reliance on simple passwords to protect data. Implementation of two factor authentication is just beginning to be seen in the healthcare industry. The final chapter in this section of the book takes another look at the use of biometric technologies as a means of controlling access to healthcare data. The author explores some of the potential benefits and challenges to using this technology.

The third section of this book focuses on some of the really tough ethical issues that are being created as a byproduct of technology adoption within the healthcare industry. Information security and other healthcare professionals face hard choices every day as to how to properly balance security controls with data availability and access.

One of the tools that are being used in a variety of ways within the healthcare industry is Radio Frequency Identification or RFID technology. This technology has been adopted as a more sophisticated replacement for older bar coding technology as a means of tracking inventory and supply chain management. These kinds of implementations that relate to tracking of inanimate objects are not seen as highly controversial. The ethical aspects of how this technology is being used relate to when it is applied to tracking or otherwise monitoring the location or activities of human beings. The author describes how this technology is being used and what some of the ethical issues are in how it is being used. Examples include tracking of patients, as well as staff, and some evidence of potential health concerns that may relate to the use of this technology that might be considered by organizations seeking to leverage the benefits of RFID technologies.

As the healthcare industry moves towards electronic collection and storage of health data there will be an increased movement towards associating this data with the Internet. This author explores the privacy implications around collection and exchange of sensitive health data and the ability, or inability, of providers to secure this information and the potential that providers currently underestimate the level of risk to privacy and overestimate their ability to protect the information from unauthorized disclosure as a consequence of associating it with the Internet.

Nurses are among those within the healthcare industry who are most impacted by technology adoption and ethical issues. This author explores ethical issues facing the nursing profession including those related to global education and migration and how technology might address nursing shortages in different parts of the world.

The final chapter of this book is an ethical opinion paper that looks at how the healthcare industry is leveraging technology or, failing to leverage technology for optimal return on investment. The industry that began in a highly segmented and locally controlled data collection and storage environment is now moving toward a more integrated environment. The author looks at how the industry might be more effective in how technology is integrated into the overall work processes to maximize the benefit that this technology adoption can provide to the industry.

The authors of the chapters within this book have documented examples for how their particular country or aspect of the healthcare system are integrating healthcare technology and how that technology may impact the security, privacy and medical ethics of patients and practitioners. The information in these chapters offers useful insights for those charged with leveraging technology to enhance and improve the healthcare system in other countries.

Acknowledgment

We would like to acknowledge the contribution of the late Dr. Jack Krichen who provided encouragement, support, and guidance throughout the course of this project.

Steven A. Brown
Capella University, USA

Mary Brown
Capella University, USA

Section 1
Trends in Global Healthcare

Chapter 1
Will Comparative Effectiveness Research Lead to Healthcare Rationing?

Mary Brown
Capella University, USA

ABSTRACT

The Affordable Healthcare for America Bill that was signed into law in March 2010 includes support for activities that come under the heading of 'comparative effectiveness' research. The bill attempts to accelerate the conversion to electronic health records by all payers and providers who participate in the healthcare payment data stream. Conversion to electronic health data collection and storage solutions will create a large amount of treatment and payment data that is increasingly standardized by health standards organizations which reduces integration issues between technologies. There are federal advisory committees at work on designing the infrastructure needed to support a National Health Information Network (NHIN) that will support the healthcare data exchange required for comparative effectiveness research. The theory behind this work is that the availability of a large portion of existing health data will make it possible for researchers to identify therapies that lead to superior patient outcomes. It is assumed that the superior therapy would become the 'best practice' approach to treating a particular ailment. Supporters of comparative effectiveness see this as a strategy for making the system more effective both in terms of good medicine and also in terms of decreased cost. Opponents of comparative effectiveness see it as healthcare rationing and an inappropriate injection of government into the healthcare decision making process. Supporters and opponents have identified both positive and negative consequences to comparative effectiveness and this chapter will analyze the impact and propose some ways to optimize the results of this work.

DOI: 10.4018/978-1-60960-174-4.ch001

INTRODUCTION

The Affordable Healthcare for America Bill that was signed into law in March 2010 includes resources and operational support for activities that come under the heading of 'comparative effectiveness' research. The high level concepts of comparative effectiveness research include the idea that it is possible, through analysis of existing transactional healthcare data, to determine which particular medication or therapy is most effective in treating a particular disease. Advocates point to the work being done on a limited and local scale in organizations, like the Mayo and Cleveland Clinics, as evidence of the ability to improve treatment while lowering costs through identification and application of medical best practices. Aston (2010) points out, however that it is equally possible that this research may discover that the most effective form of treatment turns out to be the most expensive form of treatment, in which case the quality of care may be improved but with an associated increase in cost.

Concerned practitioners express reservations that the practice of medicine includes so many variables and is so situational in nature that they need to have available to them all of the tools at their disposal. It is common sense to assume that if a particular medication is deemed to be superior by payers, who begin to limit their payment only to that particular medication, then manufacturers of competitive medications are not as likely to continue producing that product. What then is the recourse for those patients that are not fortunate to experience any benefit from receiving that particular medication? Is implementation of comparative effectiveness a cost saving measure that, over time, will reduce the role of physician judgment and will restrict the current model that includes a wide, diverse, and expensive approach to therapeutic treatment in a competitive economy? Webster (2010) identifies an additional concern that the comparative effectiveness research proposal included in the Affordable Healthcare for

America law includes formation of a governing board that includes a 20% representation by industry causing concern in some that this creates a conflict of interest that may influence the decisions they make. It is possible that if clinicians perceive undue influence by commercial interests they will be less inclined to embrace any potential recommendations that might come out of comparative effectiveness research.

The healthcare industry has been using technology for several decades in their medical specialty departments to support diagnosis and treatment activities. The result has been an eclectic mix of cardiology, radiology, clinical laboratory and other medical specialty systems that supplement a paper chart which, for many healthcare organizations, is still considered to be the official medical record. Many healthcare clinics and clinician offices, unless they are associated with a larger healthcare organization, still run their practices using completely paper based or a combination of paper and locally installed practice management systems.

The more diverse the services that are offered onsite by a particular provider, the more complicated the technologies that have been deployed to support these clinical practices. For example, some hospitals began, in the 1970's and 1980's to explore transactional systems known as 'Admission, Discharge and Transfer' (ADT) systems designed to store customer demographic and billing information. These systems did not communicate to the medical specialty systems and the medical specialty systems did not communicate with one another. Integration of this data was handled through reports generated by these systems that were then printed onto paper and filed in the paper chart which was then considered the official medical record. There has been an interim step in some organizations involving the use of interfaces to transmit data between systems in order to increase data quality and reduce the amount of duplicate entry of patient information. The use of interfaces creates the need to find and hire skilled staff so they are available to create and manage the interfaces. Freedman (2007) describes the limitations of using interface engines and why they do not constitute true 'interoperability' in the healthcare environment.

The next phase in which many health organizations today find themselves is the adoption of Electronic Medical Records (EMRs) and the integration of these records into the day to day business of providing and paying for healthcare. HIMSS (2009) latest CIO survey indicates that only 5% of participants indicated that they had not yet begun planning for a move to an electronic medical record. It is unclear the degree to which the audience at HIMSS is reflective of the general population however the survey suggests that the industry is, in general, beginning to move in the direction of automating healthcare information collection and storage.

This adoption of an EMR is perceived to be the engine necessary to supply the amount, quality, and consistency of healthcare data that will be required for comparative effectiveness research. McKinney (2010) identifies some of the limitations with existing EMR systems that will need to be addressed before the data generated by these systems can be maximized for use in comparative effectiveness research. For example, the creation of health data standards and the development of the infrastructure for data sharing are a part of the vision for a fully automated healthcare industry and are efforts that are being promoted by the federal government through both economic stimulus and health reform legislation.

The percentage of healthcare that is funded by the federal government is very high. Levey (2010) indicates this figure will, for the first time, exceed 50% of healthcare costs by 2011 if there are no changes to the present system. This makes the federal government, through health agencies such as the Centers for Medicare and Medicaid (CMS), one of the most important payment sources for the healthcare industry. The health reform debate has often included examples of how insurance companies failed to approve payment when the

policyholder became ill and submitted a claim for service; however the discussion has often failed to explore how government sponsored health programs compare with private insurers relative to the percentage of claims that are disputed or denied. The AMA Practice management Center (2008) research indicates that Medicare actually represents a higher rate of denied claims than any of the private insurance companies. Many of the current examples of denial of payment reflect a desire of the health insurer to dictate a less expensive form of medication or treatment other than what is initially recommended by the clinician. There are angry clinicians sharing with the media their plans to get out of treating patients rather than trying to make a living in a system that they perceive is increasingly mandating how they practice medicine and then failing to fund them at a level that does allows them to generate sufficient profit. Santiago (2010) cites the results of a physician survey that indicates that nearly half of participating physicians indicate that they are considering early retirement as a result of the passage of health reform legislation. There is no way of knowing if these results are applicable across the industry or the degree to which it reflects more venting than reality but it is, nonetheless, a disturbing indication of a high level of dissatisfaction with the current system among medical practitioners.

It is unknown whether or not the application of rigor and transparency in comparative effectiveness research will result in clinicians being less resistant to possible restrictions in how they diagnose and treat their patients.

The great health reform debate that went on in the United States legislatures throughout much of 2009 reflects the two commonly expressed perspectives on the impact of comparative effectiveness. The supporters of the most recent health reform legislation have stood in the wells of both chambers of government and spoke, using high level concepts, of broad benefits of comparative effectiveness without fully explaining the concepts or the details of how this work would specifically be of benefit to their constituents. Ridgely and Jarrell (1996) report on their participation in a study designed to assess the cost effectiveness of providing chemical health treatment to severely mentally ill patients. This is an example of a research project that offers the potential to both reduce costs and to improve the care of these patients.

The opponents of the bill use comparative effectiveness research in the form of healthcare rationing and death panels. These appear to have been successful political tools but they accomplish little in advancing a serious debate about how the dramatic increase in data is going to impact health research and how those changes to health research are going to impact how Americans receive and pay for healthcare. Wechsler (2009) elaborates on the concern expressed by some political and industry interests on the potential for CER to result in healthcare rationing.

There are significant barriers that yet exist to having the tools available to conduct full blown comparative effectiveness research. The Office of the National Coordinator (ONC) has created a handful of federal advisory committees that are drafting recommendations for how the ONC can advance and adopt the health technology goals outlined in the health reform and economic stimulus legislation. There are seven factors that have been identified by the ONC and the appointed federal advisory committees as contributors to the research on the primary research question. These seven factors include:

1. Construction of a National Health Information Network (NHIN)
2. Development of acceptable information security and privacy practices
3. Successful adoption by sufficient numbers of clinicians
4. Continued emphasis on legislation and incentives by the federal government
5. Successful training of sufficient numbers of researchers and technicians
6. Successful negotiation of an accepted governance model
7. Successful creation and implementation of national standards and certification processes

It is the goal of these federal advisory committees to produce recommendations that will support completion of these seven steps necessary in order to provide the framework to support the goals of comparative effectiveness research that are included in the recent health reform and economic stimulus legislation.

The American Recovery and Reinvestment Act of 2009 (ARRA) contains support and resources for the accelerated adoption of EMR systems through funding for educators to train the additional health and technology professionals that are going to be needed to support this infrastructure once it is set up. There are proposals in the legislation that include administering financial incentives to clinicians who are able to meet the legislative goals related to the adoption of automated health data collection, storage and 'meaningful use.' Brailer (2010) describes the theory behind meaningful use and addresses some of the difficulties in coming up with a commonly accepted definition. Meaningful use has become a concept that is designed to quantify specific health treatment data elements that will be collected, stored and shared with the federal government in a particular format as a means of demonstrating the ability to use health information technology in a meaningful way. The federal government will, in exchange for this proof of meaningful use, contribute financial incentives to these providers that is assumed will allow them to meet the next phase of meaningful use criteria that is currently being developed. These meaningful use data elements are being staggered with a new set of requirements being implemented every two years. The ultimate goal will be sufficient interconnectivity, standardization of data and resolution of potential privacy and security concerns to allow for sophisticated analysis of a significant percentage of all healthcare data that is created in the course of treatment, payment, operations and research in America in near real time. The data elements identified as a necessary component of the first phase of meaningful use include data related to behaviors and chemistries pertaining to diabetes and smoking which are some of the most commonly identified health problems that plague the existing health system. There are significant issues related to patient privacy and security that will need to be overcome before substantial amounts of patient identifiable data can be shared. Anonymous (2010) reported in Modern Healthcare on a privacy survey that indicated that only 24% of those surveyed believed that privacy enhancements included in the ARRA will actually result in increased privacy protections for patients. This seems a realistic perspective given that the Patriot Act, and other legislation that was enacted following the September 11, 2001 attacks, have already created significant inroads into the ability of the government to gain access to individually identifiable health data as part of a proper public health and homeland security surveillance system. This will diminish some of the barriers to accessing the data needed for comparative effectiveness research that may have existed prior to 9/11. There are still technical issues related to the creation and management of a NHIN including ownership and stewardship rules involving permission procedures, access controls, and authentication strategies for both users and administrators. There is concern in the industry that the speed at which this legislation is trying to accelerate the adoption of these technologies will result in wasted time and resources on ineffective solutions and false starts. News Staff (2010) of the American Association of Family Practitioners expressed concern that the rapid implementation of meaningful use incentives may have a negative result by discouraging small physician offices and clinics from adopting technology. They recom-

mend that the ONC spend more time advancing certification and standardization work to ensure that technology is able to meet the meaningful use requirements once they are adopted. Avorn (2009) identifies some of the political challenges that have so far created barriers to the success of widespread CER implementation. Regardless of how far supporters succeed in advancing comparative effectiveness or how successful opponents are in managing to slow it down, there is still much practical work that has to happen before it becomes truly robust and of sufficient substance to impact the healthcare industry.

PROGRESSION OF HEALTHCARE TECHNOLOGY AND RELATED LEGISLATION

The healthcare industry has been slow to adopt technology as compared to other mature industries such as manufacturing and banking. Some of the first examples of using technology in healthcare happened in the fields of radiology, cardiology and clinical laboratory analysis. The typical approach to these technological solutions involved creating a computerized interface between treatment tools such as chemistry analyzers, cardiac monitoring equipment and sophisticated scanning equipment. This interface to a computer provided a means by which to collect, store and share the results captured by these treatment tools. Prior to the creation of these interfaces all of the analysis and interpretation of results were gathered manually and in real time. This manual processing involved significant risk of human error and strictly limited the ability of a practitioner to share these results with others. In the case of radiology, a patient would have to depend on the provider to ensure that films made it from their office to the hospital or specialist to which they were directed for additional treatment. Too often this approach failed at some stage along the line resulting in the need of the hospital or specialist to repeat these same diagnostic procedures in order to have access to the information. An alternative to repeating the missing films would mean relying only on the interpretation offered in the paper report created by the original person viewing the films. Neither outcome would be considered optimal by most of the stakeholders engaged in the process. The advent of radiology management systems reduced the impact of having to manually interpret and transport radiology data and introduced alternatives including the ability to burn images on CDs that the patient can take with them or the ability for the original provider to email images or otherwise electronically transfer them to other caregivers downstream.

The experience with the radiology system described above has been repeated throughout the healthcare industry over the past few decades and across the individual departments that make up the industry as a whole. Korst, Signer, Aydin, and Fink (2008), propose a regional network specific to the work of perinatal research as an example of how the technology and research efforts have, to date, been segmented creating considerable complexity, cost and redundancy. Technology solutions within the healthcare industry developed using a silo based approach involving a patchwork of local solutions supplied and heavily supported by proprietary vendor solutions. These turnkey based solutions have often been designed to foster and promote this fractured architecture. The glue with which these silo based solutions have been held together is through printing out documents particular to orders and results and printing this data for integration into a comprehensive patient chart for every patient being seen by a particular provider. By filing reports and results in the paper chart along with physician narratives and orders it is possible to recreate or compile sufficient information to understand the medical history of a patient. These paper charts are created and held locally as property of the individual providers. When there is a need to share some of this information with other hospitals or specialists, providers

typically photocopy or fax only what appears to be directly relevant to the particular health issue at hand. This fragmented approach to patient documentation results in missing information or potentially important health implications. Inclusion of unrelated material costs both the sender and recipient and increases the risk of privacy to the patient creating the need to balance competing interests. Lassetter (2010) describes changes in practice that are expected in how health data is exchanged using the NHIN and the need to accommodate meaningful use functionality as the catalyst that will move these changes forward.

The ability for healthcare providers to print and store data from multiple medical specialty systems and to do that in a timely and accurate fashion, in order to maintain a paper chart as the official medical record, is becoming less viable. The industry is becoming more receptive to the idea of integrated health data collection and storage solutions as it becomes increasingly difficult to ensure that a complete paper chart is available at the point of care whenever it is needed. Hillestad, Bigelow, Bower, and Girosi (2005) examine some of the potential benefits to the industry that come with the move towards elimination of the use of paper based records.

One of the biggest drivers in the early days of health adoption of technology unrelated to medical treatment was the need to reduce the cost of the healthcare payment system. The number of patients who directly pay for their own care is negligible making the payment system for healthcare a complicated web of third party payers. McCormick & et al. (2009) estimates the total number of uninsured Americans in 2009 to be 47 million and, Truffer & et al. (2010) explores the percentage of public and private insurers submitting claims within the healthcare system which reveals some of the complexities for those charged with obtaining reimbursement for healthcare services provided.

Early attempts at controlling healthcare costs included n attempt to address the fact that each of these third party payers required healthcare providers to submit a proprietary healthcare reimbursement or claims form. Each individual insurer also required an often complicated set of coded data submitted using a particular data format of the insurance companies choosing. Often these requirements were meant to make the claim form compatible with the application that these insurers used to automate the payment of claims. These many unique requirements created a patchwork system and the need for healthcare providers to hire staff or contractors that could take their healthcare treatment activity information and format it into the appropriate fields that each of these proprietary insurance solutions required in order to process a claim on behalf of one of their subscribers. These 'middle men' are known as healthcare clearinghouses.

Under the best of circumstances complying with all these diverse requirements in order to be paid for services was a tedious process of typewriters and reams of paper charts that too often resulted in the identification of inaccurate, illegible or missing data that would then need to be manually researched and documented before the claim form could actually be processed. Payers would further up the ante by carefully scrubbing claims for potential defects in processing that would allow them to return or reject the claim requiring the provider to start all over again in seeking reimbursement for their services. The system soon became so heavily impacted by the whims of individual payment processes that the cost of these activities were identified by legislators as significant drivers in the increased cost of providing healthcare to Americans. The cost of care experienced by those federal agencies responsible for healthcare payment for special populations and the impact on the federal budget provided sufficient incentive for legislators to mandate that more sensible payment practices be adopted by the industry at large.

In 1996 congress passed one of the first health reform laws that addressed the need to automate

healthcare activities in order to help reduce the cost of providing healthcare. The Health Information Portability and Accountability Act of 1996 (HIPAA) was originally designed to protect Americans from losing health insurance as a result of losing their job. The focus on the healthcare industry evolved into a broader discussion with the result being that the final HIPAA rules included mandates for 'covered entities' that included healthcare providers, payers and clearinghouses and involved the use of a standardized claim form and submission format for healthcare claims. Merlis (2009) documents some of the drivers and results of this element of the federal HIPAA rules.

HIPAA further introduced guidelines for the controls necessary to support security and privacy of this electronic health information. This early effort at automating the 'business' of healthcare provided the catalyst for some health organizations to review their existing technology and information architectures and the need to redesign the infrastructure in a more rational and comprehensive manner in order to meet the new mandates and guidelines introduced in HIPAA.

Another catalyst for healthcare organizations to review and redesign their technology infrastructure was the Y2K event that created the need for early adopters of health technologies to turn their attention to how technology was being used within their organizations. The premise of Y2K was that some systems would fail at midnight on January 1, 2000 by reading the 00 to mean the year 1900. Healthcare systems were not unique, however there were instances where the software code would read a date and use that date to do a mathematical calculation to create a new data element such as age of the patient or number of days that a patient has been receiving a particular therapy. These potential points of failure had to be found and remediated before they resulted in the creation of potentially dangerous inaccuracies in the data used to treat patients. The approach that most organizations took towards accomplishing this goal was to begin the project by creating an inventory of clinical systems. This initial inventory often generated surprises at how many potential places had developed where patient information was being collected, stored and used for treatment, payment, operations and healthcare research. Many organizations became aware as a byproduct of this activity how much redundancy existed in the data that was being collected and stored. The act of revealing and sharing existing data resources and activities was helpful in bringing to the surface, for those managing these organizations, the need to include in their Y2K work a conscious step as to whether a particular data source was worthy of the cost of Y2K remediation or would be phased out of use as a more practical alternative. It was also the first step that some healthcare organizations had ever taken in creating a formal technology and information plan rather than allowing for organic and unrestrained growth of these solutions which had been typical in the early years of electronic healthcare solutions. While Y2K provided the motivation for healthcare organizations needed to do some long needed accounting and house-cleaning Morrissey (1999) points out that it also served as a distraction and created competition with important system integration objectives for time and resources.

An important contributor of redundant health data is the use of healthcare transactional data to perform local research being conducted by clinicians. Existing medical research laws create a need to comply with health privacy rules by tightly restricting the particular data elements to which the researcher will be given access based on consent of the research subject. The implementation of clinical specialty systems were an important catalyst for health researchers to begin to integrate the data from these systems along with the more common practice of manually collecting aggregate health data through review of patient charts. The ability to identify and integrate electronic data being captured in clinical systems enhanced the more traditional approaches to healthcare research. Systems were, and to a degree still are, relatively

unsophisticated in the ability to control or limit granular access to the data stored in clinical databases. This complicates the task of providing access to only Institutional Review Board (IRB) approved data and so, has typically been accomplished by assigning an information technology (IT) person to create a specialized database and populate the database with copies of the appropriate data elements. Clinical researchers are, more often, choosing to focus on medical technologies as a legitimate medical specialty. Detmer, Lumpkin, and Williamson (2009) document the work being done within the American Medical Informatics Association (AMIA) to create the framework for a medical specialization in clinical informatics. As the lines within the healthcare and health informatics industries continue to blend between clinical staff and information technology workers it is possible that the existing procedures that regulate how research datasets are created will change over time in keeping with this increase in highly skilled clinical users. In the meantime the trend continues to be creating redundant sets of research data needed in order to comply with HIPAA and other regulations that manage how research is conducted.

The third important contribution that has created redundant pools of data is the result of actions that were taken by the federal government. The federal government, as the funding source for nearly half of the healthcare in the country, is among one of the largest healthcare stakeholders and they suffered their own HIPAA and Y2K experiences. This led President George W. Bush, in 2004 to create Executive Order (EO) 13335. The EO created The Office of the National Coordinator (ONC) and assigned this office to coordinate the management of healthcare data within federal programs with the goal of making the entire system more effective and less costly. The ONC was to be visionary, mediator, architect and manager of how technology can make healthcare delivery cheaper. One of the objectives that have consumed the resources of the ONC is support for a goal that had been set by the IT agenda under President Bush to have the majority of American health care supported by Electronic Health Records (EHR) by the year 2014. The plan to advance implementation of EHRs included a dual mission of promoting more efficient and less costly healthcare with the mission of generating the infrastructure needed to promote large scale biomedical research as a form of public health. The ability of the federal government to make public health and homeland security broad exceptions to personal privacy rules has been facilitated since 9/11 by passage of a number of laws including the Patriot Act. The even more compelling events that occurred that impacted the ability and desire of the federal government to collect health data was the anthrax attacks that occurred soon after 9/11. These events promoted fear and resulted in laws that literally require providers to transfer large amounts of data to public health agencies for bioterrorism and public health surveillance. Buehler, Berkelman, Hartley, and Peters, (2003) identify syndromic surveillance sites that were established by local health departments following the anthrax attacks with the goal of establishing early warning systems that might identify disease clusters whether biological or natural in origin.

More recently Johnson (2010) documents a strategy used by the Center for Disease Control (CDC) involving the request for data from supermarkets that use customer loyalty cards for large files of data generated by these cards. The data includes a combination of user demographic and contact information along with very specific details of their purchases and the CDC was able to identify the source of tainted food for recall. These examples demonstrate some of the earlier privacy barriers to data exchange that have been overcome as a result of these high visibility attacks and suggest the opportunity for the federal government to successfully move the line when they identify a need to do so.

Among the objectives of EO 13335 is to enable the movement of data while ensuring the security and privacy of the patients, who are the subject of the data. The framework needed to support the large scale movement of healthcare data is highly complex from both a procedural and a technical perspective. From a purely technical perspective the healthcare industry has become increasingly accustomed to generating files of patient information requested by regulators and payers as part of the normal business cycle that makes up the healthcare industry. The steps to creating these files using the methodology and formatting requested by the recipient has replaced a stack of different claim forms to be filled out for the insurance companies. Instead IT staff is figuring out how to format and transfer data collected by a variety of proprietary clinical systems and merged into a single dataset. The ability to join data from multiple systems and synch it to make sure that the data is associated with the correct patient is work that has been accomplished on a smaller scale. Safran and et al. (2007) describe some of the barriers to implementing the NHIN and suggest that the concerns related to security, privacy and development of data standards will play a much larger role than resolving the technical issues involved with using the Internet to establish connectivity.

The ONC has been working towards the goals that it was assigned by President George W. Bush. They continue to play a very significant role in the plans of President Obama to advance health technology as a means to support the work of CER. An element of EO 13335 included a charge for the ONC to create a federal health information technology strategic plan. This plan was updated in June of 2008 and a new edition published that builds on the foundation with a new set of objectives that cover the years from 2008 through 2012. The document includes two goals for federal health that include a focus both on patient health but also on population (aka public) health. These goals are attained through continued progress towards four high level themes:

- Privacy and Security
- Interoperability
- Adoption
- Collaborative Governance

It is striking how similar the content in both of these documents are to the Yasnoff and et al. (2004) proposals in which a group of highly regarded experts in the field were asked to speculate on what it would take to support the creation of a National Health Information Infrastructure. While there has been progress in the areas identified, there is still considerable distance to the goal post of implementation that needs to be covered before these concepts actually become a reality.

In the most recent push towards automation of healthcare, it is the ONC that is coordinating and advancing the operations of the federal advisory groups that are influencing the direction that Health Information Technology (HIT) will take in the near future and beyond. All of these advisory groups including groups developing recommendations for standards, certification, privacy and security and the creation of the NHIN that will play an important role in creating the conditions that are necessary before widespread use of CER can actually be done on the scale that is being proposed by the new health reform laws.

The latest attempts to legislate the use of technology in the healthcare industry involves the passage of the American Recovery and Reinvestment Act of 2009 (ARRA) and the Affordable Healthcare for America Bill that was passed in 2010. The ARRA includes financial incentives for providers to adopt health technologies in general and Electronic Medical Records (EMRs) in particular. It also includes financing for twelve distinct roles within HIT that the ONC believes will be necessary to support the acceleration of the healthcare industry to computerized operations. The industry is in very diverse progress in terms of adoption of technologies with larger healthcare systems more likely to be farther along with integration of technology than smaller participants.

This variation in the existing state of technology has created within the ARRA language creating the adoption of the concept of meaningful use as the measure by which providers will have to meet in order to receive the financial incentives within the law. Blumenthal (2009), who is the current head of the ONC, outlines his plan for the implementation of meaningful use as the foundation for pushing forward the widespread use of Health Information Technology (HIT) that is necessary to support widespread use of CER. The federal advisory committees and the ONC have developed a proposal for meaningful use that involves very limited benchmarks required by providers in 2011. Those benchmarks are expanded both in breadth and depth for 2013 and are projected to be more aggressive still in 2015. There is considerable pressure from the healthcare industry on the ONC to back up, delay or reduce the demands that are on the table. It is expected that this work will continue to morph and change as practical realities meet ambition and the need to control costs. Bacon (2010), reports on a trend within the Republican Party to engage in a focused effort to 'repeal and replace' health legislation as a campaign strategy for upcoming elections.

As was the case with the HIPAA legislation, once congress began to focus on the industry the need to build in supporting legislation became apparent. The need, for example, to consider security and privacy impacts on existing HIPAA language became clear and the result was inclusion of additional controls within a section of the ARRA which is known as the HITECH Act. The primary areas where the original HIPAA language was enhanced was in the areas of mandatory reporting of data breaches and a change in the obligations of the group of business partners within HIPAA that had been identified as 'business associates.' These increased requirements were meant to address the concerns of the public that would result from a dramatic increase in the amount of sharing of personally identifiable health information (PHI).

Additional factors that were included involve the need for providers to have a reliable EMR certification process so that providers, when buying systems, would know that, in the end, they would meet the requirements of the ARRA for meaningful use. The Certification Commission for Health Information Technology (CCHIT) offers a private and non-binding certification for health technologies. The federal advisory board responsible for selecting a certification process for the ONC expressed concern that the CCHIT was not sufficiently independent from the industry to be appropriate for the purposes of meaningful use certification. Because of their current role within the industry as a non-binding certification organization paid for by private industry it is proposed that they continue to fill the role of certification body for the short term. The longer term approach that is expected to be adopted involves the use of multiple certification agencies that will use standardized evaluation criteria to make their assessments prior to issuing certifications. While this work is still unfinished it is assumed that the ISO and other existing federal standards organizations will fill this role in the long term.

THE IMPACT OF PRIVACY AND SECURITY ON CER

Comparative effectiveness research will involve making judgments that can impact the lives of many if this research is used to determine superior therapies and medications. It is important that this research is of high quality and that it can be replicated before it is adopted as truth. In order to be most assured that the results of this research is of high quality and is accurate there is a need to make available to researchers' huge pools of individually identifiable health data. When health data is collected and stored in a paper chart, the subject of that data needs only to worry about information exposure to those with physical access to that chart. As the industry begins to adopt new technologies the number of people to whom personally identifiable health (PHI) data are exposed is growing exponentially. If the NHIN that is being proposed as the supporting infrastructure for providing data to comparative effectiveness research comes into being this exposure of PHI will continue to grow. The current proposal is that local providers would transmit their data to a state run health information exchange (HIE) and the state HIEs would, in turn, share their data with regional and national HIEs.

According to the U.S. Department of Health and Human Services (2010), the current status of the NHIN is called the NHIN Exchange and is a pilot project involving some federal agencies including the Veterans Administration (VA), the Social Security Administration, MedVirginia, Department of Defense, and Kaiser Permanente. These core participants are expected to identify potential barriers and benefits with the expectation that additional participants will be added gradually until the full blown NHIN has been implemented. The NHIN itself is being described by the procedural, standards and policy framework involved rather than identifying specific technologies that will make up this national network.

Global health organizations suggest that eventually there will be need for a global HIE to handle public health emergencies such as the recent H1N1 outbreak. Brown, Cueto, and Fee, E (2006) make a case for the World Health Organization (WHO) to take the leadership role in creating this global health system. Brownstein, Freifeld, and Madoff, (2009) document the success that the WHO has had leveraging the Internet and open search tools such as Google's Insights for Search to create a public health surveillance network that were then used to try to predict and prepare for outbreaks of H1N1.

There is currently need for researchers to obtain patient permission to use their data for research which involves a healthcare researcher having to follow a complex set of rules and protocols in order to gain access to the data needed to conduct this research. Much research involving human subjects (AKA the common rule) requires approval and oversight by an Institutional Review Board (IRB) to ensure that patient privacy is protected, at least in theory. There are a number of exceptions to research that requires individual patient permission that relate to public health and safety. In order to optimize CER on the scale that is being proposed it is at most likely that the approach taken will include the ability for a patient to opt out of participation rather than putting in place a proactive approach where a patient must consciously opt in to contributing their data to the cause of comparative effectiveness research. It is even more likely that the approach will be mandatory participation for all. Gostin, and Nass (2009) make a case for elimination of consent and the creation of a universal exception for healthcare research similar to what HIPAA now allows for treatment, payment and operations (TPO) and other public health and safety exceptions that were carved out to satisfy various constituents during the public comment period. The inability to predict potential bias that may occur if patients are allowed to selectively engage combined with the potential impact of an undetected bias in the data on accuracy and safety is a compelling argument for the ONC to make in support of mandatory participation. An additional benefit to mandatory participation is the elimination of the significant operational costs that would be involved with managing all the documentation associated with obtaining and tracking permission.

The norms around privacy rules for health data seem to be changing. As social networks like Twitter and Facebook promote a trend towards personal transparency it is possible that future generations will not find personal privacy of health data to be an important concept. Until that comes into being it is important that care be taken when creating a NHIN made up of multiple HIEs that all of these repositories implement robust information security controls. Security is only as effective as the weakest link. Failure to

secure this data can result in embarrassing and damaging consequences for individuals whose personal information is exposed. Security is the means by which privacy is enabled and as a result there are increasingly severe legal penalties based on recent legislation (Blumenthal, 2010) that adds to the original HIPAA security and privacy rules in setting standards for covered entities and their business partners. There are in some states special controls put on particularly sensitive kinds of health data including things like mental health therapy notes, HIV and chemical dependency treatment. These special controls create barriers to the creation of a homogenous set of ground rules that are being sought as part of the creation of the NHIN. The federal advisory policy workgroup, under the direction of the ONC is working to create a plan for modifying these special rules in an attempt to come to agreement on a national policy instead. Limiting the potential access profiles that are included in the security plan for the NHIN may help to reduce the complexity of the security management rules for stakeholders. To that end there have been several projects charged with assessing the current status of healthcare security and privacy and with recommending how to evolve the existing system to better support the data exchange and research goals included in the health reform law. In 2006, HHS hired RTI International to lead an effort to engage in this work of assessing healthcare security and privacy within the states known as the Health Information Security and Privacy Collaboration (HISPC). The most recent effort is the appointment of a security and privacy standards group appointed by the ONC to identify existing industry standards related to security and privacy that can be applied to specifically support the exchange of the research data that has been identified as that which constitutes 'meaningful use.' McGraw, Dempsey, Harris, and Goldman, (2009) address these important issues surrounding information security and privacy from a unique position. They suggest that we stop taking the traditional approach to these issues including perception that they are barriers to progress. These authors suggest that a more productive way to think about these concepts is to think of how the development of a robust security and privacy architecture can be useful in establishing confidence in patients who will then be more comfortable that their privacy will not be put at risk.

THE IMPACT OF INTEROPERABILITY ON COMPARATIVE EFFECTIVENESS RESEARCH

Interoperability is an issue for those trying to engage in large scale data exchange activities in general. It is equally an issue in the healthcare industry. An important aspect of the ARRA that is being addressed by a federal advisory committee involves the application of standards to the health technology architecture. Standards can be applied to everything from what data security protocols, such as levels of encryption, will be required when transmitting data across the NHIN to what standard will be used for the selection and format of a patient diagnosis. Standards under consideration include the International Classification of Diseases (ICD9 and ICD10), Snomed CT, and Health Level Seven (HL7) which are currently heavily used in the healthcare billing processes. Networking standards, operating systems and setting standards, data formatting standards are among the complex set of considerations that are a part of interoperability. The more in common the hardware, software and data management and formatting procedures, the less complicated will be the work of transmitting and collecting large amounts of PHI needed for comparative effectiveness research. The industry has wrestled with some of these complexities as part of HIPAA compliance making technical standards among the least of the potential issues that might arise. It is far more likely that the complexities will come at the higher levels of the networking protocols and

within the collection and formatting of the data itself. Blumenthal (2009, 2010) writes at length on the role that standards will play in the successful adoption of the NHIN that is an important piece of successful widespread use of CER.

A concept that is gaining steam within the healthcare technology field is the idea of creating application independent pools of data. The idea of eliminating the formatting and transformation steps currently required in order to use comingled data from disparate systems is appealing in terms of potential cost reduction but also for the reduction in complexity of collecting, storing and transmitting the data. With the advent of technologies like XML and CCOW it does not seem an unrealistic long term goal however it will require cooperation and coordination of a large number of stakeholders if it is to be successful. Schwartz, Pappas, and Sandlow (2010) propose one such system that could be used for the purposes of medical education.

THE IMPACT OF ADOPTION ON COMPARATIVE EFFECTIVENESS RESEARCH (CER)

Implementation of the technical and procedural architecture necessary to support comparative effectiveness research is an expensive and complicated effort. In larger organizations there has been an effort to develop integrated solutions that includes participation by all of the business units including hospitals, clinics, and individual physicians. It is the small and mid-sized provider that is the focus of recent health technology legislation. These providers have traditionally run their business on paper and, because there is no need to scale operations in the same way that a large organization, they are relatively content to continue to run their practices on paper. The HIPAA legislation included one of the first mandates against this inertia within the small and mid-sized practitioner. Up until the HIPAA legislation it was possible for these smaller providers to submit their claims to the Center for Medicare and Medicaid (CMS) on paper claim forms. CMS, as part of HIPAA, created the infrastructure of standardized claims and format as well as the security and privacy rules designed to offset provider concern of putting patient information into a computer. CMS then issued a rule that providers were going to be required to submit all future patient claims in electronic format. States created and provided for free software that could be used by these providers to create the file in order to further eliminate any avenue of opposition that these providers may want to offer.

The current legislation includes similar kinds of incentives for smaller providers in the attempt to move them from their existing silo systems and onto a common EMR that will provide standardized data that can be easily shared. Some of these incentives include the creation of regional support centers that are, in particular, designed to support rural practitioners who may not have access to the kinds of technical support. There is federal funding being offered to providers to put towards implementation of the EMR and then added incentives into the future designed to ensure that the technology is not only purchased but that the use is maximized and expanded once the foundation has been laid. Kaushal and et al. (2009) conducted a study that attempted to identify providers that appeared likely to be early adopters of HIT. One of the factors they found had impact on early adoption was financial incentive. There are incentives worth billions of dollars in the recent economic stimulus and health reform laws that may present an opportunity to test those theories depending on how readily providers use this funding as motivation to implement HIT within their practices.

Many physicians are now employees or in some way associated with large health organizations. The number of independent physicians is unknown but is widely accepted to be getting slightly smaller each year as more and more become

employees of larger health organizations. This consolidation of physicians and clinics with Health Maintenance Organizations and other healthcare systems supports the move to HIT, particularly Electronic Health Records (EHRs). These larger health organizations are able to provide the HIT, support and training for these smaller entities at a level and quality that they could not afford as an independent entity. From the perspective of the larger health organization, Isaacs, Jellinek, and Ray (2009) point out that market pressures to absorb these assets into the organization and the benefit of increased leverage when contracting for payment represent two of the incentives that the health systems have to partner with previously independent physicians and clinics.

It has been possible for the federal government to force the transition of small providers onto electronic billing using the carrot and stick approach that is being applied to current legislative efforts to move to ubiquitous use of EMR systems. When forcing providers to move to electronic billing one approach was to provide for no or low cost the software that was required to submit those requests for payment. The incentives built into the economic stimulus and health reform laws reflect a similar approach of providing the technical tools that providers need to move forward. Margolis and Halfon (2009) describe in their article some of the ways that these health networks are changing the way that healthcare documentation is gathered and shared between health providers and partners.

There are potential barriers to progress with the existing controversy related to health reform in general and a surge in the discussion of whether the control of healthcare belongs with the states or with the federal government. Richey (2010) documents 14 states that are in the process of suing the federal government in an attempt to block the health reform law that is meant to provide the foundation for the NHIN and the ability to engage in widespread use of CER. These legal and political barriers may not be able to prevent what is a logical progression towards the use of technology in healthcare however it is possible that it may complicate progress and delay the timeline in which implementation can be achieved.

Provider adoption may be accelerated through the provision of support resources and financial incentives and it is only reasonable to assume that automating patient care is inevitable eventually regardless of how effective are the support and incentives. What will be more interesting, in addition to a potential ambivalence about the concept of healthcare rationing, is how smaller providers, who may have a closer relationship with their patients than a larger and less familiar setting, will react to the widespread sharing of their patient data that is a primary objective of this move towards automation, integration, and finally, CER to identify superior outcomes.

There are some providers that have indicated they are not willing to pay the price that comes along with receipt of federal incentives for meaningful use. Strecha, Persad, Marckmann, and Danis (2009) conducted a systematic review of three medical databases and included information specific to 16 surveys in this review. The objective of the survey was to evaluate the likelihood that physicians would be willing participants in a system of healthcare rationing. What the authors found was a very wide range of results that suggests there is significant ambivalence among physicians which may result in an unpredictable impact on the likelihood that CER will lead to healthcare rationing.

THE IMPACT OF COLLABORATIVE GOVERNANCE ON COMPARATIVE EFFECTIVENESS RESEARCH

As has been discussed throughout this paper, larger organizations are arguably already in a position technically to meet the objectives of advancing meaningful use of health data. Indeed, some of these organizations have already been engaged internally in the application of comparative ef-

fectiveness and superior outcomes research. What is lacking for these organizations are the legal and procedural aspects of the supporting architecture. The current patchwork of patient consent rules, many of which operate at the state level, must be reconciled into a cohesive plan that will make the rules consistent across the NHIN. There is an aspect of state and federal control that exists within this patchwork of consent rules in that many of the federal rules related to patient privacy indicate that if a state has rules more stringent than that in the federal rule then the state rule trumps. If the comparative effectiveness infrastructure is going to work without collapsing under the weight of bureaucracy, there is a need to develop a national policy related to patient consent that takes precedence over state laws. One of the reasons that most federal rules include the ability for the state to trump is the recognition that overriding states rights can be a tricky business that can end up mired in politics. It is possible that rather than trying to tackle this problem the ONC will instead try to design a system that will work with existing state laws which will result in increased cost, complexity and opportunity for system failures resulting in breaches of personal privacy. The federal security and privacy advisory group (Health IT, 2010) is focusing their work on creating standards in data format; file structures etc as a foundation for implementing patient consent as part of large scale health data exchanges. Much of the work being done involves applying existing technical security controls already used for secure data exchange in other industries such as finance and banking. This work will likely be included in the NHIN implementation even if the need for patient consent is successfully removed from the data exchange requirements for health research.

Another aspect of governance that will present technical and procedural changes is the practical day to day issues currently involving ownership of the data and the systems that house the data. Health information security and privacy compliance is not atypical of other organizations.

Data is protected on a trusted network behind the organizational firewall. Access controls and authentication devices are under the control of the organization that collects and stores the data and any external access to that data is tightly controlled based on federal laws, state laws and good security practices. Entities are also often part of a competitive and commercial environment and are likely to be resistant to the idea of exposing their confidential patient information to a competitor. What would then stop that competitor from mining that data for competitive purposes? These pressures are all going to complicate the kinds of governance decisions that are going to need to be made as part of creating the NHIN to support comparative effectiveness research. Shortliffe (2005), who is a former president of AMIA and one of the founders of the HIT movement, suggests that this competitive pressure will interfere with the growth and success of HIT without the kind of leadership from the government that has currently been demonstrated with recent legislation meant to advance these concepts.

Another hurdle to the development of the NHIN is the need to create a national architecture and to balance the pros and cons of the alternatives to creating that architecture. For example, is it preferable to have only a single instance of data with the provider with the networking capacity to virtually comingle that data with those of other providers for the purposes of research? Is it preferable to replicate the data into a number of instances creating larger and larger pools of comingled data until the data at a national level contains a comprehensive database of the entire set of patient data collected and stored by all of the individual providers in America? There are obvious tradeoffs to both of these approaches to creation of the NHIN. The current effort is supporting the latter approach of multiple databases that is less complicated than virtualization of this work but creates the expense and security and privacy issues related to having to store, maintain, synch and protect access to redundant data stores. This

work is being encouraged through the creation of state and regional health information exchanges as is described by Blumenthal (2009).

Another politically charged aspect of creating the infrastructure necessary for comparative effectiveness research includes the creation of a National Patient Identifier. This was a component of the HIPAA legislation that was never successful and was dropped from the planning at the time. Privacy advocates at the time had considerable support in the legislature to block this concept from being advanced couching it as just a backdoor attempt at registering everyone in the country with the federal government through the use of a National ID card. There are no current plans in the existing health reform to move towards a National Patient Identifier however it is realistic to assume that as long as patients see multiple practitioners in the pursuit of healthcare there is going to be a need to have a means by which to integrate these multiple files into a unique patient identifier. Hammond, Bailey, Boucher, Spohr, and Whitaker, P (2010) explore the issues that surround the implementation of a National Health Identifier which include both technical and social elements that will have to be solved as part of implementing such a plan.

If the work of the NHIN committee advances and becomes closer to a reality, those who are charged with making these regional and national healthcare databases work are going to soon find the need to normalize records through the use of a primary key for each patient. Whether it is possible to implement this key without publically acknowledging and assigning a National Patient Identifier is yet to be seen.

The typical perspective currently held within the healthcare industry in regards to governance or ownership of patient health data is that the provider who collects and generates the data is the owner of the media on which the data is stored. It is the patient who is considered the owner of data and, unless there is a state or federal law that mandates data sharing for public health and safety, it is generally the patient that must give overt permission to use the data for research. Rodwin (2009) proposes consideration of the potential benefit in shifting the emphasis from private to public ownership of healthcare data.

Assuming that the federal rules are able to by-pass the consent requirement it is likely that there will remain a need to apply some parameters to the use and the need to create an audit trail of how data was used. In the existing paradigms, organizations hire system administrators that control this access through the use of access controls and authentication or through the creation of specialized datasets that are then physically provided to the researcher. It is far less clear how these access, authentication and auditing procedures will work when this data is replicated in regional or national health databases. How will these database administrators who are so far removed from the patient manage the access, authentication and audit processes? Who gets to decide that a research project is of sufficient importance to allow unfettered access to this pool of data and who will be responsible for making sure that this access is not abused or the data compromised? These complexities in technology and process are some of the driving factors that are increasingly proposing the elimination of consent and the need to focus instead on privacy and security controls that protect the data from inappropriate use even though the subject of the data does not retain control of how the data is used for medical research.

The issues of governance that impact the creation of an infrastructure to support CER are possibly even more difficult and will prove more obstructive to the process than the technical challenges. With the advent of social networking and the trend towards personal transparency becoming more common it may be that over time the concept of personal privacy and control over healthcare data will become less of an issue. There remains enough support in the current culture for the concepts of personal privacy and control that make it reasonable to assume that there will be pushback

if the emphasis on public health impedes too strongly on the rights of individuals to personal privacy and control of their healthcare information.

CONCLUSION

Since the implementation of presidential Executive Order 13335 in 2004 there have been organized and well funded efforts by the federal government to accelerate and incentivize the healthcare industries adoption of HIT. Both state and federal governments have experienced large increases in the cost of administering government health programs which has provided significant incentives for these government entities to fund these efforts. These efforts began with efforts to move the industry in the direction of EHR adoption and implementation. The Veterans administration is one federal agency that has been at the forefront of developing EHR technology that is suitable for adoption by private healthcare entities.

As progress has been made in increasing the adoption of EHR technologies the focus is beginning to shift to the development of HIEs, regional and state exchanges, and the NHIN. The ONC and government health officials have identified a series of potential barriers to the successful implementation of this health data exchange infrastructure. The approach being taken to address these barriers includes the creation of federal advisory committees that are working on recommendations thought to mitigate some of these challenges. Other efforts include significant financial incentives in recent federal legislation meant to accelerate the adoption of 'meaningful use' of healthcare technology.

The Affordable Healthcare for America bill was heavily debated in congress throughout 2009. The adoption of mandatory insurance requirements was highly controversial and has resulted in numerous lawsuits by states claiming this mandate goes beyond what the federal government is legally entitled to require. This was not, however, the only controversial proposal. There were endless speeches given on the floor of the US Senate both for and against this legislation. One of the frequent topics within these speeches was the need to reduce the cost of care and how this legislation would accomplish that goal. Among the strategies for reducing the overall cost of care includes support for the work of CER. The adoption of electronic clinical systems combined with standards, procedures, and technology that support large scale exchange of this data through the state, regional and national health networks will overcome many of the practical barriers to research that have existed with paper charts and silo based clinical specialty systems. This new ability to consolidate and analyze large amounts of healthcare data provides new opportunities to measure the effectiveness of different therapies in ways that have not been previously possible.

The insurance companies and government agencies that pay for most of the healthcare provided in the US have been engaged in limited and smaller scale attempts at CER as a means of controlling their costs. These efforts have become most familiar to those who depend on these payers and who have increasingly experienced a restriction in the therapies and medications for which payers will pay. For example, there are a range of medications that are available for the treatment of high blood pressure. It is common practice for insurers and government health agencies to restrict which of these blood pressure medications are available to patients with full funding by these organizations. Proponents of this practice will suggest that these restrictions are not the result of rationing of care but are rather adoption of best practices which most properly balance the cost of a therapy with the benefit it provides. Opponents of this practice perceive this as a restriction on the ability of the practitioner to select the drug that they believe to be the most effective in treating the condition without consideration of the cost.

These current examples of ways in which CER have been implemented suggest that it is highly likely that an increase in the ability to engage in this research will result in an increase in the identification of medical best practice and an adoption of a more restricted set of therapeutic alternatives that are available to the patient and their provider. To date, the patient has the option of choosing to pay privately for the medications that are not sponsored by the agency that pays for their healthcare. This private pay option has resulted in continuation of the sale of some of these medications by those patients willing and able to do so. This creates a market for those drugs that incentivize drug makers to continue to produce these drugs and helps to keep options available to those who may not receive benefit from the approved drugs.

While it is likely that widespread adoption of CER will result in adoption of medical best practices that will be perceived by some as healthcare rationing, it is also likely that the number and severity of the barriers that must be overcome in order to bring it to reality are real and complex. It is likely that the adoption of EHR, the development of the infrastructure including state, regional and national health networks and all of the associated components of those efforts will be gradual and will be years in the making. Hopefully Americans can use this time to engage in the tough conversations needed to make sure that the system we do develop is the most effective and ethical approach to administering and paying for healthcare.

REFERENCES

AMA Practice Management Center. (2008). *2008 national health insurer report card*. AMA.

American Recovery and Reinvestment Act of 2009, (2009). *Text*.

Anonymous. (2010). *Privacy & security standards workgroup.* Retrieved Mary 30, 2010, from http://healthit.hhs.gov/portal/server.pt?open=512&objID=1481&parentname=CommunityPage&parentid=2&mode=2&in_hi_userid=10741&cached=true

Anonymous. (2010). *Privacy and security and health information technology.* Retrieved May 21, 2010, from http://healthit.hhs.gov/portal/server.pt?open=512&objID=1147&parentname=CommunityPage&parentid=16&mode=2&in_hi_userid=10741&cached=true

Anonymous,. (2010). Privacy issues still a concern. [from ProQuest Medical Library.]. *Modern Healthcare, 40*(9), 36. Retrieved May 9, 2010.

Aston, G. (2010). Comparative effectiveness. [from ProQuest Medical Library.]. *Trustee, 63*(1), 13–14, 19–21. Retrieved May 9, 2010.

Avorn, J. (2009). Debate about funding comparative effectiveness research. *The New England Journal of Medicine, 360*(19), 1927–1929. doi:10.1056/NEJMp0902427

Bacon, P., Jr. (March 18, 2010.). GOP lawmakers, candidates promise to 'repeal it', more than 100 sign pledge to back effort to overturn healthcare bill. *The Washington Post,* A04.

Blumenthal, D. (2009). Stimulating the adoption of health Information Technology. [from ProQuest Medical Library.]. *The New England Journal of Medicine, 360*(15), 1477–1479. Retrieved May 16, 2010. doi:10.1056/NEJMp0901592

Blumenthal, D. (2010). Launching HITECH. [from ProQuest Medical Library.]. *The New England Journal of Medicine, 362*(5), 382–385. Retrieved May 25, 2010. doi:10.1056/NEJMp0912825

Brailer, D. (2010). Guiding the health Information Technology agenda. [from ProQuest Medical Library.]. *Health Affairs, 29*(4), 586–594. Retrieved May 9, 2010. doi:10.1377/hlthaff.2010.0274

Brown, T. M., Cueto, M., & Fee, E. (2006). The World Health Organization and the transition from "International" to "Global" public health. [from ABI/INFORM Global.]. *American Journal of Public Health, 96*(1), 62–72. Retrieved May 16, 2010. doi:10.2105/AJPH.2004.050831

Brownstein, J., Freifeld, C., & Madoff, L. (2009). Digital disease detection-harnessing the Web for public health surveillance. [from ProQuest Medical Library.]. *The New England Journal of Medicine, 360*(21), 2153–2155, 2157. Retrieved May 17, 2010. doi:10.1056/NEJMp0900702

Buehler, J. W., Berkelman, R. L., Hartley, D. M., & Peters, C. J. (2003). Syndromic surveillance and bioterrorism-related epidemics. *Emerging Infectious Diseases, 9*(10), 1197-1204. Retrieved May 15, 2010, from http://ezproxy.library.capella.edu/login?url=http://search.ebscohost.com.library.capella.edu/login.aspx?direct=true&db=aph&AN=11063767&site=ehost-live&scope=site

Detmer, D. E., Lumpkin, J. R., & Williamson, J. J. (2009). Defining the medical subspecialty of clinical informatics. *Journal of the American Medial Informatics, 16*(2), 167–168. doi:10.1197/jamia.M3094

Executive Order 13335. (2004). Federal Register U.S.C.

Freedman, I. (2007). What does "interoperability" really mean? [from ProQuest Medical Library.]. *Health Management Technology, 28*(10), 50–51. Retrieved May 9, 2010.

Gostin, L. O., & Nass, S. (2009)... *Journal of the American Medical Association, 301*(13), 1373–1375. doi:10.1001/jama.2009.424

Hammond, W., Bailey, C., Boucher, P., Spohr, M., & Whitaker, P. (2010). Connecting information to improve health. [from ABI/INFORM Global.]. *Health Affairs, 29*(2), 284–288. Retrieved May 31, 2010. doi:10.1377/hlthaff.2009.0903

Healthcare Information Management and Systems Society. (2009). *20th annual 2009 HIMSS leadership survey (annual survey No. 20)*. HIMSS.

Hillestad, R., Bigelow, J., Bower, A., & Girosi, F. (2005). Can electronic medical record systems transform health care? Potential health benefits, savings, and costs. *Health Affairs, 24*(5), 1103. Retrieved May 11, 2010, from http://proquest.umi.com.library.capella.edu/pqdweb?did=899710741&Fmt=7&clientId=62763&RQT=309&VName=PQD

Isaacs, S., Jellinek, P., & Ray, W. (2009). The independent physician-Going, going… [from ProQuest Medical Library.]. *The New England Journal of Medicine, 360*(7), 655–657. Retrieved May 25, 2010. doi:10.1056/NEJMp0808076

Johnson, T. D. (2010). Health officials use new means to trace sources of food illness. *Nation's Health, 40*(4), 1-12. Retrieved May 16, 2010, from http://ezproxy.library.capella.edu/login?url=http://search.ebscohost.com.library.capella.edu/login.aspx?direct=true&db=aph&AN=50140933&site=ehost-live&scope=site

Kaushal, R., Bates, D., Jenter, C., Mills, S., Volk, L., & Burdick, E. (2009). Imminent adopters of electronic health records in ambulatory care. [Retrieved from Academic Search Premier database.]. *Informatics in Primary Care, 17*(1), 7–15.

Korst, L. M., Signer, J. M. K., Aydin, C., & Fink, A. (2008). Identifying organizational capacities and incentives for clinical data-sharing: The case of a regional perinatal information system. *Journal of the American Medical Informatics Association, 15*(2), 195–197. doi:10.1197/jamia.M2475

Lassetter, J. (2010). HIEs to transform. [from ProQuest Medical Library.]. *Health Management Technology, 31*(1), 18. Retrieved May 9, 2010.

Levey, N. N. (February 4, 2010). Soaring cost of healthcare sets a record: Spending was 17.3% of the economy last year. The share paid by the U.S. will soon exceed 50%, a study says. *Los Angeles Times,* pp. 1.

Margolis, P., & Halfon, N. (2009). Innovation networks. A strategy to transform primary health care. *Journal of the American Medical Association, 302*(13), 1461–1462. doi:10.1001/jama.2009.1428

McCormick, D., Woolhandler, S., Bose-Kolanu, A., Germann, A., Bor, D. H., & Himmelstein, D. U. (2009). U.S. physicians' views on financing options to expand health insurance coverage: A national survey. *JGIM: Journal of General Internal Medicine, 24*(4), 526–531. doi:10.1007/s11606-009-0916-x

McGraw, D., Dempsey, J., Harris, L., & Goldman, J. (2009). Privacy as an enabler, not an impediment: Building trust into health information exchange. [from ABI/INFORM Global.]. *Health Affairs, 28*(2), 416–427. Retrieved May 25, 2010. doi:10.1377/hlthaff.28.2.416

McKinney, M. (2010, April). 'Huge potential' for EHRs and comparative effectiveness. [from ProQuest Medical Library.]. *Hospitals & Health Networks, 84*(4), 41–42. Retrieved May 9, 2010.

Merlis, M. (2009). *Simplifying administration of health insurance.* Retrieved May 11, 2010, from http://www.rwjf.org/files/research/merlisadmin.pdf

Morrissey, J. (1999). Integration sacrificed for Y2K preparation. [Retrieved from CINAHL with Full Text database.]. *Modern Healthcare, 29*(18), 31.

News Staff. (2010). *'Meaningful use' rule needs significant modifications, says AAFP.* Retrieved from http://www.aafp.org/online/en/home/publications/news/news-now/practice-management/20100304mean-use-ltr.html

Richey, W. (March 23, 2010). Attorneys General in 14 states sue to block healthcare reform law. *The Christian Science Monitor.*

Ridgely, M. S., & Jerrell, J. M. (1996). Analysis of three interventions for substance abuse treatment of severely mentally ill people. *Community Mental Health Journal, 32*(6), 561. Retrieved May 8, 2010, from http://proquest.umi.com.library.capella.edu/pqdweb?did=10347436&Fmt=7&clientId=62763&RQT=309&VName=PQD

Rodwin, M. A. (2009). The case for public ownership of data. *Journal of the American Medical Association, 302*(1), 86–88. doi:10.1001/jama.2009.965

Safran, C., Bloomrosen, M., Hammond, E., Labkoff, S., Markel-Fox, S., & Tang, P. C. (2007). Toward a national framework for the secondary use of health data: An American Medical Informatics Association White Paper. *Journal of the American Medical Informatics Association, 14*(1), 1–9. doi:10.1197/jamia.M2273

Santiago, A. (2010). *The medicus firm physician survey: Health reform may lead to significant reduction in physician workforce.* Retrieved May 9, 2010, from http://www.themedicusfirm.com/pages/medicus-media-survey-reveals-impact-health-reform

Schwartz, A., Pappas, C., & Sandlow, L. J. (2010). Data repositories for medical education research: Issues and recommendations. *Academic Medicine, 85*(5), 837–843. doi:10.1097/ACM.0b013e3181d74562

Shortliffe, E. H. (2005). Strategic action in health Information Technology: Why the obvious has taken so long. [from ABI/INFORM Global.]. *Health Affairs, 24*(5), 1222–1233. Retrieved May 31, 2010. doi:10.1377/hlthaff.24.5.1222

Strecha, D., Persad, G., Marckmann, G., & Danis, M. (2009). Are physicians willing to ration health care? Conflicting findings in a systematic review of survey research. *Health Policy Journal, 95*(2), 113–124. doi:10.1016/j.healthpol.2008.10.013

Truffer, C., Keehan, S., Smith, S., Cylus, J., Sisko, A., & Poisal, J. (2010). Health spending projections through 2019: The recession's impact continues. [from ABI/INFORM Global.]. *Health Affairs, 29*(3), 522–529. Retrieved May 13, 2010. doi:10.1377/hlthaff.2009.1074

U.S. Department of Health and Human Services. (2010). *NHIN exchange.* Retrieved 2010, May 17, from http://healthit.hhs.gov/portal/server.pt?open=512&objID=1407&parentname=CommunityPage&parentid=8&mode=2&in_hi_userid=11113&cached=true

U.S. Department of Health and Human Services. (2010). *Health information security and privacy collaboration.* Retrieved 2010, May 17, from http://healthit.hhs.gov/portal/server.pt?open=512&mode=2&cached=true&objID=1240

Webster, P. (2010). Concern raised over control of cost-benefit research in United States. [from ProQuest Medical Library.]. *Canadian Medical Association Journal, 182*(2), E127–E128. Retrieved May 9, 2010. doi:10.1503/cmaj.109-3140

Wechsler, J. (2009). Pharma girds for healthcare reform. *Pharmaceutical Technology, 33*(8), 22, 24, 26-27. Retrieved May 8, 2010, from ABI/INFORM Global.

Yasnoff, W. A., Humphreys, B. L., Overhage, J. M., & Detmer, D. E. (2004). A consensus action agenda for achieving the national health information infrastructure. [from ProQuest Medical Library.]. *Journal of the American Medical Informatics Association, 11*(4), 332–338. Retrieved May 16, 2010. doi:10.1197/jamia.M1616

Chapter 2
Health Care Information Systems and the Risk of Privacy Issues for the Disabled

John Beswetherick
Capella University, USA

ABSTRACT

The healthcare industry is moving towards adoption of electronic health records. There are associated privacy and security implications to this move towards electronic collection and storage of sensitive health information. This chapter suggests that the impact on the privacy and security of health information for disabled individuals is greater than that for the general populace. Contributors to this increased risk are related to the increase in dependence on the clinical care system and the related increase in volume of the data that is collected, stored and exchanged as a function of providing care to this population.

INTRODUCTION

Recent technological advances in online healthcare services are providing patients and care providers' unprecedented access to medical records. Consequently with expanded online availability of medical records, the potential for privacy and security issues increases dramatically. Medical records can contain detailed information regarding

a wide variety of personal medical data regarding disease information, family histories, genetics, substance abuse and even mental health issues. Patient sentiment is echoed by a Harris Interactive (2005) survey on medical privacy revealing that over 70 percent of patients were concerned that their private medical information might be compromised.

Patients with disabilities generally have a greater need for medical specialty care and the ability to access online medical records delivers

DOI: 10.4018/978-1-60960-174-4.ch002

many added benefits. Because disabled individuals amass a higher than average volume of medical data, they naturally have a statistically higher exposure to privacy and security violations. When online medical records are available, healthcare communication and information access is made more efficient for referrals, prescriptions, appointment scheduling, obtaining specialty consultation and other medical information. Additional efficiency is provided for disabled patients who need to rely on guardians, caregivers and family members to help administer medical records, billing and insurance claims.

This unprecedented access to medical data is not without risks, as privacy violations frequently occur at odds with the rigid requirements of the Health Insurance Portability and Accountability Act of 1996 (HIPAA 2009). In the Conn (2007) interview with Paul Tang of the Medical Foundation, Tang asserts that vendor IT contracts have provisions that counter HIPAA guidelines. "There are contracts that say they will have real-time access to the database, that they will have exclusive access to the data, that they can resell the data. I think it would be unlawful that covered entities abide by that."

Leveraging and commoditizing patient medical information have become common practice by employers, insurers and medical providers to help manage risk and maximize profits. D'Allegro (2000) reports from a study by California Health-Care that 6 out of 21 companies surveyed, forwarded results of online health assessment survey to outside companies for analysis, disregarding privacy consent requirements. In quote from the D'Allegro article, Sam Karp CIO of California HealthCare states, "Information is being collected without consumers' knowledge and consumers are not being told and some companies that say they don't transfer information to third parties do."

There is continued pressure in the insurance markets to reduce costs and limit exposure. Access to confidential patient data can help make actuarial decisions about a patients potential for

generating insurance claims. Compromised genetic information can provide insurance companies with definitive information about the potential for acquiring a disease later in life or even the potential for children of the insured to develop any of over 6,000 known single gene disorder currently known in the medical field (Center for Disease Control, 2009).

Genetic testing is now becoming much more common and such information can be stored in the patient history and used for profiling susceptibility to illnesses. Other information such as participation in pharmaceutical clinical trials, exposure to environmental hazards, even applications for life, disability or accident insurance can be included.

Our disabled population is put at great risk for continuity of care when medical and insurance decisions are made using private medical information. Furthermore, employers and insurance companies may ask applicants to grant access to private medical information in the conditional application process. Any employment and insurance decisions under these guidelines can constitute unfair privacy practices. If an employer offers a position conditionally in a non-binding contract for employment, they can ask the prospective employee to sign an insurance waiver granting access to their private medical records. Loopholes in privacy law may allow for third parties to circumvent privacy legislation by outsourcing patient data to Managed Care Organizations (MCOs) operating outside HIPAA guidelines. Soon after HIPAA was introduced in 1996, Acuff (1999) discusses the dilemma faced by mental health providers in regards to the ethical access of private patient data. This is especially problematic for the developmentally disabled population that may have limited understanding of their privacy rights.

Acuff (1999) states that "Many practitioners are experiencing dilemmas or are raising questions about their ethical obligations because some MCOs deny authorization for needed treatment, fail to respect patient privacy, restrict communications between psychologists and their patients, or are perceived as attempting to intimidate psychologists through the use of "no cause termination" clauses. Although these practices are not engaged in by every MCO, they are clearly problematic when they occur."

The continued trend to outsource health care information services to areas outside of HIPAA and World Trade Organization (WTO 2009) protective guidelines further erodes privacy guidelines for intellectual property. Anand and Data (2004) discuss the nondeterministic legal protection of outsourced medical data; "European data directives insist that if data relating to EU citizens is being transferred to an outsourcing destination such as India for processing then India must accord a commensurate level of protection or else the data cannot be transferred."

Many pharmaceutical companies are outsourcing clinical trials to India. One of the questions being examined by an Indian government advisory group is whether Article 39 of TRIPs (WTO 2009) envisages a specific period for data protection, irrespective of the confidentiality of the data. One view is that the obligations of Article 39 arise in the context of "undisclosed information" or trade secrets only. In other words if the data is available on the internet then it need not be protected by a body in charge of giving marketing approval for pharmaceuticals.

Patients funded by government health and human services agencies have an increased level of administrative overhead required to process payments and document care. Online transactions and storage of files in large government hosted databases are attractive targets for would be hackers and identity thieves. Also, because of the nature of some disabilities, many patients require guardian or third parties to help administrate their medical transactions, further opening up private information to other caregivers.

Compromised patient information has a punctuated effect on the disabled population, as they have a higher level of online medical transactions and are more vulnerable to the effects of agencies who may scope or deny coverage based on patient care data. Once compromised, illegally accessed patient data can continue to have ripple effects at many levels, including insurance and employment opportunities. The instances of identity theft has risen consistently each year even though security technology and efforts have also increased. The Federal Trade Commission (2006) reports as many as 8 million Americans (3.7%) were victims of identity theft in 2005, this number increased to 9.9 million in 2008.

With so much at stake, clearly protecting our most medically vulnerable citizens from illegal access to their private information, needs to be a high priority for future and enhanced privacy legislation.

BACKGROUND

Throughout history individuals with disabilities have been treated as second-rate citizens in most world cultures. Many were labeled as outcasts and kept from enjoying the same privileges afforded to the non-disabled population. Prior to modern medical advances, little was known about therapeutic and rehabilitative practices. Individuals with disabilities or developmental impairments were typically unable to get the medical help needed to live full mainstream lives. This type of prejudice went on for much of recorded history.

The Disability Social History Project (2009) chronicles the long historical journey disabled individuals have travelled to obtain equal rights under the law. It was not until the 16th century that legal scholars even began accepting the right of deaf and mute individuals to marry and have children. Other notable milestones in obtaining equal rights for disabled individuals were: The establishment of the first school for the deaf in 1755, Louis Braille invents raised text in 1829, and the first wheelchair is patented in 1869, the first elevator for the disabled built in 1912 and the

American Foundation for the Blind was formed in 1921.

Eventually governments began to officially recognize different classifications of disabilities and began to award benefits on a limited basis. Helander (1999) states that "In many developing countries, efforts have started to provide services for certain recognized groups of disabled people. At the very beginning, these groups often included injured freedom fighters or war heroes. Efforts focused frequently on providing rehabilitation, as well as on paying disability pensions to make up for the loss of income which such persons might have incurred as a result of a serious disability. Other groups, which have received official recognition, services and benefits, are traffic injury victims, military personnel and government civil servants. In many cases, an insurance system or a social security system has been set up for these categories of people."

PRIVACY AND DISABILITY LEGISLATION

In the latter half of the 20th century the disability rights movement started to make progress, gradually giving disabled individuals in the United States more equal access to society. Social Security Disability Insurance (SSDI) was established in 1956, followed by concurrent pioneering work for the developmentally disabled by Eunice Kennedy Shriver creating multiple agencies for the disabled, including establishment of the Special Olympics in 1968. Passage of the Rehabilitation Act of 1973 was a major precursor to the most sweeping doctrine on disabled rights, the Americans with Disabilities Act (ADA), passed into law in 1990.

In an unprecedented milestone for individuals with disabilities, the United Nations passed the Rights of Persons with Disabilities and its associated Optional Protocol on December 13th, 2006 with almost unanimous approval by UN member nations. This legislation declares comprehensive

individual rights for the disabled. A key element of the legislation is equal access to health care and mandate of privacy rights for adults with disabilities. U.N. Office of Legal Affairs (2006) suggests banning all forms of discrimination against persons with disabilities specific to privacy, through the adoption of article 22 "Respect for Privacy". The UN legislation specifically states:

1. No person with disabilities, regardless of place of residence or living arrangements, shall be subjected to arbitrary or unlawful interference with his or her privacy, family, home or correspondence or other types of communication or to unlawful attacks on his or her honour and reputation. Persons with disabilities have the right to the protection of the law against such interference or attacks.

2. States Parties shall protect the privacy of personal, health and rehabilitation information of persons with disabilities on an equal basis with others.

Kanter (2007) discusses the gravity and importance of the legislation. "As to the important issue of access, the Convention requires State Parties to identify and eliminate obstacles and barriers, in order to ensure that persons with disabilities may access their environment, transportation, public facilities, services, information, and communications.' The Convention also affirms the equal rights and advancement of women and children with disabilities."

Hendriks (2007) points out a key unenforceable aspect of the legislation, allowing nation states to continue prejudicial practices against the disabled members of society. Hendriks (2007) states that "The Convention, above all, imposes duties upon States, instead of bestowing individuals with rights. At the same time, it should be noted that this provision - and the Convention in general - builds on the classical typology of State obligations first described by UN Special Rapporteur and Norwegian human rights scholar Asbjorn

Eide, seemingly aware of the fact that obligations to ensure and protect typically correspond with justifiable rights, whereas obligations to promote can - dependent on the particularities of the situation - only under certain circumstances be enforced by individuals."

Even with firm rights and guidelines in place, Smith (2009) reports employers have put together an impressive litigation record fighting disability-based cases, "From 1992 to 1997, employers won 92 percent of the ADA cases tried and 86 percent of the administrative complaints ruled on by the Equal Employment Opportunity Commission (EEOC), according to an American Bar Association Commission on Mental and Physical Disability Law... The vast majority of the employers successfully argued that the employee was not disabled and, therefore, not covered by the Act."

Based on this impressive showing by employer legal departments, Congress amended the ADA in 2008 to broaden the classification of disabilities and determine the level of disability afforded to an individual even if they have rehabilitated to a fully functional condition. According to Smith (2009) "Determination of disability will be made in the "uncorrected" state so that even if the impairment is controlled, in remission, or episodic in nature, if it would substantially limit major activity if it were active it would be considered a disability."

While we now live in an era, where the inalienable rights of person's with disabilities are recognized by the vast majority of nations on Earth, the legislation necessary to enforce these rights are still in their infancy. Requiring individuals to be aware of their rights and mandated to take action when rights are compromised. However, knowing when privacy rights are infringed upon can be a difficult proposition, as access to privacy information is not necessarily a reportable offense under multiple circumstances (Rothstein and Talbott 2007, Hendriks 2007). Even though individual remedies through litigation may be possible, bringing on change that has profound effect on the disabled population as a whole is not as realistic.

THE HIGH POTENTIAL FOR SECURITY BREACHES

Medical records contain the most sensitive personnel data we own. Security breaches can lead to billing fraud, privacy violations, indentify theft and other forms of information disclosure. Black market entities seek out account information, insurance cards and other personal collateral on a continuing basis. Even more shocking, is the rise in criminal activity related to ransoming of sensitive information. A recent incident reported by Wikileaks (2009) describes a security breach in Virginia were eight million confidential prescription drug records were sequestered. A subsequent ransom attempt to collect ten million dollars for return of the data is ongoing.

While it is essential to control unauthorized records access by hackers and through other illegal activities, there are cases where patient files can be legally compromised. Rothstein and Talbott (2007) elaborate further, "the authorized access to health information pursuant to a compelled authorization represents a significant and largely overlooked threat to privacy and confidentiality. In short, it is lawful for employers, insurers and other third-parties to require that individuals sign authorizations of unlimited scope for the release of their health records as a condition of applying for or obtaining employment, insurance, or benefits under numerous essential programs and services."

An individual's medical condition can have a profound effect on the level of privacy afforded their medical and personal records. If classified with a life threatening or infectious condition, disabled patients can relinquish many of their inherent privacy rights even in countries with ADA like protections. Societies without inherent protections for individuals with disabilities routinely institutionalize the disabled. Through stronger privacy legislation, the China Daily (2001) reported that Chinese government lost its first lawsuit regarding leaking of personal medical data, as up through 2001 it was common place for medical officials in China to release the names of HIV patients.

Worldwide the vast majority of disabled patients do not have access to networked computer systems. According to a study by the Pew Internet and American Life Project (2003) "Just 38 percent of disabled Americans use the Internet...This compares to the 58% of all Americans who use the Internet." Rarely are computer systems provided to disabled patients in institutional settings. Those systems that are available can be monitored under the auspices of protecting the disabled patient from outside networks. Medical records thus become one of the primary sources of privacy information exposure for disabled individuals.

Most disabled patients are dependent on their health care providers and governmental agencies to secure personal healthcare data. While secure and private access to medical data is mandated by HIPAA and ADA decree in the United States, online medical data utilized and accessed by legitimate entities has a significant potential for error. Kuehn (2009) documents to the impact of errors in patient records at the Veterans Administration, "Nine VA medical centers reported another type of problem related to their electronic records system: physician orders to stop medication were missed, causing some patients to receive intravenous medications longer than necessary. The problem occurred because after the software upgrade, physician orders to discontinue such medications, which had previously appeared at the top of the screen, were not displayed."

Elizabeth Freeman (2004), Director of the VA Palo Alto Health Care System, reveals the broad reach of the VA services in the United States and potential impact of such errors, "About a quarter of the nation's population, approximately 70 million people, are potentially eligible for VA benefits and services because they are veterans, family members or survivors of veterans." Freeman adds that a large percent of the disabled veterans use VA services annually, "In 2002, more than 4.5 million people received care in VA health care facilities, which are used annually by approximately 75 percent of all disabled and low income veterans."

In another well-documented software defect in the VA system, patient medical data was merged with other patient records, when healthcare workers progressively scanned through files. This error was detected in 41 of 153 agencies, allowing medical and administrative personnel to access patient data for individuals they were not caring for. Subsequently this privacy violation was fixed with a software patch in late 2008, limiting the period of the defect to about 6 months.

Privately administered databases through local care providers are potentially less vulnerable to hacker attacks since they are not considered high value targets, however, their level of IT proficiency is typically lower than large managed government run institutions. Ideally all agencies would house medical information securely, but there remains a substantial risk to data compromise by unwanted attackers or unauthorized data access by affiliated agencies.

Meeting the rigid requirements of HIPAA and the Medical Information Privacy and Security Act (MIPSA, 1999) is a continuing uphill battle for IT professionals serving the medical community. MIPSA is the follow-on legislature designed to tighten up HIPAA requirements. Key provisions of HIPAA include generation of audit trails with all medical transactions. Also, MIPSA (1999) provides options for other key components of patient privacy;

- "Gives individuals the right to view their medical records without exception unless they elect to waive that right as part of a clinic trial.
- Allows an individual to self pay if they do not want their personal health informa-

tion to be disclosed to a health insurer for payment.

• Allows individuals to segregate portions of their medical record from broader viewing."

Unfortunately many of the specific steps that consumers can take to view, conceal and correct their medical information has currently not been established by any legislative body. We are still in our infancy in securing online medical data.

INCREASED PRIVACY EXPOSURE IN THE NETWORK FOR DISABILITY CARE

Continuity of care for disabled individuals can be quite extensive, with data storage extending from the government health care databases, to the physical records of the patient's locals personal physician and out to any number of specialists in the medical community. Each office, lab and administrative building has their own computer network and security protocols.

The full chain of patient records is only as strong as the weakest link in the data stream. Because of the extraordinary volume of medical data, institutions and specialists that the disabled community interacts with, there is a much higher level of data activity that can be exposed to infiltration. Communicating across multiple agencies with such volumes, exposes patient records to more frequent security attacks and increases opportunities for private data disclosure.

Prior to HIPAA enactment there was a wide range of disparate data management requirements that evolved in the United States. After establishment of HIPAA in 1996, the transition was not immediate to meet medical data management requirements. Even today in the United States not all government and private healthcare agencies have the same levels of privacy, training, network security and data protection protocols necessary to

be HIPAA compliant. Medical offices are required by HIPAA law to manage medical data professionally, by securing, backing up and protecting patient protected healthcare information. Not all health care entities can carry their own IT departments and often look to outside data management groups to administer their patient data. More complex data management requirements include; multiple site storage, incremental backup of medical data, automated scheduled data maintenance tasks and self documenting data processing to meet the rigid privacy requirements of HIPAA.

Onsite data management solutions are now being supplanted by web-based solutions, allowing for central protected storage of medical data. Online warehousing and processing of data allows medical offices to contract out their medical needs on systems designed to be HIPAA compliant. Disabled patients, especially those that have government funding options, have their records exposed in data warehouses that are considered high value targets. These large government and healthcare databases contain extremely sensitive patient data, when compromised can have disastrous effects.

In 2006 a VA employee's laptop was stolen containing healthcare data for 26 millions United States veterans. While the laptop did not contain health records, it did contain patient name, social security numbers and disability codes. Lubell (2006) discusses the potential impact on effected veterans, "The simple release of a diagnostic or *disability* code leading to sensitive and private *medical* information could damage a person's ability to get a job or insurance in the private sector", said Deborah Peel, chairwoman of the Patient Privacy Rights Foundation, a national watchdog organization based in Austin, Texas. "This is about public shame and humiliation, even extortion and bribery. Someone for example could threaten to reveal that a veteran who was now living and working in some town as an elected official has HIV, or post-traumatic stress disorder, to damage his public image."

While most developed countries have national based healthcare systems, the United States is somewhat unique in their health care system, as it's a combination of public, private and corporate based funding. This structure leads to more dynamic dataflow relationships and opens up additional potential for health data compromise. Typical patient/provider insurance claims require a series of information requests between agencies to pre-authorize care. Disabled individuals typically have more complex relationships with health care providers. Medical authorizations may range across multiple agencies from State departments of Developmental Disabilities, to federal levels like Medicare/Medicaid and the Veterans Administration.

All these transactions start at the patient provider and work their way through a complex set of relationships which typically include interaction between physicians, home healthcare providers, employers, pharmacies, insurance companies, state and federal agencies. Auxiliary support staffs that are outside of the HIPAA boundaries are often called in for medical diagnostic and imaging support. Ongoing palliative and therapeutic care rounds out a wide array of health care providers that need access to patient data. The more systems the patient data passes through the greater the risk for information compromise.

GLOBAL PRIVACY CONSIDERATIONS AND THE DISABLED

The National Health Service (NHS) of the United Kingdom has been criticized for not having rigid enough security on their national health care databases, potentially allowing open access by healthcare workers to patient data, as millions of government workers can access UK health care records at anytime. Privacy provisions in the United Kingdom are based on the Data Protection Act 1998 (2009). Like MIPSA, the NHS does have

protocols for viewing and correcting patient data, but the procedures are not widely established and few patients have to date been successful in correcting and cordoning off their sensitive data. A recent movement established by the TheBigOptOut.org (2009) is pushing the provisions of NHS charter, to allow for UK patients to block large portions of sensitive medical data from view.

In New Zealand the Health Information Privacy Code 1994 (2009) is similar in structure to the UK Data Protection Act, again providing legislation and open allowances for correcting personal data. According to the Human Rights Commission (2009), "The Health Information Code 1994 applies to providers of health services and services for disabled people. It addresses the collection, storage and security of personal health information, and protects the right of consumers to access and correct information about themselves, as well as restricting its use to the purpose for which the information is obtained."

In countries, without similar protections and less focus on maintaining secured record systems, the potential for privacy abuses continue to increase. In many third world countries, records are not yet electronically stored. As their online systems develop, the core requirements must be to safeguard patient data and protect citizenry from the potential devastating effects of medical file compromise.

For example, Burris (2002) discusses the status loss and discrimination an individual may endure if sensitive medical information is not fully protected. Moreover, Burris acknowledges the limitations of protections for the disabled in respect to privacy issues. Burris (2002) states that "we have to confront the current weakness of U.S. protective law, particularly the Americans with Disabilities Act (ADA). Under the U.S. Supreme Court's most recent cases, the protection actually available to a range of traditionally stigmatized diseases, including epilepsy and cancer, is uncertain Privacy law is also an often slender reed. We have tended to concentrate protection of medical information in the public sphere and medical practice, but more risk of disclosure may lie in the insurance, pharmacy, and other commercial uses of data."

The African Charter on Human and People's Rights (the African Charter), 1981 was established in 1981 and is clear on its focus on protection of woman's rights in the region. Even with the passing of the United Nations Rights of Persons with Disabilities, at continued risk are the privacy rights of disabled women in certain regions of Africa. Numerous critics continue to cite the reality of the situation for woman's rights in Africa. Olowu (2006) states that "From access to land and commercial credit, to employment, labor and training, to health, reproductive and family life, to equal participation in governance and development processes, African women have continued to face particularly great obstacles in the realization of the promise of human rights."

Public assistance for the disabled population has been slow to manifest in China. Even up through the latter half of the 20th century (Leung 2006) indicates that China operated a limited relief program in the cities, catering mainly to the disabled and a few other underprivileged classes in major cities. In total only 2 million Chinese received any additional assistance from the central Chinese government in 1997. Then as part of a movement to support the disadvantaged population, assistance from the central government increased to 22 million by 2003, serving more people outside large cities. Leung (2006) indicates that "About 34 per cent of them (households receiving assistance) had disabled persons, and 64.9 per cent had chronically sick members in their family."

With this increase in government support for the disabled and infirmed, a call for increased patient privacy protection has grown in China. Together with the growing level of support for the disabled population in the home, a large percentage of the severely disabled population is also institutionalized. Leung (2006) character-

izes the Chinese support system as disjoint and decentralized. According to Leung (2006), "All benefits are means-tested, stringent, low level and heavily stigmatized. Complementary support in housing, medical care, education, employment and personal social services is largely underdeveloped, inadequate and not institutionalized. The role of private charity is extremely limited. With these features, Chinese social assistance does not seem to fit neatly into any one of the typologies of social assistance regimes categorized by Gough et al. (1997). Accordingly, it is still premature to group the Chinese social welfare system conceptually together with those of other countries.

White (1998), states that "Given the growing and decentralized support for disabled care and assistance, there is a marked increase in risk of privacy violations." Without clear guidelines in place in China, the effect on patient privacy is also magnified. China recognizes the inherent level of medical privacy rights and in 2001 ruled on the countries first case involving the leaking of sensitive medical information, involving a patient that had their HIV/AIDS diagnosis revealed. The China Daily (2001) reveals that "Officials from the Ministry of Health have called for more attention to the protection of the right to privacy of HIV/AIDS patients, following a court ruling that a hospital damaged a patient's reputation by releasing false HIV-related information about her. The Xinzhou Intermediate People's Court of Shanxi Province rejected the appeal of the Xinzhou Prefectural People's Hospital against the original ruling by a district court, in the country's first such case."

Chinese law tends to recognize the rights of society over individual privacy rights. Specific to the HIV/AIDS privacy rights Ye and Wei (2005) provide specific insight into the damaging potentials of being labeled at HIV positive. According to Ye and Wei (2005), "Starting from the beginning of the 1990s, China has made the viral test of surface antigens and antibodies a must, which rules out the possibility of privacy protection (anyone who handles the physical checkup form, when there is not any restriction, may get to know who is an HVB carrier). This, plus the misunderstanding of HVB carriers, has made HVB carriers universally excluded by employer units. For those who have been screened out to carry HVB, they are often discriminated against in work or even dismissed due to the lack of corresponding privacy protection mechanism."

Yet the potential for addressing patient privacy issues in developing countries and those with centralized medical systems is positive according to (Bristol, 2005) who indicates, "Countries that are farthest along in privacy protections are those with more centralized health systems, comprehensive strategic plans, and the willingness to make the necessary investment. Leaders include many European countries, Canada, Australia, China, South Korea, and Japan."

In this millennium positive advances for disabled rights has been made, starting to bring privacy levels on par with non-disabled patients. Recognizing the inherent rights of the disabled to privacy is a monumental step forward. However, until insurance companies, governments and employers recognize the additional pressures that are faced by the disabled population in forfeiting privacy rights, individuals with disabilities will continue to be discriminated against in the employment opportunities, insurance coverage and other issues which have medical care as a major decision point. Release of sensitive medical information can have profound effects on individuals, especially those with conditions that are shunned by society or genetic defects that insurance companies rule out for coverage.

MEDICAL RECORDS ACCESS AND PATIENT RIGHTS

Employment opportunities are limited for the Developmentally Disabled, yet State governments are committed to providing developmentally disabled individuals with opportunities to achieve meaningful lifestyles (Washington State DDD 2009). Employment health screening and insurance requirements can alienate developmentally disabled individuals from mainstream occupational choices. Having online access to health care records further exacerbates this experience, as employers can find out through investigations if a prospective employee is a net health care liability. As such, tight controls need to be put in place to prevent unauthorized access or request for health care information.

Fuhrmans (2005) indicates as many as 60 million individuals needing to buy their own health insurance and some 8% are rejected because of pre-existing conditions. As we evolve as a society and take part in a complete transformation to a digital medical record paradigm, developmentally disabled individuals, while protected under law by HIPAA, are constantly being subjected to requests for personal medical information disclosure. Whether it is admissions to a medical facility, applying for life insurance, or as part of a job application, loop holes are available to insurers, employers and medical institutions to access confidential medical records.

This needless intrusion on privacy rights is on its face illegal, but rarely is the behavior investigated, much less prosecuted. Everyday developmentally disabled individuals are subjected to institutionalized prejudice and reckless disregard to patient rights due to ignorance of the law. It is our obligation as a society to protect the infirmed and disabled from such violations.

HIPAA requires that the release of any patient information be accompanied by signed documentation specifying which parties can receive what information. Individuals with developmental disabilities may have limited knowledge of the rules of HIPAA or AMA's Code of Ethics, yet as a population are routinely asked to provide medical information for a wide variety of situations. There are a relatively small number of institutionalized patients that have individual authority over the release of their patient files. Most developmentally disabled patients have been assigned care-givers with proxy authorization, yet the number of proxy representatives with full knowledge of HIPAA and other information release protocols, is unclear according to Erlen (2004), "Patients and their families may have heard of HIPAA and the Privacy Rule, but they may be uncertain about what these regulations are and how they apply to their situation. They may have been given privacy rights documents and asked to sign consent forms, but they may not know why."

Leaving the patient open to multiple information exposure risks, in the most serious cases can potentially interrupt patient care, reduce or remove insurance benefits. A basic requirement in protecting individual privacy rights is informing people of their rights so they know when a violation has occurred and can be remedied.

DEVELOPMENTALLY DISABLED EMPLOYMENT PRACTICES

When a disabled individual shows up for a job interview, they are required by law to be treated the exact same as every other applicant. Specifically there is no box to check that the person being interviewed is disabled. Yet after a conditional offer of employment, perspective employees can be asked to go through a health screening. The American Management Association (2004) states that, "Employers long have been interested in selecting healthy employees because these employees are likely to be more productive, have lower rates of absenteeism and turnover, and cost less money for sick leave and health benefits. Under the Americans with Disabilities Act (ADA), employers with 15 or more employees are prohibited from asking health-related questions to applicants or requiring them to undergo a pre-employment medical examination… The American Management Association conducts employer surveys on medical testing of employees. According to the

2004 survey, 35.8% of employers required medical examinations to assess fitness for duty"

Not only are medical examinations possible for developmentally disabled applications for companies with less than 15 employees, employers in large companies can also subject applicants to medical information disclosure as part of pre-employment screening. For larger companies a conditional offer of employment puts the prospective employee in an awkward legal situation. Applicants are not assured of the new position until they relinquish their privacy rights to have their medical records assessed by insurance underwriters.

If a request was made to access patent's medical history, procedures could be put in place to log the request through a central service that would process the request with respect to the most up-to-date privacy laws. Any requests out of the realm of standard medical practice could be routed to the appropriate parties for additional consideration. Instead of full information disclosure, the system could negotiate a subset of information required to only meet the records request.

Any patient subscribing to such a privacy clearinghouse service, may initially be met with prejudice from requesting authorities until this type of advanced information access is made more mainstream, otherwise requesting entities may raise additional concern as to why an individual is associated with a medical information privacy protection service.

HEALTH CARE PRE-EMPLOYMENT INFORMATION REQUESTS AND PATIENT PRIVACY

The Bioethics Committee for the California Department of Developmental Services (DDS) is cognizant of the undercurrent of prejudice towards developmentally disabled individuals in the employment and medical setting. "It is the duty of the Department to protect fragile and vulnerable citizens, to serve those who are most often devalued by society in various ways. Prejudice starts with simple perception of difference, whether that difference is physical or psychological."

One way to combat this prejudice is not to label applicants and have them apply online. Leveling the playing field starts at the employment referral and application, but also extends to medical information disclosure. Employers should only be allowed to ask generic questions regarding an applicants physical and cognitive ability. For instance, can they read, use an computer input device, travel short distances unassisted. This would at least allow developmentally disabled applicants to have a fair shake at getting selected to participate in a real interview process. Once in the interview, then there are a myriad of other prejudices to overcome, but these are protected the Fair Hiring laws.

In addition, a compromised medical record, in the hands of a would be insurance provider, can affect the decision to insure a patient and lead to increased insurance premiums. While in some cases a pre-existing a condition diagnosis may legally be available to insurance providers and potential employers, specific diagnosis and levels of care need to be protected. Prescription records are readily available by insurers as soon as the patient gives consent to have their health history analyzed as part of the underwriting process.

In an interview with Deborah C. Peel, MD, founder of Patient Privacy Rights (Macios, 2009), Peel provides insight into the potential for private medical data to be accessed by unauthorized individuals, "The worst part, according to Peel, is that these entities are not required to keep an audit trail, so there is no way to know how far data travels and to what extent". "Plus," she says, "there is no requirement of breech reporting."

What kind of personal health information may be misused? Peel says everything from lab tests and genetic records, to medical and claims records, are subject to data mining because businesses that originally store or transfer the information later find that they can make money from selling it. For example, information is sold to medical device manufacturers, marketers, drug companies, and even to employers who want the information for making decisions regarding hiring and promotion. She also points out that data mining creates the perfect scenario for identity theft because health records also include all the necessary information (Social Security number, birth date, address, etc) to open a bank account."

Safeguarding private medical data from data mining interests that are in compliance with current HIPAA law, can be difficult. Limiting the amount of patient data medical providers can access, to just the data necessary for medical will help protect patient privacy. Also periodic follow-up with personal healthcare providers to make sure they are respecting all HIPAA requirements is an essential requirement. Disabled individuals typically have a much broader network of medical records to protect. When tied in with large institutional databases such as Medicare and HHS, these entities become high impact targets for hackers. As such, it is essential for governments to make it the highest possible priority to protect and monitor their healthcare databases on a continuous basis.

DEPENDENT CARE

Developmentally disabled individuals frequently require family members or guardians to provide proxy health service authorization. Giving guardians training on patient rights and responsibilities is essential to protecting a developmentally disabled individual from privacy violations. Guardian responsibility typically falls to a family member, however, Wikler and Hirschfeld (2003) and Jecker (2002) point out that there is no law on the books "…compelling family member to personally provide direct, hands-on care to dependent relatives."

Advances in medical, communication and robotic technologies will allow advanced remote monitoring of disabled patients from their own homes. With the advent of these smart technologies comes the increased need for information security. Implementation of remote sensing, RFID (Radio Frequency Identification) and tele-presence are highly dependent on wireless technologies, which have added security requirements beyond hard-wired systems. RFID embedded documentation can pose a serious privacy risk if medical alert information is placed in the RFID tag (Allan 2005). Hackers with RFID scanners can browse passersby undetected in crowded areas, reading contents of passports, driver licenses and employee access badges. If contents are not encrypted or shielded, private medical information is especially vulnerable for disabled individuals.

Cheek (2005) discusses the need for maintaining a level of technologic subtlety in the home environment to mitigate privacy concerns, especially when sensitive medical information is readily available to house guests via in home medical equipment display. "Integrity, security, and privacy are important concerns when designing such proactive systems. Unobtrusive placement of such systems would accommodate the need for privacy. It is important that people do not feel as if "Big Brother" is lurking about in their home but view the technology as something "being available" in time of need."

Our disabled population is gaining more independence with advances in computer system interfaces, better transportation and communication. But even in today's culture there is a mindset that people with disabilities are fully dependent on others for care. Those that provide help may feel obligated to provide personal assistance for every aspect of disabled individual's life. Doing so quickly erodes the boundaries of privacy. Any hint of not being self-sufficient seems to be a de facto invitation for another person to insert oneself directly in the life of a disabled individual. Those that take it upon themselves to manage others affairs are clearly making extraordinary privacy violations. There needs to be new protocols of behavior in place to allow our disabled popula-

tion to accept required help from others, without having to erode any sense of privacy.

Caring for individuals in group home or home health care settings provide excellent living environments for the developmentally disabled. Without the rigid IT requirements of a hospital or modern doctor's office, additional privacy issues could arise. For example homes using unsecured wireless networks could easily be compromised by local cyber criminals. Furthermore, the use of unencrypted 900 MHz phones to communicate with health care providers and insurance companies, could easily have health care, financial and personal data compromised

DEVELOPMENTAL EDUCATION AND PRIVACY

Prior to the passing of the Rehabilitation Act (1973) disabled students were routinely excluded from mainstream schools. Special education programs where not provided by the government, parents were expected to provide the funding for any special education needs. After World War II there was some movement to bring disabled children into the classroom. However, without the proper curriculum, teachers and counseling, disabled children during this era traditionally fell behind fellow students and in a majority of cases did not matriculate through to graduation.

Section 504 of the Rehabilitation Act mandated that disabled individuals cannot be excluded from any federally funded program based on their disability. Then in 1975 the Individuals with Disabilities Education Act (IDEA) was passed assuring individuals with disabilities a free and public education. Together with ADA mandates, disabled children in the United States are assured of being provided appropriate education for their disability.

Entry into these programs generates a large amount of medical, psychological and personal family data for each student. The amount of detailed medical and privacy information far exceeds the documentation level of non-disabled students in the educational system. Legislators recognized this and passed the Family Education Rights and Privacy Act (FERPA) and its follow-on legislation the Improving America's School Act (1994), to assure privacy of student records and establish clear criteria for release of sensitive data.

While these laws provide a huge level of privacy protection for disabled students, the National Center for Education Statistics (1997) reports there are some aspects of FERPA legislation that allows private records to be released to law enforcement and student disciplinary actions to be shared, "Information about disciplinary actions taken against students may be shared, without prior consent of the parent, with officials in other education institutions. Schools may release records in compliance with certain law enforcement judicial orders and subpoenas without notifying parents."

Aside from these potential privacy rights infringements, the past few decades have provided disabled students in the United States enhanced privacy protection. The remaining issue to be solved is the tightening of network security and file access by unauthorized individuals. Unlike mainstream students in the educational system, disabled students have details of their medical history, family backgrounds and even genetic diagnostic information. These records require extra protection from infiltration by unauthorized personnel; doing so is mandated by a number of high profile pieces of legislation.

ACCURATE AND SECURE CONVERSION OF PATIENT FILES

The art of maintaining a manual patient file in the primary care office had been perfected to some level in the latter half of the 20th century. With the push to an online-centralized patient record system, overall quality of patient record keeping was initially less efficient and prone to data transcription errors. As providers move to fully digitized record systems, error levels will decline. However, as a stopgap medical offices may opt to keep separate record systems, one using the old manual methodology and the other maintained through electronic databases. The process of maintaining records in parallel is in itself a process that contributes to added errors.

The number of disabled individuals living in home health care facilities has risen dramatically in the past 30 years. Many disabled people that were once institutionalized have now found more friendly living conditions in group home settings. Unlike government run treatment centers or private hospitals, home health care systems are more apt to keep paper based record systems and have primitive electronic medical record systems. In some respects it safer for small-localized agencies to keep their written record system in place and wait for fully secure affordable turn-key EMR's to come available. However, the disabled population can have a higher frequency of urgent care, hospitalization, medical appointments and administrative communication. As a result, medical histories, authorizations and administrative information have to be available at a moment's notice in order to receive the most effective emergency care. Any delay in authorization of records release can have profound effects on treatment.

When moving a patient to a temporary facility, bringing the right set of medical data is extremely important to assure precise continuity of care. If online records are relied upon, the records may be incomplete or important aspects of the medical information inaccessible due to mixed data access privileges. Additionally, stringent privacy policies may prevent emergency medical staff from understanding the full medical history of a patient, potentially compromising quality of care. Knowing what data to keep protected and what to be authorized for view, is an essential balance that must be optimized by care providers, for the individual medical situation of each disabled patient.

Until all these data access issues are resolved, each patient will have a challenge in securely sharing their records with the appropriate medical personnel. As a result, care facilities need to transport patients with full medical histories, along with doctor's orders in emergency situations. Transport has risks in losing information, detailing the wrong information and increasing diagnostic time in the event an unexpected medical condition is uncovered. Clearly online records would be a huge benefit for developmentally disabled patients with long and complex medical histories, but not at the cost of compromising patient privacy.

SECURING ONLINE ACCESS TO MEDICAL RECORDS

Securing our online medical resources is a difficult task and needs to be optimized around patient care, completeness of history, privacy and security of records. Privacy and security of records can only be assured when robust data access protocols are in place to assure immediate and secure access by authorized personnel. Medical access systems powered by a variety of vendors including Microsoft Healthcare (2008) focus on Single Sign-on (SSO) security and authentication using Active Directory technology. "Single sign-on (SSO) is the brass ring of Web security. It can help untangle the thickets of password prompts that frustrate clinicians and lead to security lapses, especially on easy-to-view shared workstations. More important, healthcare workers can share patient information securely across the entire continuum of care. By making it easier for clinicians to use digital records, SSO eliminates barriers to true collaborative patient care. Federal guidelines are also motivating the adoption of SSO, requiring most businesses with regulated data to use multi-factor authentication."

Beyond patient care for the developmentally disabled, the health care industry as a whole is concerned about privacy and security of patient records. A Health Industry Insights (2006) study shows that 85.5% of respondents are either concerned or very concerned about protecting privacy of personal health care information.

As Electronic Medical Records (EMR) systems proliferate across the health care environment, additional benefits will be accorded to the disabled. For example, a study by McLaughlin et al (1984) shows the difficulty in even tracking developmentally disabled infants over time. Without the proper record keeping in place and archived, something as simple as locating a patient for follow-up care was difficult. In their study the researchers tracked 237 developmentally disabled infants hospitalized in the first month of their lives, were attempted to be tracked at a mean age of 20 months. Researchers found that over half of the infants could no longer be located by the State or medical authorities. The study concluded that "Many infants likely to have major disabilities are hard to track using simple retrospective techniques." What is unknown from the study is the percent of patients that were uncovered in the research that had their birth medical records intact.

CONCLUSION

The United States and European Union have led the way in reforming patient privacy legislation. These last three decades have brought about great change in the way disabled individuals are treated in the world. After so many centuries and lifetimes of neglect and mistreatment, with the passing of the UN charter on the Rights of Persons with Disabilities, the rights of all disabled individuals in the world have finally been brought up to par with all citizens of our planet. While some societies will continue to treat people with disabilities as second class citizens, the framework has been established to provide the disabled population with a more level playing field to live their lives.

Because disabilities tend to require more extensive medical treatment over the lifetime of a patient, the risk for privacy breaches increases substantially for our disabled population due to the sheer volume of the medical data. Furthermore, if a disabled patient has their medical data compromised, it has the likelihood of revealing a serious condition that may be highly leveraged by data pirates. With these added risks, comes the potential for being excluded from employment opportunities and paying higher premiums if insurance is available at all.

The effects of a privacy breach can manifest beyond the disabled individual, especially if genetic patient data is compromised. As knowing the genetic signature of a disabled parent can provide deterministic and probabilistic data on the future of their children's health. As an example, testing newborn's for HIV or genetic defect, is an indirect violation of the mother's medical privacy. Knowing an offspring's medical condition can provide direct evidence of the parents medical condition. Once genetic or infectious disease information is tagged on an individual's medical record, it can be very difficult to remove from one's record or even detected that the onerous data has been recorded in the first place.

Disabled children are one of the few classes of individuals that have a full documented medical history in their expanded student file. Key legislations have been passed to limit the access to student files, but there is real potential for hackers compromising large educational databases. Once compromised the data can be ransomed, sold or made public at the expense of an individual's privacy. There are lawful exclusions to privacy laws that give authorities access to private medical data, all the way from reporting of infectious diseases to informing authorities of disciplinary actions of disabled students in the school.

The current set of privacy laws, legislations and guidelines in North America and Europe are the model for the rest of the world. Many nations are just now enacting their own privacy legislations, but all countries are now mandated by the Rights of persons with Disabilities to fully support privacy for the disabled population, a sharp contrast to the treatment of disabled individuals less than half a century ago. While penalties are in place for compromising the privacy information of disabled individuals, there are multiple loopholes around privacy legislation that allow access to the most sensitive data we own as individuals. Future legislation, coupled with continued advances in information technology in medical records databases and auditing technologies, will help to protect and inform us of privacy violations. This is especially critical for disabled individuals who have greater exposure to medical information and are most impacted by unauthorized access to personal medical records.

REFERENCES

Allan, R. (2005). Biometrics wields a double-edged sword. [from Academic Search Premier Database.]. *Electronic Design, 53*(14), 77–81. Retrieved September 10, 2009.

Allen, K. (1999). *Adults with severe disabilities: Federal and state approaches for personal care and other services: HEHS-99-101*. GAO Reports.

American Management Association. 2004. *AMA 2004 workplace testing survey: Medical testing*. Retrieved on July 29, 2009 from http://www.amanet.org/research/pdfs/medicaltesting04.pdf

Anand, P., & Datta, A. (2004). Protect your IP when outsourcing to India and managing intellectual property. Retrieved September 5, 2009, from Business Source Complete Database.

Bioethics Committee in Long-Term Care Institutions for the Developmentally Disabled. (2004)...*HEC Forum, 4*(3), 163–173. doi:10.1007/BF00057869

Blitz, C., & Mechanic, D. (2006). Facilitators and barriers to employment among individuals with psychiatric disabilities: A job coach perspective. *Work (Reading, Mass.), 26*(4), 407–419.

Blum, D. (2004). Weigh risks of offshore outsourcing. [from Business Source Complete Database.]. *New World (New Orleans, La.)*, *21*(10), 35–35. Retrieved September 6, 2009.

Bristol, N. (2005). The muddle of US electronic medical records. [from Academic Search Premier Database.]. *Lancet*, *365*(9471), 1610–1611. Retrieved September 6, 2009. doi:10.1016/S0140-6736(05)66492-6

Britz, J. (2008, May). Making the global information society good: A social justice perspective on the ethical dimensions of the global information society. *Journal of the American Society for Information Science and Technology*, *59*(7), 1171–1183. Retrieved September 6, 2009. doi:10.1002/asi.20848

Brooker, R. (2004). Consumers and IT: Setting policy priorities. [from Business Source Complete Database.]. *Consumer Policy Review*, *14*(4), 116–125. Retrieved September 6, 2009.

Burris, S. (2002). Disease stigma in U.S. public health law. [from Academic Search Premier Database.]. *The Journal of Law, Medicine & Ethics*, *30*(2), 179–190. Retrieved September 6, 2009. doi:10.1111/j.1748-720X.2002.tb00385.x

Cats-Baril, W., & Jelassi, T. (1994). The French Videotex system Minitel: A successful implementation of a national Information Technology infrastructure. [from Business Source Complete Database.]. *Management Information Systems Quarterly*, *18*(1), 1–20. Retrieved September 6, 2009. doi:10.2307/249607

Chan, V., Ray, P., & Parameswaran, N. (2008). Mobile e-Health monitoring: An agent-based approach. *IET Communications*, *2*(2), 223–230. Retrieved September 6, 2009. doi:10.1049/iet-com:20060646

Cheek, P., Nikpour, L., & Nowlin, H. (2005). Aging well with smart technology. [from CINAHL with Full Text Database.]. *Nursing Administration Quarterly*, *29*(4), 329–338. Retrieved September 6, 2009.

China Daily. (2001). *Patient's privacy rights become an issue in China*. Retrieved September 6, 2009, from http://www.china.org.cn/english/2001/Jul/16178.htm

Cintron, A., & Hamel, M. (2006). The effect of a Web-based, patient-directed intervention on knowledge, discussion, and completion of a healthcare proxy. *Journal of Palliative Medicine*, *9*(6), 1320–1328. doi:10.1089/jpm.2006.9.1320

Conn, J. (2007). Invasion of privacy? [from Business Source Complete Database.]. *Modern Healthcare*, *37*(29), 20. Retrieved September 12, 2009.

Curran, K., & Canning, P. (2007). Wireless handheld devices become trusted network devices. *Information Systems Security*, *16*(3), 134–146. Retrieved September 6, 2009. doi:10.1080/10658980701401686

D'Allegro, J. (2000). Study: Health websites divulge personal information. *National Underwriter / Life & Health Financial Services*, *104*(8), 3. Retrieved September 2, 2009, from Business Source Complete Database.

Data Protection Act. (1998) *Data protection act*. Retrieved August 17, 2009, from http://www.opsi.gov.uk/ACTS/acts1998/ukpga_19980029_en_1

Davis, K., Schoenbaum, M., & Audet, A. (2005). A 2020 vision of patient-centered primary care. *JGIM: Journal of General Internal Medicine*, *20*(10), 953–957. doi:10.1111/j.1525-1497.2005.0178.x

Erlen, J. (2004). HIPAA-clinical and ethical considerations for nurses. *Orthopedic Nursing, 23*(6), 410–414. doi:10.1097/00006416-200411000-00014

Federal Trade Commission. (2007). *2006 Identity theft survey report*. Retrieved September 2, 2009, from http://www.ftc.gov/os/2007/11/SynovateFinalReportIDTheft2006.pdf

Freeman, E. (2004). *Veterans Administration Palo Alto healthcare system*. Retrieved August 15, 2009, from www.csahq.org/pdf/bulletin/issue_6/va_freeman043.pdf

Fuhrmans, V. (May 31, 2005). Health insurers' new target. *Wall Street Journal*, B1, B4.

Harris Interactive. (2004). Survey on medical privacy. Retrieved from http://www.harrisinteractive.com/news/newsletters/healthnews/HI_HealthCareNews2004Vol4 Iss13.pdf

Hayes, J., & Hannold, E. (2007). The road to empowerment: Historical perspective on the medicalization of disability. *Journal of Health and Human Services Administration, 30*(3), 352–377.

Health Information Privacy Code. (1994). *HIPC*. Retrieved August 30, 2009, from http://www.privacy.org.nz/health-information-privacy-code-1994/

Health Insurance Portability and Accountability Act. (1996). *Health information privacy*. Retrieved September 1, 2009, from http://www.hhs.gov/ocr/privacy/hipaa/understanding/index.html

Helping Hands for the Disabled. (2008). *July 2008 board meeting proceedings*.

Hendriks, A. (2007). UN convention on the rights of persons with disabilities. *European Journal of Health Law, 14*(3), 273–298. Retrieved September 8, 2009. doi:10.1163/092902707X240620

Hirschfeld, M., & Wikler, D. (2003). An ethics perspective on family caregiving worldwide. *Generations (San Francisco, Calif.), 27*(4), 56–60.

Human Rights Commission. (2009). Human rights in New Zealand today. Retrieved September 10, 2009, from http://www.hrc.co.nz/report/chapters/chapter05/disabled02.html

Jecker, N. (2002). Taking care of one's own: Justice and family caregiving. *Theoretical Medicine and Bioethics, 23*(2), 117–133. doi:10.1023/A:1020323828931

Kanter, A. (2007). The promise and challenge of the United Nations convention on the rights of persons with disabilities. [from Business Source Complete Database.]. *Syracuse Journal of International Law & Commerce, 34*(2), 287–321. Retrieved September 7, 2009.

Kaplan-Leiserson, E. (2001). The tremendous issues of technology. *T+D, 55*(11), 27. Retrieved September 6, 2009, from Academic Search Premier Database.

Knapp, K., & Boulton, W. (2006). Cyber-warfare threatens corporations: Expansion into commercial environment. [from Business Source Complete Database.]. *Information Systems Management, 23*(2), 76–87. Retrieved September 6, 2009. doi:10.1201/1078.10580530/45925.23.2.20060301/92675.8

Kuehn, B. (2009). IT vulnerabilities highlighted by errors, malfunctions at veterans' medical centers. [from CINAHL.]. *JAMA: Journal of the American Medical Association, 301*(9), 919–920. Retrieved September 10, 2009. doi:10.1001/jama.2009.239

Leung, J. (2006). The emergence of social assistance in China. *International Journal of Social Welfare, 15*(3), 188–198. doi:10.1111/j.1468-2397.2006.00434.x

Lobree, B. (2003). IT security: A tactical war. [from Academic Search Premier Database.]. *Information Systems Security, 12*(3), 9. Retrieved September 6, 2009. doi:10.1201/1086/43327.12 .3.20030701/43622.3

Logue, K., & Selmrod, J. (2008). Genes as tags: The tax implications of widely available Genetic information. [from Business Source Complete Database.]. *National Tax Journal, 61*(4), 843–863. Retrieved September 6, 2009.

Lorenzi, N., Kouroubali, A., Detmer, D., & Bloomrosen, M. (2009). How to successfully select and implement electronic health records (EHR) in small ambulatory practice settings. *BMC Medical Informatics and Decision Making, 9*, 1–13. doi:10.1186/1472-6947-9-15

Lueng (2006) characterizes the Chinese support system as disjoint and decentralized.

Macios, A. (2009). Who's watching what? Data mining raises privacy issues. *Radiology Today, 10*(1), 20.

Mavhunga, C. (2009). The glass fortress: Zimbabwe's cyber-guerilla warfare. [from Academic Search Premier Database.]. *Journal of International Affairs, 62*(2), 159–173. Retrieved September 6, 2009.

McLaughlin, J. Gustafson, C., Sutton, M., Stone, E., & Davis, N. (1984). *Developmentally disabled infants can be hard to trace.* Retrieved August 20 2009 from http://www.ncbi.nlm.nih.gov/pubmed/6199152

Microsoft Corporation. (2008). *Securing a better future for electronic medical records.* Retrieved July 24, 2009, from http://www.microsoft.com/business/peopleready/business/relationshps/insight/digitalrecords.aspx

MIPSA. (1999). *Setting information age parameters for medical privacy.* Retrieved September 1, 2009 from http://leahy.senate.gov/press/199903/990310b.html

Morin, D., Tourigny, A., Pelletier, D., Robichaud, L., Mathieu, L., & Vézina, A. (2005). Seniors' views on the use of electronic health records. *Informatics in Primary Care, 13*(2), 125–133.

Mullaney, J. (2006). The digital doctor logs off. *Business Week, 3983*, p12-15.

Network World. (2007, January 8). *Year ahead to bring risks, opportunities.* Retrieved September 6, 2009, from Business Source Complete Database.

Olmsted, S., Grabenstein, J., Jain, A., & Lurie, N. (2006). Patient experience with, and use of, an electronic monitoring system to assess vaccination responses. *Health Expectations, 9*(2), 110–117. doi:10.1111/j.1369-7625.2006.00378.x

Olowu, D. (2006). A critique of the rhetoric, ambivalence, and promise in the protocol to the African Charter on Human and People's Rights on the Rights of Women in Africa. [from Academic Search Premier Database.]. *Human Rights Review, 8*(1), 78–101. Retrieved September 6, 2009. doi:10.1007/s12142-006-1017-4

Patient Handoffs. (2008). *H&HN: Hospitals & Health Networks.* Retrieved September 14, 2009, from Academic Search Premier Database.

Pew Internet and American Life Project. (2003). *Who's not online: Several demographic factors are strong predictors of Internet use.* Retrieved September 7, 2009, from http://www.pewinternet.org/Reports/2003/The-EverShifting-Internet-Population-A-new-look-at-Internet-access-and-the-digital-divide/02-Who-is-not-online/03-Several-demographic-factors-are-strong-predictors-of-Internet-use.aspx

Powner, D. (2006). *Health Information Technology: HHS is continuing efforts to define its national strategy: GAO-06-1071T.* GAO Reports. Retrieved September 6, 2009, from Business Source Complete Database.

Quibria, M., Tschang, T., & Reyes-Macasaquit, M. (2002). New information and communication technologies and poverty: Some evidence from developing Asia. *Journal of the Asia Pacific Economy*, 7(3), 285–309. doi:10.1080/1354786022000007852

GAO Reports. (2007). *Health Information Technology: Early efforts initiated but comprehensive privacy approach needed for national strategy: GAO-07-238.* Retrieved September 6, 2009, from Business Source Complete Database.

Riemer-Reiss, M. (2000). Vocational rehabilitation counseling at a distance: Challenges, strategies and ethics to consider. [from Academic Search Premier Database.]. *Journal of Rehabilitation*, 66(1), 11–17. Retrieved September 6, 2009.

Robertson, L., Smith, M., Castle, D., & Tannenbaum, D. (2006). Using the Internet to enhance the treatment of depression. *Australasian Psychiatry*, 14(4), 413–417.

Robeznieks, A., & Conn, J. (2006). GAO blasts HHS on IT, privacy. [from Academic Search Premier Database.]. *Modern Healthcare*, 36(36), 8–9. Retrieved September 6, 2009.

Rothstein, M., & Talbott, M. (2007). Compelled authorizations for disclosure of health records: Magnitude and implications. *The American Journal of Bioethics*, 7(3), 38–45. doi:10.1080/15265160601171887

Slattery, F. (2008). Medicine and the Internet. *The OECD Observer. Organisation for Economic Co-Operation and Development*, 268, 31–32.

Swartz, N. (2008). Partnerships advance e-health records. *Information Management Journal*, 42(3), 10–14.

The Disability Social History Project. (2009). Disability history timeline. Retreived August 15, 2009, from http://www.disabilityhistory.org/timeline_new.html

The Economist. (2005). The no-computer virus - IT in the health-care industry. *The Economist, 375*(8424), 65-67.

TheBigOptOut.org. (2009). *About the campaign.* Retrieved September 10, 2009, from http://www.thebigoptout.com/?page_id=3

United Nations Office of Legal Affairs. Convention on the Rights of Persons with Disabilities, (2006). *U.N. Doc A/RES/61/.* Retrieved September 1, 2009, from http://www.un.org/esa/socdiv/enable/opsigola.htm

United States Department of Education Family Educational Rights and Privacy Act (FERPA). (1974). *Family Policy Compliance Office (FPCO) home.* Retrieved September 7, 2009, from http://www.ed.gov/policy/gen/guid/fpco/ferpa/index.html

United States Department of Education - Individuals with Disabilities Education Act. (2004). *Building the legacy: IDEA 2004.* Retrieved September 7, 2009, from http://idea.ed.gov/

United States Department of Health and Human Services - Center for Disease Control and Prevention. (2009). *Single gene disorders and disability.* Retrieved September 7, 2009, from http://www.cdc.gov/ncbddd/single_gene/default.htm

United States Department of Health and Human Services - Office for Civil Rights. (2009). *Your rights under section 504 of the rehabilitation act.* Retrieved September 7, 2009, from http://www.hhs.gov/ocr/civilrights/resources/factsheets/504.pdf

Vaas, L. (2001). Disability laws take flight. *eWeek, 18*(9), 50. Retrieved September 6, 2009, from Academic Search Premier Database.

Verheijden, M., Bakx, J., Van Weel, C., & Van Staveren, W. (2005). Potentials and pitfalls for nutrition counseling in general practice. *European Journal of Clinical Nutrition, 59,* S122–S129. doi:10.1038/sj.ejcn.1602185

Vijayann, J. (2003). Offshore ops to get stronger privacy lock. [from Academic Search Premier Database.]. *Computerworld, 37*(22), 1. Retrieved September 6, 2009.

Washington Division of Developmental Disabilities. (2009). *Vision statement.* Retrieved July 12, 2009, from http://www1.dshs.wa.gov/pdf/adsa/ddd/reports/Overview2_03.pdf

Wasko, N. (2001). Internet Technology makes clinical data systems technically and economically practical: Are they politically feasible? [from SocINDEX with Full Text Database.]. *Journal of Technology in Human Services, 18*(3/4), 41–62. Retrieved September 6, 2009. doi:10.1300/J017v18n03_04

Weiner, M. (2003). Using Information Technology to improve the healthcare of older adults. *Annals of Internal Medicine, 139*(5), 430–436.

Wikileaks. (2009). *Over 8M Virginian patient records held to ransom.* Retrieved August 17, 2009, from http://wikileaks.org/wiki/Over_8M_Virginian_patient_records_held_to_ransom,_30_Apr_2009

World Trade Organization. (2009). *Standards concerning the availability, scope and use of intellectual property rights.* Retrieved September 10, 2009 from http://www.wto.org/english/tratop_e/trips_e/t_agm3_e.htm

Ye, J., & Wei, Q. (2004). *Legal problems concerning health discrimination in employment.* Retrieved from http://www.humanrights.cn/zt/magazine/200402004921170301.htm

Yu-Che, C., & Thurmaier, K. (2008). Financing e-government business transactions: An enterprise pricing framework for G2B services. *Public Administration Review, 68*(3), 537–548.

Chapter 3
Hippocratic Database and Active Enforcement

Terry Dillard
Dillard Systems, LLC

ABSTRACT

There are an increasing number of laws and statutes being passed globally to protect the privacy of sensitive healthcare information. This complexity of legislation creates legal concerns for those stakeholders in the healthcare systems that collect and store this sensitive data. This chapter seeks to explore some technology based solutions for managing these complexities and that aim to mitigate some of the potential legal concerns associated with these activities.

INTRODUCTION

Governments across the globe are establishing data protection laws that constrain the disclosure and processing of personally identifiable information. These laws impose custodial and pecuniary burdens upon organizations that manage personal information, and may hinder the legitimate sharing and examination of information (Johnson & Grandison, 2007).

Member states within the European Union are required under the Directive on Data Protection to establish laws that impose rigorous limitations upon the processing of personally identifiable information (European Union, 1995). The United States, Canada, Australia, and Japan also followed suit to protect the privacy and security of personal data. These laws play a major and defining role in the management, sharing, and analysis of electronic health records (Agrawal & Johnson, 2007).

As the number of organizations and governments collecting personal information continues to grow at an unprecedented rate, individuals are

DOI: 10.4018/978-1-60960-174-4.ch003

ever more exposed to the unauthorized disclosure, misuse, or abuse of their personal information, which increases the risk of medical or financial identity theft, injury to their reputation, or loss of personal privacy. Failure to adequately protect information could lead to organizations exposing themselves to civil and governmental liabilities due to negligence. However, failure to protect personal information within electronic health records could also restrain researchers from having access to data, therefore diminishing the potential for innovation, efficiencies, and medical breakthroughs (Solove, 2004).

Despite the growing number of countries that have enacted data and privacy protection laws, security breaches resulting in data, privacy loss, and identity theft seems to be at an all time high. This is primarily due to ineffective enforcement or execution of data protection policies within organizations, may they be within government or the private sector. Also, due to differing constitutional standards and cultural attitudes on the need to protect privacy, disparities exists within legal protections between different countries, which poses obstacles to the free flow of information to researchers, as well as the global economy (Johnson & Grandison, 2007).

Technology-based privacy solutions can be employed to address many of these obstacles by restricting the access and exposure of sensitive personal information stored within information systems. Such privacy technologies must have the ability to accommodate or adapt the complexities of heterogeneous data protection laws, by discretely handling each information element. To be effective, solutions need to accomplish this task without egregiously constraining legitimate or bona fide disclosure of information. Effective solutions must also be cost-effective and computationally compatible with existing information systems infrastructure, which reduces the overall burden of solution implementation and execution (Grandison, Ganta, Braun, & Kaufman, 2007).

HIPPOCRATIC OATH, CONFIDENTIALITY AND BENEFICENCE

The Hippocratic oath is a solemn promise that was required of physicians entering the medical profession, which can be trailed back to the Greek physician and teacher, Hippocrates (403 B.C.). Within the oath, physicians were firmly admonished to maintain appropriate decorum and privacy in the execution of their calling as physicians by refraining from the practice of disseminating what they saw or heard regarding the treatment of patients. Maintaining the confidentiality of the physician-patient relationship was essential to the ethical exercise of the profession (Eliot, 1910).

Confidentiality is most conspicuous within medical ethics, and is inextricably linked to the four founding principles of the Hippocratic oath, which are: (1) autonomy, the principle that expresses that personal data must not be disseminated in an unauthorized fashion. Each individual has the sovereign right to determine who may receive, store, and transmit their personal information; (2) Self-determination, which is the ability to circumscribe or restrict access to one's personal data; (3) Informed consent is the courtesy that must be extended to individuals prior to distributing any medical data to others; and (4) Non-malfeasance, which is the principle of doing no harm. Disclosing private information about patients could violate individual rights, and could produce harmful consequences, such as family members, friends, health care organizations, insurance companies, employers, or researchers misusing data in such a way as to violate individual preferences (Beauchamp & Childress, 2001). Therefore, the Hippocratic oath seeks to uphold confidentiality through the overarching principle of beneficence, which encapsulates all four founding principles (Neitzke, 2007).

HIPPOCRATIC DATABASE AND ACTIVE ENFORCEMENT OVERVIEW

One solution that addresses the problem of distributed privacy policy enforcement is the Hippocratic Database (HDB) and Active Enforcement (AE). HDB and AE are an integrated set of privacy solutions that seamlessly implements granular-level enforcement of privacy controls at the data level, and prevents unlawful data disclosure, while permitting legitimate information flow (Agrawal & Johnson, 2007). The Hippocratic Database is a centralized, federated technology that provides cell-level, policy-based disclosure administration capabilities, where databases can only yield data that is compliant with organizational policies, relevant legislation, and the individual's preferences. The Active Enforcement element guarantees that enterprise applications accessing data within the enterprise architecture are adherent to fine or granular-level data disclosure policies. HDB-AE is capable of aggregating and enforcing an organization's security, privacy, and data protection policies, as well as legal, regulatory requirements, and individual preferences (Johnson & Grandison, 2007).

Within Active Enforcement, user queries are transparently re-written in a layer above the database in order to execute granular-level access to various disclosure policies. This is atypical of most existing privacy enforcement solutions that handle policy execution at the application level. HDB's Compliance Auditing function provides accounting capabilities that allow for policy compliance tracking and accountability without degrading system performance (Grandison, Ganta, Braun, & Kaufman, 2007).

EUROPEAN UNION DATA PROTECTION DIRECTIVE

The European Union Data Protection Directive (EUDPD) is the most comprehensive effort legally, for protecting privacy and security of personal information around the world. EUDPD established rules that traverse various industries throughout the EU that member states are required to follow. EUDPD is noteworthy in that it circumscribes the processing, rather than merely the disclosure, of personal data. It places a greater burden upon data processors, in that, it mandates that data collectors will (1) forewarn individuals that their data will be collected, (2) permit individuals to examine and correct errors within their personal data, (3) procure opt-in consent from individuals prior to furnishing their personal data to third parties, (4) obtain clear, understandable opt-in consent from individuals prior to providing any sensitive or delicate personal data, such as race, ethnic origin, political affiliations, or religious beliefs, (5) protect all personal information within their custody, (6) confine processing of personal data to the purposes for which it was gathered or allowed, and (7) be answerable for all divulgences of personal data (European Union, 1995; Johnson & Grandison, 2007).

The Directive also requires member states to administer enforcement measures and countermeasures for infractions of data protection laws. Comparable cross-industry privacy statutes were constituted in Canada, Japan, Australia, and Argentina to govern the aggregation, processing, and disclosure of personal information. These laws were inspired by the Organization for Economic Cooperation and Development (OECD) Guidelines on the Protection of Privacy and Transborder Flows of Personal Data. OECD Guidelines promote a platform of eight privacy protection principles, which were designed to foster the free flow of information and eliminate social and economic obstacles between member countries (European Union, 1995).

ORGANIZATION OF ECONOMIC COOPERATION AND DEVELOPMENT

The development of automatic data processing, which allows vast amounts of data to be conveyed within seconds across national boundaries, as well as continents, has made the consideration of privacy protection of personal data necessary. Various privacy protection laws have been introduced within approximately one half of OECD Member countries (Austria, Belgium, Canada, Denmark, France, Germany, Iceland, Luxembourg, Netherlands, Norway, Spain, Sweden, Switzerland, and the United States) to dissuade violations of basic human rights, such as the illegal storage of personal data, the warehousing of incorrect personal data, or the abuse or unauthorized divulgence of personal data. Privacy and security notwithstanding, there is the risk that differences in national legislation or statutes could encumber the free flow of personal data across borders. Transborder data transmissions have increased considerably with advances in information communication technologies [ICT](OECD, 1980).

Within the Organization of Economic Co-Operation and Development, Member countries recognize that, despite variations in national laws and policies concerning the protection of individual privacy and freedoms, shared interests exists in maintaining fundamental but competing values such as privacy and the free flow of information. Because automatic processing and transborder transmission of personal data generates new relationships between countries that contributes to economic development and societal progress, new rules and procedures (protocols) must be established to address these relationships. Domestic or national privacy protection protocols must not impede transborder data flow between OECD members. Members must be resolute in discouraging unwarranted obstructions to economic and social interchange between countries (OECD, 1980).

Personal data should be germane to the purpose for which it was acquired, and should not be disclosed for any other purposes. Reasonable protection measures should be taken to ensure the confidentiality, integrity and availability of data (OECD, 1980).

HEALTH INSURANCE PORTABILITY AND ACCOUNTABILITY ACT

Rather than instituting a singular cross-industry privacy ordinance, the United States took a markedly different approach, by separating privacy protection into two distinct sectors, health care and financial services. The Health Insurance Portability and Accountability Act (HIPAA) addresses privacy by requiring covered entities (health care plans, health care providers, or health care clearinghouses) to enact necessary measures that ensure the privacy and security of patient's personally identifiable information. HIPAA requires covered entities to inform patients of their privacy policies, as well as furnishing patients the opportunity to abstain from third party disclosure of their personal information. In the absence of patient authorization, HIPAA restricts the parties to whom personal information may be revealed, the reasons for which information may be revealed, and the circumstances for information disclosure. The burden of reasonable protection is placed upon all covered entities, to safeguard personally identifiable information, as well as answer for any illegitimate or wrongful disclosures upon the patient's or lawful government agency's request. However, patient information that has been appropriately de-identified in accordance with the HIPAA Privacy Rule may be processed and divulged without limitation (104Th Congress Of The United States Of America, 1996).

Privacy of financial services data is regulated by the Gramm-Leach-Bliley Act (GLBA), which mandates that financial services organizations provide clients with notification of their privacy policies as well as the opportunity to abstain from third party disclosure of their non-public information (FTC, 1999).

Market forces within the global economy, as well as the value of unrestrained information flow are challenging countries to work out legal discrepancies encompassing privacy, and agree upon a common set of data protection principles, such as Article 25 of the European Union Data Protection Directive, which requires members to limit sharing of personal data only to countries that demonstrate an acceptable measure of privacy protection (European Union, 1995). To settle disagreements and legalities between the United States and the European Union on the legitimateness of cross-border sharing between organizations, the United States Department of Commerce and the European Commission established an agreement, known as the Safe Harbor Agreement, which closely conforms to OECD Guidelines on the Protection of Privacy and Trans-border Flows of Personal Data (U.S. Department of Commerce, 2009). The common privacy principles specified within the OECD Guidelines and the Safe Harbor Agreement are the basis of the Hippocratic Database (Agrawal & Johnson, 2007).

HDB ACTIVE ENFORCEMENT

With respect to privacy laws, one commonality that seems to exist between various nations is the issue of how data is to be used, as well as the ability to enforce appropriate usage of data. For instance, under the provisions of the European Union Data Protection Directive, a European bank would be forbidden from using customer personal data for purposes other than the primary reason for which it was originally gathered. HDB AE captures and transposes queries to constrain them into compliance with organizational or governmental privacy policies, as well as customer opt-in / opt-out preferences. Transposed or rewritten queries are then submitted to the database, which retrieves results that are compliant with prevailing mandates. Further, HDB is capable of managing the complexity of roles within organizations. From an operational perspective, Active Enforcement is capable of controlling and enforcing role-based access control (RBAC) to information assets based upon clearance level and roles of data requesters, as well as sensitivity of data being requested (Johnson & Grandison, 2007).

HDB Active Enforcement has many clear benefits over other privacy solutions. To begin with, it functions at the middleware level of data processing operations, merging seamlessly with enterprise applications. This alleviates the need to re-code ERP, CRM, or Health IT systems to conform to policy controls. Secondly, due to HDB's compatibility with Structured Query Language or SQL, it places minimal burden or impact upon query processing, thus allowing all queries to occur directly within the database, leveraging the full performance capabilities of the database management system. Third, HDB enforces policies at the individual or granular level within the database, which obviates unnecessary restrictions upon data that might be beneficial to research or other domains. Fourth, HDB supports sophisticated or complex policies, such as roles, purpose, recipient, or a host of other unconstrained conditions. In other words, HDB AE is extremely powerful, capable of seamlessly interfacing with any SQL enabled relational database environment using Open Database Connectivity (ODBC) or Java Database Connectivity (JDBC) (Lefevre et al. 2004).

The Hippocratic Database provides a refined (fine-grained) compliance auditing capability that allows administrators to observe the level of conformity to privacy and data disclosure policies. Within the audit application, administrators can specify an audit query to detect whether sensitive information has been exposed. In return, HDB produces an itemized list of suspicious queries requesting specific data, along with the issuer, time, purpose, and recipient for each query. The compliance-auditing tool assists in maintaining accountability of organizations that handle personally identifiable information, as well as enforcement of data protection laws. The EU Data Protection Directive, as well as the Safe Harbor Agreement mandates that governments and organizations furnish legal recourse to individuals whose privacy data has been violated. Within the United States, the HIPAA Privacy Rule mandates that covered entities supply a written explanation, giving an account of disclosures. This is done upon request by the patient or authorized government agency (Agrawal et al. 2004).

HDB's method of logging offers enormous performance and storage benefits over other systems. HDB only stores updates or changes, also known as deltas, which are typically kept within the infrastructure of the database, thus minimizing costs generally associated with read accesses within databases. HDB inflicts minimal overhead upon query processing, as it only requires query string and meta data to be logged during standard query processing. HDB's flexible audit query language allows administrators to declaratively stipulate the exact information that they would like to examine. And finally, HDB's storage overhead allows auditors or administrators to preserve audit logs for extended periods of time, which could allow the auditing of data access or disclosure activity of preceding years (IBM Corporation, 2006).

CONCLUSION

This chapter has underscored how Hippocratic Database enforcement and auditing capabilities can achieve many of the common principles contained within various data protection laws around the world. Organizations and governments must have the ability to automatically enforce security and privacy controls, while simultaneously ensuring compliance with common principles. HDB

delivers a scalable design that enables enforcement of such controls with minimal impingement upon performance (Johnson & Grandison, 2007).

REFERENCES

(104Th Congress Of The United States Of America 1996 Health Insurance Portability and Accountability Act of 1996)Johnson, C.M., & Grandison, T.W. (2007). Compliance with data protection laws using Hippocratic Database active enforcement and auditing. IBM Systems Journal, 46(2), 255-264.

104.th Congress of the United States Of America. (1996). Public Law 104-191. In Health Insurance Portability and Accountability Act of 1996. Retrieved July 28, 2009, from http://www.cms.hhs.gov/ HIPAAGenInfo/Downloads/HIPAALaw.pdf

Agrawal, R. B., Faloutsos, R., Kiernan, C., Rantzau, J. R., & Srikant, R. (2004). Auditing compliance with a Hippocratic Database. Proceedings of the 30th International Conference on Very Large Databases, 30, 516-527.

(Agrawal R Johnson C 2007 Securing electronic health records without impeding the flow of information)Agrawal, R. & Johnson, C. (2007). Securing electronic health records without impeding the flow of information. International Journal of Medical Informatics, 76(5-6), 471-479.

(Beauchamp T L Childress J F 2001 Principles of biomedical ethics)

Corporation, I. B. M. (2006). IBM Hippocratic Database auditing user guide, Version 1.0. Retrieved August 7, 2009, from IBM Corporation Web site: http://www.almaden.ibm.com/cs/projects/iis/hdb/Publications/papers/HDBAuditingUserGuide.pdf

Eliot, C. W. (1910). Oath of Hippocrates. In P.F. Collier and Son (Ed.), Harvard Classics (vol 38). Boston: Harvard Press.

(Eliot C W 1910 Oath of Hippocrates)Solove, D. (2004). The digital person. New York: NYU Press.

European Union. (1995, November 23). Directive 95/46/EC of the European Parliament and of the Council of 24 October 1995 on the Protection of Individuals with Regard to the Processing of Personal Data and on the Free Movement of Such Data. Official Journal of the European Communities of, L(281), 31–50.

(FTC 1999 Gramm-Leach-Bliley Act: Disclosure of nonpublic personal information)FTC. (1999). Gramm-Leach-Bliley Act: Disclosure of nonpublic personal information. Retrieved July 28, 2009, from Federal Trade Commission Web site: http://www.ftc.gov/privacy/glbact/glbsub1.htm

(Grandison T Ganta S R Braun U Kaufman J 20070823 Protecting privacy while sharing medical data between regional healthcare entities)Grandison, T., Ganta, S.R., Braun, U., & Kaufman, J. (2007). Protecting privacy while sharing medical data between regional healthcare entities. Paper presented at the meeting of the Session S113: Sharing Data. Brisbane, Australia.

(Johnson C M Grandison T W 2007 Compliance with data protection laws using Hippocratic Database active enforcement and auditing)

Lefevre, K., Agrawal, R., Ercegovac, V., Ramakrishnan, R., Xu, Y., & Dewitt, D. (2004). Limiting disclosure in Hippocratic Databases. Proceedings of the 30th International Conference on Very Large Databases, 30, 108-119.

(OECD 19800923 OECD guidelines on the protection of privacy and transborder flows of personal data)OECD. (1980, September 23). OECD guidelines on the protection of privacy and transborder flows of personal data. Retrieved July 30, 2009, from http://www.oecd.org/documentprint/0,3455,en_2649_34255_1815186_1_1_1_1,00.html

(Solove D 2004 digital (European Union 1995 Directive 95/46/EC of the European Parliament and of the Council of 24 October 1995 on the Protection of Individuals with Regard to the Processing of Personal Data and on the Free Movement of Such Data(Neitzke G 2007 Confidentiality, secrecy and privacy in ethics consultation)Neitzke, G. (2007). Confidentiality, secrecy and privacy in ethics consultation. HEC Forum, 19(4), 293-302.

U.S. Department Of Commerce. (2009). Safe Harbor privacy principles.

(US Department Of Commerce 20090301 Safe Harbor Privacy Principles)Beauchamp, T.L., & Childress, J.F. (2001). Principles of biomedical ethics (5th ed.). Oxford: Oxford University Press.

Chapter 4

Implementation Issues on a National Electronic Health Record Network

John McGaha
Capella University, USA

ABSTRACT

The United States congress and the past several administrations have dedicated considerable funding for incentives focused on accelerating the adoption by the healthcare industry of Health Information Technology (HIT) solutions. The most recent effort towards these objectives includes a focus on the creation of a National Health Information Network that will support large scale exchange of health information. This chapter explores the technical, security and privacy implications of the advent of such an integrated network and the steps towards its successful completion.

INTRODUCTION

An electronic health record (EHR) contains a patient's medical history in electronic format. Access to an EHR with Internet technologies has the potential for early detection and response to bioterrorist attacks; nation-wide and global monitoring and treatment of communicable disease; and

DOI: 10.4018/978-1-60960-174-4.ch004

monitoring, detecting, and treating exposures to biochemical agents (Teich, Wagner, Mackenzie, & Schafer, 2002).

Information security is vital to the operation, success, and sustainability of today's information-centric organizations, such as those in the health-care business, and is now a top business concern on a global scale (Filipek, 2007). There are many obstacles preventing the implementation of a national electronic health record (EHR) infrastructure. This project examines the issues stakeholders have with the adoption of an EHR network and identifies some effective measures that can be taken to minimize the security risks inherent to sensitive information shared across a national network. Common obstacles at the local and national level include funding, privacy, security and accuracy of sensitive data. Common obstacles on a global level include communication, standardization, funding and interoperability (Arnold et al., 2007).

BACKGROUND OF REGULATORY CONTROLS IN HEALTH CARE

In an information system, controls are actions taken by people or software to minimize security risks. Controls also serve to direct desirable behavior and processes in an organization (Carter, Cobb, Earhart, & Noblett, 2008). The healthcare and financial industries are compelled to comply with several government imposed regulations (controls). While many organizations have developed and implemented their own sets of controls, the federal government enacted the Health Insurance Portability and Accountability Act (HIPAA) in 1996. The Act requires security and privacy controls on managing medical data. Organizations are required to comply to HIPAA regulations if the organization provides a health plan for employees, provides healthcare to patients, or provides healthcare insurance. Compliance to HIPAA is enforced by the US Health and Human Services (HHS) Department. The law requires the HHS to establish national standards for electronic health care transactions and national identifiers for providers, health plans, and employers (HISPC, 2007).

Failure to properly apply HIPAA security controls can result in civil monetary penalties imposed by the HHS. The Security of Treasury is empowered to impose tax penalties on organizations that are not in compliance (Foultz, 2004).

After February 18, 2010, the HHS is authorized to penalize HIPAA violators up to $1.5 million, a 60% increase of current limits (CMIO, 2009). This new authorization is problematic because many healthcare providers are not in compliance with HIPAA primarily due to the lack of funds and understanding the regulations (Netchert, 2008; Foultz, 2004).

In 2004, President Bush directed the HHS to develop, plan, and guide the implementation of nation-wide health information technology (GAO-07-988T, 2007). As part of the directive, the HHS is responsible for the protection of personal health information that will populate a nation-wide healthcare database. The GAO report identifies key challenges that have yet to be addressed by the HHS. Challenges associated with the safeguarding the exchange of electronic health information include: understanding and resolving legal and policy issues; ensuring appropriate disclosure; ensuring individual's rights to request access and amendments to health information; and implementing adequate security measures for protecting health information.

The Health IT for Economic and Clinical Health (HITECH) Act enacted in 2009 gives the HHS authority to impose increased financial penalties on organizations in non-compliance to HIPAA. Maximum fines outlined in HIPAA are a maximum of $25,000. According to HITECH regulations, the HHS can fine organizations up to $1.5 million (HHS, 2009) for HIPAA violations. The Health Information Technology for Economic and Clinical Health (HITECH) Act is part of the contested stimulus legislation. HITECH authorizes limited funding of EHR implementation.

HEALTH INFORMATION EXCHANGE

A prelude to a national EHR network (and global network) is the Health Information Exchange (HIE). At least 35 states are actively involved with creating state-wide electronic medical record systems that will exchange health information (Dimitropoulos & Rizk, 2009). The technical architecture of a national health information exchange (HIE) is yet to be developed. However, in early 2010, the federal government will begin distributing $564 million to states to fund state-level HIE networks (McBride, 2009). This grant supports state programs for only three years. States will be forced to fund the operation and maintenance in 2014. Iowa is the first state that with approval to receive funds for their EHR incentive program (Merrill, 2009). Iowa plans to use the $1.6 million grant to study barriers to EHR adoption and create a health information technology plan for its Medicaid program.

The state of Nebraska instituted a body, Health Information Security and Privacy Committee (HISPC), to investigate and recommend how the state can create a health information exchange. A main focus of the research is the issue of privacy because HISPC understands that security in a nation-wide HIE is beyond the ability of any state's control (HISPC, 2007).

In 2006, researchers at Beth Israel Deaconess Medical Center in Boston successfully exchanged data among three network sites located in Massachusetts, Indiana, and California in what the researchers hope will become a prototype for a national healthcare information network (Monegain, 2006). The data exchange used a record locator service instead of a unique, single patient identifier method. A record locator service finds the record based upon the record's location thereby eliminating the need to centrally store clinical data. The exchange uses a specially developed a record locator service rather than a single patient identifier. The locator service does not store any clinical data centrally; instead, the service identifies the location of records wherever they are stored. Researchers claim the tests demonstrate that a national identifier is unnecessary for the exchange of medical information across a national healthcare network (Monegain, 2006). However, researchers at the RAND Corporation claim that

unique patient IDs are necessary to eliminate errors in EHRs (Anonymous, 2009a).

A standardized protocol for data exchange in software development is lacking (Davidson & Heslinga, 2004). This is significant because data will be shared by physicians, pharmacies, laboratories, and hospitals in the new national HIE. Standardization is also a key obstacle on the global scale (Arnold, Wagner, Hyatt & Klein, 2007).

A committee chartered by the American National Standards Institute (ANSI) is tasked to develop standards for electronic data interchange. The HHS contracted ANSI develop and implement a set of standards that will support interoperability among EHR systems and other healthcare software applications (HISPC, 2007).

If the HIEs are properly implemented and integrated nation-wide, then global sharing of data may become a reality. The American Medical Informatics Association urges the federal government to fund and implement a national health information infrastructure needed to detect and monitor global threats to health (Tang, 2002).

During the 2009 outbreak of the H1N1 influenza, the Center of Disease Control (CDC) reviewed vaccine results by using the U.S. Vaccine Safety Datalink database (CDC, 2009). Administrative and electronic medical records contained and managed in this database are the collaborative effort between the CDC and several managed-care organizations. The CDC acknowledges that since the data reporting is voluntary the database may not have all reports and the data may only contain preliminary diagnoses.

Recognizing that a pandemic threat could halt national and global air traffic, the airline industry is using enterprise risk management (ERM) strategies to collaborate with the CDC (Beasley, Frigo, & Litman, 2007). It is technologically possible that the CDC can share meaningful data with the airlines and other mass transportation entities.

OBSTACLES TO THE IMPLEMENTATION OF ELECTRONIC HEALTH RECORDS

The U.S. federal government plans to enforce universal adoption of the use of EHRs by 2014 (Galt & Johnson, 2007). A major concern in the adoption of EHR is how such a massive system of networks can protect the privacy and security of individual health information. Opponents of the digitization of health records are concerned with security of their private medical information (Angst & Agarwal, 2009). News reports of hackers penetrating a top nuclear lab facility and stealing personal information (including social security numbers) of employees and visitors (Paul, 2007) substantiate the fears of national EHR with government oversight. Risk management strategies, discussed later, may solve most non-monetary concerns.

Countless individuals have access to electronic health records – from initial data entry to medical personnel administering care. Since control and accuracy of this sensitive information relies upon people, it is surmised that people pose the greatest threat to security in electronic health record (EHR) management. A recent study examines the relationship between electronic medical record (EMR) systems and integrated healthcare delivery systems. Results of the study indicate there is a positive correlation between the allocation of operating budget and annual productivity measures (Richardson, 2009). The findings support earlier research that purports investments in electronic medical records lower the cost per patient while increasing the number of patients.

Large pharmaceutical companies have been using electronic records since the 1980s Stamatiadis (2005). Lessons in governance, oversight, and security of sensitive data may be gained from reviewing the practices used in the pharmaceutical industry.

Based on a statistical model developed by the RAND Corporation, if 90% of the nation's healthcare providers adopt a nation-wide EHR network, then $81 billion can be saved annually. RAND also predicts that it would cost hospitals $98 billion and doctors $17 billion to adopt a nation-wide EHR network. Hospitals and doctors would receive little benefit from their investment (Anonymous, 2009a). However, it is estimated that Medicare would enjoy $23 billion of the annual savings while other insurance providers would save $31 billion. Swartz (2005) emphasizes that healthcare providers have little incentive to make such an investment when others reap the financial benefit.

Swartz (2005) reports that roughly 25% of healthcare providers (doctors and hospitals) use EHR systems. Thielst (2007) contradicts this assessment. She claims that a 2005 survey by the Healthcare Information and Management Systems Society states that 87% of the hospitals surveyed have an EHR system or would soon develop a system. While referring to HIPAA privacy and security regulations, Thielst may be overly optimistic or naïve in her assertion "break the glass mechanisms and automatic audit trails will keep the honest people honest and will identify those who choose to abuse public trust and misuse private health information" (p. 9). Compliance to HIPAA requirements in the state of Washington (Zineddine, 2008), Pennsylvania (Maharaja, 2009), Nebraska (HISPC, 2007) and South Dakota (HISPC, 2007) show physicians share the same monetary and productivity concerns.

PHYSICIAN CONCERNS

Maharaja (2009) surveyed doctors in two Pennsylvania counties about their use or non-use of EHR in their practices. During the study, Maharaja determined that there is a relationship between the practices and EHR adoption. According to Maharaja, adoption of EHR is related to education and the doctors' opinion about productivity and profitability of implementing EHR. Cost is the major obstacle in the adoption by these doctors. This is consistent with findings of Netchert (2008) and Foultz (2004) that claim many healthcare providers are not in compliance with HIPAA because a lack of understanding of the security regulations and funding.

Young medical students may have a better understanding of the requirements. Reynolds (2008) surveyed 155 first year medical students to determine their opinion of EHRs and if they intend to use EHR in their practices. Reynolds concludes that the respondents plan on using EHR in their practices and have positive attitudes toward EHRs.

Some practicing physicians realize there are concerns with an EHR system other than costly compliance. Schackow, Palmer & Epperly (2008) describe a recent EHR crisis that almost ended their medical practice. Due to an incompetent IT director, four months of patient visits recorded in EHRs, was lost because of improper backups. The doctors report the data amounts to around 12,000 patient visits. Almost all of the data was recovered after 3 months of data recovery attempts by various vendors across the country and over $10,000 spent on recovery efforts.

Estimates show that 60% of physicians in small practices across the U.S. lack sufficient financial resources to invest in EHR applications (Davidson & Heslinga, 2004). The same report warns that IT investments in small practices have a high potential to fail or underperform.

The Office of the National Coordinator (ONC) for Health Information Technology estimates that 17-25% of medical doctors are using EHR systems (Galt & Johnson, 2007). The majority of those doctors are in practices with 10 or more other physicians. The ONC identifies several barriers that prevent implementation of an EHR system. These barriers include: start-up costs, maintenance costs, loss of productivity, lack of technical skills, and lack of technical support.

PATIENT CONCERNS

According to McGraw et al. (2009), 80% of those surveyed in a 2006 national survey are very concerned about identify theft and fraud, 77% are very concerned about someone marketing their medical information, 56% are concerned about their employers accessing their medical information, and 55% are concerned about insurance providers accessing their medical information (p. 417). McGraw et al. (2009) believe that privacy concerns, an obstacle to health information exchange, can be overcome by implementing oversight, accountability, and trusted network designs.

Dr. Susan Marden, a clinical nurse scientist at the National Institute of Health, presents a model that may explain the relationship between patient reliance of technology with health-related quality of life (Marden, 2005). She describes health-related quality of life issues and its relationship with therapeutic technology. The research proposes a new model that examines this relationship, but calls for continuing research. According to Marden, age and gender affects the attitude of technology dependence. In general, women "tend to be more perceptive about their health" (p. 193) and are likely to be more dependent upon technology. Her well-written article calls for more focused research to investigate the validity of her new model.

A recent qualitative study by a research team at Beth Israel Deaconess Medical Center (BIDMC) attempts to address what patients want in electronic medical record system (Prescott, 2009). Results from focus groups held in four major cities suggest that patients are willing to give up some privacy to gain full access to their records. Prescott (2009) reiterates the research claims that aging patients that experience more illnesses are not overly concerned with privacy issues. Validity of the findings may be questionable because 80-100 participants were selected from four geographic areas and some of the participants are healthcare workers – not patients.

In qualitative research, narrative and non-numerical data is collected, analyzed, and interpreted to gain insight into a given phenomenon (Gay et al., 2006). Data collected in a qualitative study addresses meaning (Swanson & Holton, 2005) and causes the researchers to "think deeply about the data" (p. 239). In other words, a major purpose of a qualitative study is to understand and describe the research from the participant's viewpoint (Trochim, 2006). This increases the credibility (validity) of the qualitative study. Validity of the findings may be questionable because 80-100 participants were selected from four geographic areas and some of the participants are healthcare workers – not patients.

McCaughey (2009) warns that provisions in the new healthcare bill before congress will allow government bureaucracy to use a patient's electronic health record to limit treatment. According to McCaughey, if the new legislation becomes law, a patient may be denied treatment if the patient's condition is atypical or experimental treatment is needed. Electronic healthcare records facilitate this type of micro-management of healthcare.

GLOBAL CONCERNS

Commonalities among different local and national efforts to implement healthcare are not yet clearly defined (Arnold et al., 2007). The Health Information Management Systems Society (HIMSS) Global Task Force identifies four common obstacles that 15 countries in North America, Europe, Asia Pacific and the Middle East face while implementing electronic health records. The obstacles include communication, standardization, funding and interoperability (Arnold et al., 2007).

The Office of the National Coordinator for Health Information Technology (ONC) identifies two major obstacles the hinder interoperability of health information; consensus is lacking on how to transmit the data; and lack of a nation-wide network (Heubusch, 2006). For interoperability

to be successful from a Canadian perspective, social benefits, quality of care, and economics cannot be ignored (Nikolai, 2008).

In Canada, the Deputy Health Ministers in the Canada Health Infoway are the catalysts in achieving interoperability of health information and implementing EHRs (Nikolai, 2008). In 2003, Canada invested $1.2 billion into Infoway (Arnold et al., 2007).

Security, privacy, and standardization are key issues in interoperability. Security and privacy of medical information are lesser concerns for Canadians since participation in the government controlled health care programs is mandatory (Nikolai, 2008). However, privacy of Canadian's medical information is protected by Personal Information Protection and Electronic Documents Act (PIPEDA).

Standardization of technologies and protocols is more of a challenge in the U.S. than it is in Canada since the Canadians already have a national framework. Australia, Canada, New Zealand, and the United Kingdom already have agreed upon standards (Arnold et al., 2007). However, interoperability challenges in the United Kingdom, a pioneer in socialized national health services, have become very complex because of the multi-levels of the system (Nikolai, 2008).

SENSITIVE DATA CONCERNS

Security risk assessment is essential to the security of any organization, especially when sensitive information is involved. Foultz (2004) examines how sensitive healthcare information is protected by organizations in accordance with HIPAA regulations. Research findings are base on the results of 303 healthcare workers responding to a survey. According to Foultz, over 36% of the respondents claim that the enactment of HIPAA increased protection of sensitive records in their organizations. However, the results also indicate that only 5 of 24 specific HIPAA regulations were reported as implemented. COBIT may be useful in managing the exchange of sensitive data. Control objective DS 5-11 in COBIT's Deliver and Support Domain provides this framework (ITGI, 2008).

Countries in the European Union define sensitive data by taking one of two approaches - purpose based or contextual based (Wong, 2007). A contextual based approach means that data is sensitive depending on its context of use. For example, Germany does not necessarily consider religious beliefs or political opinions are sensitive data. Wong states that purpose based approach addresses the "purpose underlying the processing of personal data" (p. 13). Wong emphasizes that personal data that reveals race, religious preference, health, and sexual lifestyles are not adequately protected in the European Union. It seems that the Europeans view the sensitivity issue as one that is open for interpretation. Prince (2008) discusses the impact of security breaches in the health care which includes sensitive data defined as social security numbers, driver's license numbers, account numbers, and health issues. These types of data are generally accepted as sensitive data.

According to Prince (2008), security incidents in healthcare organizations are increasing at an alarming rate. Nearly 50% of the incidents reported during 2000 to 2007 occurred at hospitals while insurance companies comprised 7% of the incidents. However, the insurance companies experienced the highest number of breached records. During the seven-year period, 1,739,397 medical records were compromised. The majority of the breaches (40%) were malicious in nature resulting from hackers, theft, or malevolent employees.

SECURITY CONCERNS

Elliot (2005) describes the information lifecycle as four sequential phases: (1) information request, (2) transfer to endpoint, (3) consumption, and (4) disposition. IT personnel are challenged in balancing the needs of the users with risk and exposure in all steps in the information lifecycle. However, IT personnel cannot act alone. Welander (2007) suggests that security should involve everyone involved with the system.

Remote access to patient information by healthcare professionals is problematic and has many security issues. A policy that can be enforced with software tools can decrease risks inherent in remote access of sensitive health information (Elliot, 2005). Usage of a policy as a security control is consistent with Welander (2007).

As Welander (2007) suggests, remote access without appropriate access control can produce devastating results. Healthcare workers require remote access to patient data. According to Elliot (2005), in the first two phases in the information lifecycle, users can remotely request and receive information by using a SSL VPN (secure socket level virtual private network). This is because the connection is made at the application layer. However, the last two phases in the lifecycle require different security controls.

Information in the consumption and disposition phases is "outside the box." That is, data is in the remote computer's memory and cache. Elliot (2005) urges healthcare IT personnel to implement client-based malware protection, information controls, and client activity audits (p. 34). Even though these three actions are not a panacea for end-point security, they help protect the remote workstation from unauthorized access by Trojans and unsavory users.

He & Yang (2009) assert that current controls focus on single systems and/or single organizations. They propose a Policy Driven Authorization Control framework to meet the challenges of cross-domain healthcare systems and providers.

According to Jin et al. (2009), healthcare providers require seamless access to patient health records. Their research proposes an access control scheme which claims to help alleviate concerns or privacy and theft of sensitive data contained in EHRs. The model purports to unify EHRs that are shared across a wide-spectrum of users.

Hoerbst & Ammenwerth (2009) introduce a "model-based approach to structure and describe quality requirements of EHRs" (p. 34). It is unclear if this model will actually work with complex data in a real system.

The healthcare industry must have confidence in the reliability of the medical data contained in electronic health records (EHRs). Alhaqhani, Josang, & Fidge (2009) warn of the negative consequences that may occur if reliability is not included in design of the EHR system. They propose a new model, Medical Data Reliability Assessment, to validate the reliability of the medical data included in an EHR.

Ameri (2004) identifies five pillars that are fundamental to information security; protection, detection, reaction, documentation, and prevention. Without the protection pillar the remaining pillars are unnecessary. A detection pillar is a vital benchmark of sorts. Reaction, documentation, and prevention pillars are consistent with the outer security layer described by Ciampa (2005). Ciampa states that "information security protects the integrity, confidentiality, and availability of information on the devices that store, manipulate, and transmit the information through products, people, and procedures" (p. 6). According to Ciampa, products, people, and procedures provide the outer security layer of an information system; products provide a physical layer, people provide a personnel security layer, and procedures provide organizational security.

Amir (2004) identifies five risk management practices that every information system should incorporate into the foundation of the system – this includes electronic health record system. Risk management practices identify critical processes, data, and vulnerabilities (Radack, 2009).

Many healthcare workers face is the security of medical data when the data is remotely accessed. Many in the healthcare industry routinely access patient information from remote locations. Welander (2007) argues that remote access without appropriate access control can produce devastating results. Therefore, it is imperative that administrators, regulators, healthcare and technology professionals work together to solve the remote access issue to avoid non-compliance to HIPAA.

Under new security breach requirements in the HITECH Act, healthcare providers and associated businesses are required to notify HHS and individuals when health records are compromised (Freedman, 2009). If the breach involves over 500 individuals, the law allows the use of media to make notifications.

This was not the case in December, 2002, when several computers were stolen from a government contracted healthcare management group, TriWest. Dozens of computers containing medical data and social security numbers of thousands of retired military personnel and their dependents were stolen from a TriWest facility (Sample, 2003). After the breach was released to the new media, it took several months before TriWest contacted the individuals whose records were stolen.

Dixon (2005) reports that during the first eight months of 2005, 12 of the 94 known security breaches relate specifically to medical information. Moreover, Dixon claims that more breaches are expected when EHRs are more widely adopted and shared across networks (p. 9). Although Dixon is an advocate of EHR implementation, she cautions that patients must be provided a voice in the formulation of policies designed to protect their sensitive medical data.

Between 2005 and 2007, over 100 million people in the US were victims to identify theft (Anonymous, 2007). The victim may have been notified if they live in a state or US territory that has laws requiring notification of such breaches. Crowell (2008) identifies 42 states that have enacted laws governing security breach notification. That is, information material compromise or likelihood of harm before notification is required. Moreover, only 25 states require more stringent pre-breach measures.

The California Security Breach Act (SBIA) allows residents to sue for damages when personal data is compromised due to negligence (Johnson, 2008). However, the law stops short of defining unreasonable negligence and a quantified amount for damages. The law does require immediate notification in all cases.

Likewise, Nevada's NRS 603A and Nebraska's Statute 87-801 require notification of security breaches (Crowell, 2008). Nevada (2009) defines breach of security as "unauthorized acquisition of computerized data that materially compromises the security, confidentiality or integrity of personal information maintained by the data collector."

Consumer advocates and several members of congress agree that the HHS is violating congressional intent of the requirement of notification when security breaches occur in electronic medical records (Consumer, 2009). The HHS views compromises in security to include substantial harm. Moreover, the HHS allows the entity causing the security breach to determine whether the breach is disclosed.

Indiana University received a $538,595 grant to fund a two-year study for the purpose of discovering how the HHS can exempt health research from the HIPAA privacy rule (NIH, 2009).

Schwartz & Janger (2007) argue that consumers need better protection and notification when their personal information is breached. Moreover, they call for better coordination when sharing information about a security breach and improvements in oversight of those breaches.

Schwartz & Janger (2007) discuss data security breach notification statutes from a legal perspective. They emphasize that regulations contained in HIPAA require healthcare facilities, health insurers, and other medical entities to have reasonable data security. Organizations that process personal data for a healthcare facility are also subject to the same security regulations under HIPAA (p. 922). HIPAA also requires "health plans, healthcare clearinghouses, and healthcare providers, to designate an individual as a "privacy official," who will be responsible for the implementation

and development of the entity's privacy policies and procedures" (p. 930).

On July, 29, 2009, Congressman Edolphus Towns called for an end to what he calls a self-regulation of the file sharing industry (Poirier, 2009). As Chairman of the House Oversight and Government Reform Committee, Towns announced his intentions to propose legislation to regulate file sharing services after several security breaches that involved file sharing services provide by the Lime Group. The nature of the security breaches are unauthorized access.

Reuters News reported that the security breaches included unauthorized persons having the ability to access private medical records, social security numbers, FBI files, and information about a location reserved for the safety of the President of the United States (Poirier, 2009). The number of breaches or how the breaches were discovered is not mentioned in the article.

LEGAL ISSUES

Sondheimer, Katsh, Clarke, Osterweil, & Rainey (2009) claim that over 40% of the textual information contained in the HITECH Act addresses privacy and security. Accuracy of EHR content concerns many healthcare providers because of potential misdiagnosis and malpractice lawsuits. Other concerns include ownership of the medical data, disclosure, government use of the data, access by insurance providers, and rights of the patient (p. 240). The healthcare industry is the target of very expensive lawsuits. Sondheimer et al. (2009) warn that introducing new technologies into healthcare may likely increase the numbers and range of new litigation.

Lawsuits continue to be filed that counter the current pro-regulatory U.S. congress. A recently filed lawsuit contends that the accounting board established by the Sarbanes-Oxley Act of 2002 is unfair to small auditing firms (Francis, 2009). This lawsuit may potentially impact other regulatory bills, such as HIPAA or HITECH, if the ruling is in favor of the small business plaintiffs.

Another lawsuit filed by a registered nurse, claims that HITECH violates the privacy of personal health information and violates HIPAA. According to the lawsuit, the executive branch of the government can use and distribute a person's private health information without permission of the individual (Anonymous, 2009c).

Under California law, the legal duties of the data possessor to protect the data subjects' personal information from unauthorized access are clearly defined (Johnson, 2008) and enforced. California recently imposed the maximum fine allowed under state law, $250,000, to a hospital that did not adequately protect sensitive patient information (Anonymous, 2009b).

In 1974, the US Congress passed legislation to enact the Privacy Act of 1974. This law was in response to the Watergate scandal in Washington and growing concerns that personal information stored in large databases is subject to compromise (McCain, 2009). The article claims that the US Government is circumventing its own law, Privacy Act of 1974, by purchasing personal information about US citizens from data brokers.

EFFECTIVE MEASURES TO COUNTER OBSTACLES

The nine best practices reported by Keller et al. (2005) are common sense approaches that everyone should consider using – even with home computers with Internet access. Gordon, Loeb, Lucyshyn, & Richardson (2006) identify viruses, unauthorized access and stolen laptops as the sources of greatest financial loss to the participants in the annual CSI/FBI Computer Crime and Security Survey. Using the practices identified by Keller et al (2005) are designed to counter those types of losses – except stolen computers. Therefore, physical security of hardware should be added to the short list of best practices.

Information security is vital to the operation, success, and sustainability of today's information-centric organizations. Information security is now a top business concern on a global scale (Filipek, 2007). The National Institute of Standards and Technology (NIST) emphasize that managing the risks that threaten information systems should be an essential aspect of information security programs in all organizations (NIST, July 2009).

Capturing and analyzing data that pertains to the security of that data is vital to an organization's survival. The questions asked during the analysis and the quantification of the results become the metrics that enable organizations to improve security. Results are typically translated into numeric quantifications such as, ratios, percentages, scores, averages, frequencies, and other types of statistical measures (Swanson, et al., 2003). An organization can use the metrics to improve information security thereby protecting the integrity, confidentiality, and availability of their information.

Employing risk management strategies may remedy many of the privacy, security, and sensitive data issues. A generic risk management framework establishes a set of related processes to make decision that assess, measure, and mitigate risk (Herrod, 2006). These processes are interrelated and cyclical.

Herrod (2006) claims that information security lays the foundation to information technology (IT) risk management program and ISO 17779 and ISO 27001 standards help build this relationship (Brenner, 2007). Therefore, protecting information is the first step in developing a viable risk management program at the university. As noted above, cost is an important factor to consider when developing the program.

Risk management is an art (Herrod, 2006) and refers to the future; therefore, it becomes problematic while trying to quantify (Adams, 2007). Moreover, Adams suggests that risk is a predictive activity based on the perception of past events or experience rather than based on fact. It is apparent that Adams views risk management as an exercise in common sense.

Traditional risk management typically addresses risk in isolation; that is, each business unit manages their own risks without considering how other business units within the same organization may be impacted (Beasley, Frigo, & Litman, 2007). A strength of Enterprise Risk Management (ERM) is that managers at all levels collaborate in identifying, assessing and managing risks (Barton, Shenkir, & Walker, 2009). Even though ERM is strategic in nature it should be embedded into goals at all levels of the organization. A top-down approach is required to make ERM successful (Beasley et al., 2007).

Risk refers to the future; therefore, it becomes problematic while trying to quantify (Adams, 2007). Moreover, Adams suggests that risk is a predictive activity based on the perception of past events or experience rather than based on fact. It is apparent that Adams views risk management as an exercise in common sense. However, it is possible to assess and manage risk. According to Ross, Katzke, Johnson, Swanson, & Stoneburner (2008) the National Institute of Standards and Technology (NIST) agrees with Adams that "managing risk is not an exact science" (p. 1). However, the NIST has spent considerable funds and time creating risk assessment manuals. Reflecting on lessons learned from previous security breaches, managers can implement policies or physical measures to prevent the breach from recurring. Speculation of future events cannot guarantee predictive results; however, a lackluster attitude in risk assessment can guarantee eventual disaster.

According to Barton et al.(2009) five firms - Chase Manhattan, E.I. du Pont de Neours, Microsoft, United Grain Growers Ltd., and Unocal - were singled out as champions of ERM in 2001. These major firms had common characteristics in the way in which they implemented ERM and were hailed as champions in the ERM movement. They were driven to provide "better corporate management and value creation" (p. 12). Since

2001, large corporate failures and frauds evident in Enron, WorldCom, and Tyco, changed the way corporations address risk.

Barton et al. (2009) describes what went right at the five previously identified organizations. The measures include: "a formal dedicated effort to identify all significant risks; the ranking of risks by severity and frequency; the development and implementation of sophisticated and relevant risk metrics; and a senior management committed to drilling ERM into the decision-making processes at all levels of their organizations" (p. 11).

CONCLUSION

The digitization of health records and building a nation-wide healthcare network in the U.S. is inevitable. Politicians and health care industry workers are proponents of a universal, digital method of storing patient medical records. Concerns of the physicians and patients must be addressed by the government before the healthcare industry and its patients will have confidence in the reliability, accessibility, and security of the medical data contained in a network EHR system. Extending and integrating the national network to a global network is likely once international standards for the exchange of data are adopted.

REFERENCES

Adams, J. (2007). Risk management: It's not rocket science... It's much more. *Risk Management, 54*(5), 36–40.

Alhaqbani, B., Jøsang, A., & Fidge, C. (2009). A medical data reliability assessment model. [from ABI/INFORM Global.]. *Journal of Theoretical and Applied Electronic Commerce Research, 4*(2), 64–78. Retrieved October 11, 2009. doi:10.4067/S0718-18762009000200006

Ameri, A. (2004). The five pillars of information security. [from ABI/INFORM Global.]. *Risk Management, 51*(7), 48. Retrieved October 5, 2009.

Angst, C., & Agarwal, R. (2009). Adoption of electronic health records in the presence of privacy concerns: The elaboration likelihood model and individual persuasion. [from Business Source Complete Database.]. *Management Information Systems Quarterly, 33*(2), 339–370. Retrieved August 12, 2009.

Anonymous. (2007). ID thieves targeting universities. *Information Management Journal, 41*(2), 7. Retrieved from http://search.ebscohost.com. library.capella.edu

Anonymous,. (2008). Information infrastructure cornerstone of national patient record archive. [from ABI/INFORM Global.]. *International Journal of Micrographics & Optical Technology, 26*(1/2), 2. Retrieved August 12, 2009.

Anonymous,. (2009a). Patient IDs would improve healthcare. [from ABI/INFORM Global.]. *Information Management Journal, 43*(1), 11. Retrieved October 11, 2009.

Anonymous,. (2009b). California fines hospital $250,000 for snooping. [from ABI/INFORM Global]. *Information Management Journal, 43*(5), 12. Retrieved October 11, 2009.

Anonymous,. (2009c). Lawsuit claims stimulus violates HIPAA. [from ABI/INFORM Global.]. *Information Management Journal, 43*(5), 20. Retrieved October 11, 2009.

Arnold, S., Wagner, J., Hyatt, S., & Klein, G. (2007). Electronic health records: A global perspective. *Healthcare Information and Management Systems Society* (HIMSS). Retrieved December 12, 2009, from http://www.providersedge. com/ehdocs/ehr_articles/Electronic_Health_Records-A_Global_Perspective-Exec_Summary.pdf

Barton, T., Shenkir, W., & Walker, P. (2009). The evolution of a balancing act. *Financial Executive, 25*(10), S10-S12, S14. Retrieved January 13, 2010, from ABI/INFORM Global.

Beasley, M., Frigo, M., & Litman, J. (2007). Strategic risk management: Creating and protecting value. *Strategic Finance, 88*(11), 24-31, 53.

Brenner, J. (2007). ISO 27001: Risk management and compliance. *Risk Management, 54*(1), 24–29.

California, H. C. F. (2009). *An unprecedented opportunity: Using federal stimulus funds to advance health IT in California.* California Healthcare Foundation. Retrieved October 12, 2009, from http://www.chcf.org/

Carter, R., Cobb, J., Earhart, L., & Noblett, A. (2008). *IT compliance management guide: Version 1.0.* Microsoft Corporation. Retrieved October 31, 2009, from http://technet.microsoft.com/en-us/solutionaccelerators/default.aspx

CDC. (2009). Safety of influenza A (H1N1) 2009 monovalent vaccines - United States, October 1 - November 24, 2009. *Morbidity and Mortality Weekly Report, 58,* 1-6. Retrieved December 13, 2009 from http://www.cdc.gov/mmwr/preview/mmwrhtml/mm58e1204a1. htm?s_cid=mm58e1204a1_e#tab1

Ciampa, M. (2005). *Security+ guide to network security fundamentals* (2nd ed.). Boston: Course Technology.

CMIO. (2009). *HHS requests comments on beefed up HIPAA enforcement abilities.* CMIO Online. Retrieved November 3, 2009, from http://www.cmio.net/index.php?option=com_articles&view=article&id=19372&division=cmio

Consumer. (2009, October). *Harm standard violates congressional legislative intent in protecting privacy.* Consumer Watchdog Organization. Retrieved November 3, 2009, from http://www.consumerwatchdog.org/patients/articles/?storyId=30367

Crowell. (2008). *State laws governing security breach notification.* Crowell & Moring International Law Firm. Retrieved October 21, 2009, from http://www.crowell.com/

Dimitropoulos, L., & Rizk, S. (2009). A state-based approach to privacy and security for interoperable health information exchange. [from ABI/INFORM Global.]. *Health Affairs, 28*(2), 428–434. Retrieved October 10, 2009. doi:10.1377/hlthaff.28.2.428

Dixon, P. (2005). Electronic health records and the national health information network: Patient choice, privacy, and security in digitized environments. In *testimonial before the NCVHS Subcommittee on Privacy and Confidentiality,* San Francisco.

Elliott, M. (2005). Securing the healthcare border. [from ABI/INFORM Global.]. *Health Management Technology, 26*(9), 32, 34–35. Retrieved November 2, 2009.

Fickenscher, K. (2005). The new frontier of data mining. [from ABI/INFORM Global.]. *Health Management Technology, 26*(10), 26, 28, 30. Retrieved August 12, 2009.

Filipek, R. (2007). Information security becomes a business priority. *The Internal Auditor, 64*(1), 18.

Foultz, W. (2004). *The impact of the HIPAA regulation on information technology security in the healthcare industry.* D.P.A. dissertation, University of La Verne, California.

Francis, T. (2009). These men could kill sarbox. *Business Week.* 40-43

Galt, K., & Johnson, S. (2007). *How many physicians have adopted electronic health records in Nebraska?* EHRNebraska. Retrieved October 17, 2009, from http://ehrnebraska.org/interact/

Gay, L., Mills, G., & Airasian, P. (2006). *Educational research: Competencies for analysis and applications* (8th ed.). Upper Saddle Creek, NJ: Prentice Hall.

Gordon, L., Loeb, M., Lucyshyn, W., & Richardson, R. (2006). CSI/FBI computer crime and security survey. Retrieved November 11, 2009, from http://i.cmpnet.com/gocsi/db_area/pdfs/fbi/FBI2006.pdf

He, D., & Yang, J. (2009). Authorization control in collaborative healthcare systems. [from ABI/INFORM Global.]. *Journal of Theoretical and Applied Electronic Commerce Research, 4*(2), 88–109. Retrieved October 11, 2009.

Herrod, C. (2006). The role of information security and its relationship to information technology risk management. In M.E. Whitman & H.J. Mattord (Eds.), *Readings and cases in the management of information security* (45-61). Boston: Course Technology.

Heubusch, K. (2006). Interoperability: What it means, why it matters. *Journal of American Health Information Management Association, 77*(1), 26-30. Retrieved January 11, 2010, from http://library.ahima.org/xpedio/groups/public/documents/ahima/bok1_028957.hcsp?dDocName=bok1_028957

HISPC. (2007, June). *Security and privacy barriers to health information interoperability: Final report for the state of Nebraska.* Health Information Security and Privacy Committee, State of Nebraska. Retrieved October 17, 2009, from http://chrp.creighton.edu/

Hoerbst, A., & Ammenwerth, E. (2009). A structural model for quality requirements regarding electronic health records-state of the art and first concepts. In *Proceedings of the 2009 ICSE Workshop on Software Engineering in Health Care,* (pp. 34-41). Washington, DC.

ITGI. (2008). *Aligning COBIT 4.1, ITIL V3 and ISO/IES 27002 for business benefits*. Retrieved August 16, 2009, from http://www.itgi.org

Jin, J., Ahn, G., Hu, H., Covington, M. J., & Zhang, X. (2009). Patient-centric authorization framework for sharing electronic health records. In *Proceedings of the 14th ACM Symposium on Access Control Models and Technologies*, (125-134). Stresa, Italy. NY: ACM.

Johnson, V. (2008). Data security and tort liability. *Journal of Internet Law, 11*(7), 22–31. Retrieved from http://search.ebscohost.com.library.capella.edu.

Kahn, J., Aulakh, V., & Bosworth, A. (2009). What it takes: Characteristics of the ideal personal health record. *Health Affairs, 28*(2), 369–376. doi:10.1377/hlthaff.28.2.369

Keller, S., Powell, A., Horstmann, B., Predmore, C., & Crawford, M. (2005). Information security threats and practices in small businesses. *Information Systems Management, 22*(2), 7–19. Retrieved from http://search.ebscohost.com.library.capella.edu. doi:10.1201/1078/45099.22.2.20050301/87273.2

Maharaja, A. (2009). *Use of the electronic health record in private medical practices*. Ed.D. dissertation, Duquesne University.

Marden, S. (2005). Technology dependence and health-related quality of life: A model. *Journal of Advanced Nursing, 50*(2), 187–195. doi:10.1111/j.1365-2648.2005.03378.x

McBride, R. (2009). Health information exchanges the health IT inside. *CIMO.net Online Magazine*. Retrieved November 29, 2009, from http://epubs.democratprinting.com/publication/?i=26411

McCain, J. (2009). Applying the privacy act of 1974 to data brokers contracting with the government. [from ABI/INFORM Global.]. *Public Contract Law Journal, 38*(4), 935–953. Retrieved October 11, 2009.

McCaughey, B. (2009). *Ruin your health with the Obama stimulus plan*. Bloomberg. Retrieved October 18, 2009 from http://www.bloomberg.com/apps/news?pid=20601039&sid=aLzfDxfbwhzs# McGraw, D., Dempsey, J., Harris, L., & Goldman, J. (2009). Privacy as an enabler, not an impediment: Building trust into health information exchange. *Health Affairs, 28*(2), 416-27. Retrieved October 10, 2009, from ABI/INFORM Global.

Merrill, M. (2009, November). Iowa first to receive matching funds for EHR incentive program. *Healthcare Finance News*. Retrieved November 29, 2009, from http://www.healthcarefinancenews.com/news/iowa-first-receive-matching-funds-ehr-incentive-program

Monegain, B. (2006, March). Healthcare data exchange moves from theory to proof. *Healthcare IT News*. Retrieved November 3, 2009, from http://www.healthcareitnews.com/news/healthcare-data-exchange-moves-theory-proof

Netschert, B. (2008). *Information security readiness and compliance in the healthcare industry*. Ph.D. dissertation, Stevens Institute of Technology, New Jersey.

Nevada, N. R. S. (2009). *Chapter 603A: Security of personal information*. Retrieved October 21, 2009, from http://www.leg.state.nv.us/NRS/NRS-603A.html#NRS603ASec010

NIH. (2009). *Protecting privacy in health research*. Research portfolio online reporting tool, U.S. Department of Health and Human Services. Retrieved November 3, 2009, from http://projectreporter.nih.gov/project_info_description.cfm

Nikolai, B. (2008). *Medical records: The interoperability conundrum*. University of British Columbia - School of Library, Archival & Information Studies. Retrieved January 11, 2010, from http://www.bound2leap.com/media/med_records.pdf

NIST. (July, 2009). *Risk management framework: Helping organizations implement effective information security programs.* ITL Security Bulletin. Retrieved October, 10, 2009, from http://csrc.nist. gov/publications/PubsITLSB.html

Paul, R. (2007). *Top US government research labs infiltrated by hackers.* Retrieved October 12, 2009, from http://arstechnica.com

Poirier, J. (2009). *Lawmaker urges regulations for file-sharing.* Thomson Reuters Wire Service. Retrieved August 1, 2009, from http://www. reuters.com

Prescott, B. (2009, May). *Patients reveal a willingness to trade hands-on medical care for computer consultations.* Beth Israel Deaconess Medical Center Web Site. Retrieved November 3, 2009, from http://www.bidmc.org/News/In-Research/2009/May/PatientsandComputers.aspx

Prince, K. (2008). *A comprehensive study of healthcare data security breaches in the United States from 2000-2007.* Perimeter eSecurity. Retrieved October 21, 2009, from http://www. privacyrights.org/ar/ChronDataBreaches.htm.

Reynolds, R. (2008). *A study to determine first year medical students' intention to use electronic health records.* Ed.D. dissertation, Memphis State University.

Richardson, D. (2009). *Correlationally assessing the relationship of information technology investments in electronic medical records to business value.* Ph.D. dissertation, Capella University.

Ross, Katzke, Johnson, Swanson, & Stoneburner (2008). Managing risk from information systems: An organizational perspective. *National Institute of Standards and Technology. NIST Special Publication 800-39.* U.S. Department of Commerce.

Sample, D. (2003). *TriWest answers questions on stolen computer info, increased security.* American Forces Press Service. Retrieved November, 8. 2009, from http://www.defenselink.mil/news/newsarticle.aspx?id=29491

Schackow, T., Palmer, T., & Epperly, T. (2008). EHR meltdown: How to protect your patient data. [from ABI/INFORM Global.]. *Family Practice Management, 15*(6), A3–A8. Retrieved October 10, 2009.

Schwartz, P., & Janger, E. (2007). Notification of data security breaches. *Michigan Law Review, 105*(5), 913–984. Retrieved from http://search. ebscohost.com.library.capella.edu.

Schwartz, P., & Janger, E. (2007). Notification of data security breaches. *Michigan Law Review, 105*(5), 913–984. Retrieved from http://search. ebscohost.com.library.capella.edu.

Sondheimer, N., Katsh, E., Clarke, L., Osterweil, L., & Rainey, D. (2009). Dispute prevention and dispute resolution in networked health information technology. In S. A. Chun, R. Sandoval, and P. Regan (Eds.) *Proceedings of the 10th Annual international Conference on Digital Government Research: Social Networks: Making Connections between Citizens, Data and Government.* (pp. 240-243).

Stamatiadis, D. (2005). Digital archiving in the pharmaceutical industry. *Information Management Journal, 39*(4), 54-56, 59. Retrieved October 15, 2009, from ABI/INFORM Global.

Stevenson, G. (2007). *HIPAA security: Intercultural perspectives of health information technology professionals and clinicians.* Ph.D. dissertation, University of Illinois at Chicago, Health Sciences Center.

Swanson, M., Bartol, N., Sabato, J., Hash, J., & Graffo, L. (2003). *Security metrics guide for information technology systems.* NIST Special Publication 800-55. Retrieved October 12, 2009, from http://webharvest.gov/peth04/20041027033844/csrc.nist.gov/publications/nistpubs/800-55/sp800-55.pdf

Swanson, R., & Holton, E. (2005). *Research in organizations: Foundations and methods of inquiry.* San Francisco: Berrett-Koehler.

Swartz, N. (2005). Electronic health records could save $81 billion. [from ABI/INFORM Global.]. *Information Management Journal, 39*(6), 6. Retrieved October 15, 2009.

Tang, P. (2002). AMIA advocates national health information system in fight against national health threats. *Journal of the American Medical Informatics Association, 9*(2), 123-124. Retrieved January 10, 2010, from http://jamia.bmj.com/content/9/2/123.full

Teich, J., Wagner, M., Mackenzie, C., & Schafer, K. (2002). The informatics response in disaster, terrorism, and war. *Journal of the American Medical Informatics Association, 9*(2), 97-104. Retrieved January 10, 2010, from http://jamia.bmj.com/content/9/2/202.full

Thielst, C. (2007). The future of healthcare technology. [from ABI/INFORM Global.]. *Journal of Healthcare Management, 52*(1), 7–9. Retrieved October 10, 2009.

Trochim, W. (2006). *Qualitative validity.* Research Methods Knowledge Base. Retrieved October 20, 2009, from http://www.socialresearchmethods.net/kb/qualval.htm

Welander, P. (2007). 10 control system security threats. *Control Engineering, 54*(4), 38-44. Retrieved from http://search.ebscohost.com.library.capella.edu

Wong, R. (2007). Sensitive data in the online environment: Time for a change? *Journal of Internet Law, 10*(9), 11–17. Retrieved from http://search.ebscohost.com.library.capella.edu.

Zineddine, M. (2008). *Compliance of the healthcare industry with the health insurance portability and accountability act security regulations in Washington state: A quantitative study two years after mandatory compliance.* Ph.D. dissertation, Capella University.

Chapter 5
Health Kiosk Technologies

Robert S. McIndoe
Logica UK, UK

ABSTRACT

This chapter examines the recent rise in the adoption and spread of kiosks in UK healthcare: The leading players in the healthcare market, their technologies, the main uses of the kiosks and software, including possible future developments into clinical care.

INTRODUCTION

Health kiosks can be used to deliver a wide range of personal health services as they enable patients to carry out administrative tasks themselves and have the functionality to dispense printed information or medications.

ADMINISTRATIVE AND INFORMATION GATHERING

The major worldwide technology vendor NCR offers an extensive range of healthcare self-service solutions with software modules that cover pa-

tient self-registration, patient demographic self-update, clinic management, hospital wayfinding and patient surveying which run on its robust kiosk hardware. The systems integrator Logica has deployed four patient self-registration kiosks and four hospital wayfinding kiosks with NCR at City Hospitals Sunderland NHS Foundation Trust. NCR is also deploying kiosks at King's College Hospital NHS Foundation Trust in London and Heart of England NHS Foundation Trust in the Midlands.

Other smaller, health-focused kiosk and systems vendors have deployed their packaged healthcare systems into other Trusts. So, for example, Intouch with Health Ltd – which has its own software and chooses to use kiosk hardware from the larger vendors like NCR – has deployed

DOI: 10.4018/978-1-60960-174-4.ch005

a whole out-patient flow and kiosk patient self-registration and clinic calling system at the Mid Yorkshire Hospitals NHS Foundation Trust and at University Hospitals Birmingham NHS Foundation Trust in the Midlands. It is currently deploying its patient self-registration and calling system at North Bristol Healthcare NHS Foundation Trust.

Savience is another smaller operator that has achieved a market leading position having deployed its patient self-service system at Shrewsbury and Telford, Salford Royal, Countess of Chester, Sherwood Forest, Hereford Hospitals, Rotherham General, Chesterfield Royal, Liverpool Womens', Hillingdon, Lancashire Teaching, and Blackpool, Fylde & Wyre, NHS Foundation Trusts amongst other sites. Further deployments are ongoing at Barking, Havering and Redbridge, Morecombe Bay and Sandwell and West Birmingham NHS Foundation Trusts. Other small vendors are now forming and storming the market. There is about to be a wave of adoption of kiosks in UK out-patient departments for these functions, particularly patient self-registration, patient wayfinding and patient calling and flow management which will occur prior to other kiosk functions being discovered and deployed, some of a more clinical nature. This is the 'thin end of the wedge' in administrative and clinical robotics. Let us hope the multi-functional healthcare robot turns out to be 'The Rejuvinator' rather than 'The Terminator'. However, looking ahead, it may not be too long before kiosks are able to adminster injections or plaster broken limbs in fracture clinics, particularly bearing in mind that we already have 'robot surgeons', where surgeons can digitally operate on patients using inter-hospital and inter-continental telecare.

DISPENSING

Intouch with Health Ltd has specialised in producing a comprehensive hosted web service that can be delivered to its own or other vendors' kiosks in a wide range of languages that offers the patient a public health information service on a touch-screen. The information has been validated by the Department of Health and the Intouch with Health Public Health Information Service is now in over 70 NHS Trusts in the UK. Logica is deploying four NCR touchscreen kiosks with the Intouch with Health Public Health Information Service on them at the City Hospitals Sunderland NHS Foundation Trust. This is an example of public health information 'dispensing' with patients empowered to surf the web service while awaiting their clinic appointment, and enabled to print out an 'information prescription' about their condition to read in preparation for their clinic appointment. The hope is that this will lead to a more interactive consultation with the doctor or nurse and a more informed patient.

However, kiosks can also dispense other types of goods and services, other than pure information. In the banking sector, this is evidently cash and account statements, in healthcare this can be discharge medications, or even prostheses or dressings, if they are integrated to 'robot pickers'.

City Hospitals Sunderland NHS Foundation Trust has just installed a 'robot picker' into its out-patient department for the purpose of dispensing out-patient medications to patients. When married to a kiosk such a 'robot picker' can automatically dispense discharge medications on presentation by the patient of a barcoded prescription, code, PIN or token, or, indeed, payment.

PERSONAL HEALTH SERVICES AND WELLBEING

The Wellpoint 6000 is the leading technology for kiosk-based provision of personal health 'MOTs'. Wellpoint Group Ltd is an entrepreneurial start-up company marketing citizen and employee wellbeing kiosks into UK healthcare and the wider 'public health' community. The Wellpoint 6000 offers citizens the opportunity to monitor their own health status by checking their height, weight, heart rate, diastolic and systolic blood pressure, Body Mass Index and tissue fat content. With enhanced functionality it can also measure lung function and with on board camera technology, can offer GPs the opportunity to engage in 'virtual consultations' with their patients. The Systems Integrator Logica has deployed ten Wellpoints into the nine community centres around Sunderland, of which there is one in each borough, and the Sunderland Civic Centre. Booler (2009) is an example of the considerable local press interest in the implementation of these new technologies. The latest Wellpoint deployment has been of two kiosks as part of a 'community health pod' in Hull in the north-east of England offering a range of citizen well-being and screening services of which the kiosks are a central facet, opened by the Secretary of State for Health in England, Ian Johnson.

The only serious competitor to Wellpoint at this time is Savience, which offers a 'sit-down' kiosk to measure health status, which is of benefit to the elderly in particular. Wellpoint are currently investigating the possibility of adding a sit-down version as part of a planned extension to the Wellpoint range.

There is currently one Wellpoint in the English Department of Health at Richmond House and one Wellpoint in the English Department of Health at Skipton House. Wellpoint has been appointed as a sub-contractor to the Systems Integrator and Outsourcer Capita for the NHS Choices project and Wellpoints will be used as a franchised portal for the dissemination of NHS Choices in the English community and local government areas. This is a web portal offering the citizen a very complete picture of the NHS health service options open to them both nationally and locally.

Wellpoint also have contracts with the supermarket chain Morrisons and a number of other organisations including IBM, National Grid, EDF, Mars, Kimberly Clark, Serco and Oracle.

Looking across the technology industry more widely other big players in the technology market have invested in kiosk-related technologies.

Tenczar, Lemme, and Stanfield (2009) describe a project that Microsoft is currently investing in which redefines the customer relationship with the product in a retail setting. Microsoft Surface is a glass/perspex table that contains a computer able to offer an enhanced customer experience in the retail sector, via a touchscreen/touch table-top interface.

Similarly companies such as Nike and Apple (2010) have partnered to deliver their customers an integrated experience that allows the user to track their fitness regime using a combination of standard gym equipment and the classic apple technologies such as the iPhone and the iPod.

Thus a typical health kiosk can have a range of functionality as it is essentially a networked computer that is able to collect information about the person who uses it in a variety of ways, however when used it delivers a brand new interaction experience for the user and can reduce the need for administrative staffing in particular in hospitals, and in particular in out-patient departments.

This technology began to emerge in the UK in 1989 in Glasgow where fairly primitive kiosks have been developed and evaluated. Since then the devices have evolved and become a lot more sophisticated, like the Wellpoint, first exhibited by the Systems Integrator Logica at the Scottish Exhibition and Conference Centre on the 16th and 17th June, 2009, at the NHS Scotland conference: 'Working Towards a Healthier Scotland'.

Health kiosks have not been an overnight success and have emerged from a long period of research and development, re-design and improvement. Now the technology is stable and proven in clinical and healthcare environments around the world. Self-service solutions have had great success in the United States, helping healthcare establishments cut down on their administrative costs and shorten the patient processing times. The company Galvanon, formed in 2002 and acquired

Figure 1. Projected numbers of kiosks deployed into UK healthcare/community settings as at June, 2010. (Source: The role of health kiosks in 2009 – international journal of Environmental Research and Public Health ISSN 1660-4601 (Jones, 2009) and primary research by Robert McIndoe with kiosks vendors).

Kiosk Name/Vendor	Max Numbers Approximately	Dates	Sources
NCR	120 kiosks running the NCR self-service application	2005-2010	NCR
Savience	97 kiosks	2006-2010	Savience
Intouch with Health	46 self-service only 200 Public Health Information Kiosks	2006-2010	Intouch with Health
Wellpoint	335 Wellpoints	2003-2010	Wellpoint
NHS Kiosks	136 kiosks	2000-2005	NHS Choices
Elephant Kiosks	164 kiosks	2005-2010	Elephant Kiosks
StartHere BT Street Kiosks	130 kiosks	2004-2007	StartHere
Colorama – iStop	50	2007-2008	

by NCR in December, 2005, grew the patient self-service market in North America to a point where they had around 50 healthcare customers in their portfolio.

Over 100 healthcare organizations now use NCR's solutions in North America and they have deployed more than 1,200 kiosks. To date in excess of 6.5 million patients have checked in for medical appointments using NCR's self-service technology. In the United States clearly the kiosk is ideal not only for patient self-registration, wayfinding and information provision but also for treatment closure and payment where needed.

The health kiosk is particularly useful as a tool for identifying potentially serious illnesses early on in their development and can thus be used as a preventive measure in order to reduce chronic and even life-threatening illnesses. For example, the Wellpoint 6000 can shortly offer 'chest-mapping' functionality and this renders it useful along the respiratory disease care pathway.

The Systems Integrator Logica is currently partnering with three kiosk providers that have very differing functionality from one another. NCR (2009); Wellpoint (Kabler, 2010) and, Intouch with Health (2009), are the providers involved and the three taken together cover the range of functionality kiosks can offer in healthcare almost entirely. Other small kiosk vendors are arriving in the UK healthcare market.

It is envisaged that the importance and profile of these kiosks will grow considerably in the near future especially considering the importance of the Green Agenda (2009), Digital Britain (2008), Reeves (2010), Disease prevention (2010) and other impending policy programmes in UK health and UK government.

Also the latest research funded by the Digital Economy Programme (2009) is looking at how technology can be used in new and innovative ways to improve our overall wellbeing and quality of life.

Jirotka, Luff, and Buscher, (2009) are among researcher participating in the Innovative Media for Digital Economy (IMDE) which is just one of the areas of research that looks at this topic. Government research programmes have begun to look with great interest at how NHS institutions, arts and transport can all work together to deliver the best possible care and improve the overall public wellbeing and health. The new public health agenda in the UK is emphasising 'wellness' as opposed to 'illness'.

ADOPTION AND SPREAD

Thus far a relatively small number of kiosks has been sold and deployed (see Figure 1).

The rate of adoption is increasing however and this table will be out of date for the UK by the time you are reading it. With significant deployments into the major NHS Foundation Trusts of England such as City Hospitals Sunderland (Logica/NCR/Intouch), King's College Hospital (NCR), University Hospitals Birmingham (Intouch with Health) and Heart of England (Intouch with NCR hardware) the pressure will mount on all the major acute Trusts to deploy. This will result in significant qualitative patient benefits and quantifiable administrative cost savings which need to be researched and measured as they occur. However, as is common in the UK, there is likely to be a wave of technology adoption but little or no simultaneous benefits realisation programme put in place.

DEDICATION

In memory of Mr. Robert S. McIndoe, a man of many interests who dedicated most of his life to improve healthcare. His life was too short but the trace is deep.

REFERENCES

Anonymous. (2009). *Green agenda.* Retrieved June 16, 2010, from http://www.greenagenda.com/

Anonymous. (2009). *In touch with health, limited.* Retrieved June 16, 2010, from http://www.intouchwithhealth.co.uk/

Anonymous. (2009). *Introduction to digital economy programme.* Retrieved June 16, 2010, from http://www.epsrc.ac.uk/ResearchFunding/Programmes/DE/default.htm

Anonymous. (2009). *NCR: Experience a new world of interaction.* Retrieved June 16, 2010, from http://www.ncr.com/

Anonymous. (2010). *Boost your health in 2010.* Retrieved June 16, 2010, from http://www.nhs.uk/livewell/Pages/Livewellhub.aspx

Anonymous. (2010). *Nike plus iPod: Meet your new personal trainer.* Retrieved June 16, 2010, from http://www.apple.com/ipod/nike/

Booler, T. (June 16th, 2009). Self-service check. *Sunderland Echo,* 1.

Department for Culture. Media and Sports. (2008). *Digital Britain: The future of communications.* Retrieved June 16, 2010, from http://webarchive.nationalarchives.gov.uk/+/http://www.culture.gov.uk/reference_library/media_releases/5548.aspx/

Jirotka, M., Luff, P., & Buscher, M. (2009). *EPSRC: Research cluster on innovative media for a digital economy.* Retrieved June 16, 2010, from http://www.oerc.ox.ac.uk/research/digital-economy

Jones, R. (2009). The role of health kiosks in 2009. *International Journal of Environmental Research and Public Health,* 6(6), 1818–1855. doi:10.3390/ijerph6061818

Kabler, J. (2010). *Wellpoint kiosks: Instant access to health.* Retrieved June 16, 2010, from http://www.wellpointgroup.com/

O'Hara, P. (2009). *Joined-up health and social care: Challenging times.*

Reeves, R. (2010). *Heath and well being: The role of the state.* Retrieved June 16, 2010, from http://www.dh.gov.uk/en/Publichealth/index.htm

Tenczar, J., Lemme, M., & Stanfield, S. (2009). *Microsoft surface, experience it, showcase.* Retrieved June 9, 2010, 2010, from http://www.microsoft.com/surface/en/us/Pages/Experience/Showcase.aspx

Chapter 6

eHealth Governance, A Key Factor for Better Health Care:
Implementation of IT Governance to Ensure Better care through Better eHealth

Elena Beratarbide
CISA, National Health Service Fife, Scotland

Tom Kelsey
University of St. Andrews, Scotland

ABSTRACT

In this chapter, a set of recommendations for aligning eHealth with healthcare strategies is developed. After introducing the key concepts IT governance as a key enabler of successful alignment is discussed and described. Taking outcomes from a study conducted in Scotland, this chapter compares & contrasts preliminary results with those from similar studies in other countries. This analysis forms the basis of the chapter's recommendations, the most important of which are: (a) to employ a well-known and well-developed IT governance standard, (b) to ensure that the healthcare organisation has a high level of readiness for the transformation towards strategic alignment, and (c) to utilize experts to direct and monitor both the organisational change and the eHealth alignment.

Importantly, the results presented in relation to perceived eHealth-NHS alignment are preliminary, but significant deviations compared with the results presented in advance on this chapter are not expected.

DOI: 10.4018/978-1-60960-174-4.ch006

For you Jon, my precious son, and your greatly missed and beloved brother. Wishing all the effort around eHealth will provide you and your future generations with better health care opportunities and quality of life.

Elena, your Mom, mainly.

INTRODUCTION

The central claim of this chapter is that eHealth governance is a key factor for improved health services. Many people involved in some way with patient and health care would disagree with this claim, since IT is not always seen as one of the main components of health services, or at least is not perceived to be as crucial as, say, clinical factors. IT in the health sector is commonly regarded as a support for people to help other people. However, there is an expectation that eHealth will become more and more important in the delivery of modern health care, in areas such as preventative and curative health care, mobility, telemedicine and virtual healthcare. eHealth is expected to improve the health service in the future, adding value for practitioners, patients and carers, researchers and government in different stages of the health care journey. These expectations are introducing new pressures to ensure successful delivery of eHealth; this can be obtained by implementing IT governance approaches based on proven best practices, not only to get assurance but also to show how these expectations are to be realised.

Adopting IT Governance can help health care organisations delivering eHealth; it requires commitment and support at all levels across the health care boards. This is a medium to long term process that involves series of improvement cycles that are transitions requiring careful management of the organisational change involved.

Successful delivery of eHealth in this highly demanding scenario not only requires commitment but also determination and investment that involve all types of health care organisations, together with other stakeholders, such as patients, carers, researchers, suppliers of health informatics and government.

In countries like the UK and others in the European Union, where the health care service is mostly provided via central and local public funds, there is a risk that eHealth won't get the level of investment required to grow at an acceptable pace, as it is competing for resources with other elements of the care system which are traditionally seen as more important for patient care. Moreover, eHealth is also commonly regarded as a net investment with a negative financial return. The good news is that this is only a narrow view of the whole financial picture. eHealth can be seen as one of the best candidates for funding in a competitive financial environment by demonstrating returns on investments based on savings in other areas of the health care system by implementing eHealth solutions.

IT governance standards and methodologies are used in non-healthcare industries and enterprises to provide a careful alignment of IT technologies and capabilities with the business goals of the enterprise. Levels of alignment can be measured; plans for improvement can be devised and implemented, with a monitoring framework in place to ensure a culture of continuous improvement. In this chapter we show how these standards and methods can be applied within a healthcare environment. We demonstrate the use of IT governance for eHealth to improve the alignment of eHealth with organisational targets, together with a monitoring process that measures what has been achieved, not only from the eHealth service balance scorecard point of view, but also working with Finance Departments to measure eHealth contribution to specific health care savings. This, then, is the challenge for eHealth: how best to adopt IT Governance for eHealth so that the necessary alignment is ensured, and so that measurable and predicted savings can be achieved.

After this introduction we present some fundamental concepts involving eHealth, health informatics, ICT, Information and Knowledge. Unfortunately there is no global consensus on many of these definitions and concepts, which increases the complexity of any attempt to "sell" eHealth in competitions for funding – or, indeed, to demonstrate expected levels of savings. It is difficult for all the involved stakeholders to accurately represent their positions without using a common speech.

Using this foundational terminology we go on to present the importance of getting alignment between eHealth and the goals of Health Care Organisations (HCOs). We also discuss the perceptions of some public boards, comparing and contrasting with the perceptions other industries and countries regarding IT-Business alignment. We then analyse the drivers, triggers, catalysts and conditions that determine the "momentum" to implement IT Governance, and describe the standards, frameworks and tools that can be useful when implementing IT Governance, based on the experiences across different health care organisations. We then relate some lessons learned from our experience in Scotland of implementing IT Governance as part of a demonstrator eHealth project. The aim of this project is to assess the approaches, tools and recommendations needed to roll out the IT governance in other health care boards across Scotland. Some of these are clearly applicable to other industries and to health care in countries having different models of health care funding to that of the United Kingdom. The final section of the chapter is a summary of these recommendations, with notes regarding their wider applicability.

Let's Talk eHealth

IT Governance in the health sector is a controversial topic as the boundaries between IT, information, eHealth, health informatics, ICT and health care are not crystal clear. An important factor is the lack of consensus between groups of professional who traditionally talk in either business, clinical or technical speech.| We first describe the independent concepts of health care and ICT, and then associated these through the definition of "Health Informatics". This will be added on to, so as to build a wider view of what eHealth is understood to be for our purposes. Then we describe IT Governance in general, and this is contrasted with and compared to eHealth Governance.

HEALTHCARE & HEALTHCARE SYSTEM

We start with the observation that health care is one of the fundamental human rights as recognized through the Universal Declaration. This may be overly philosophical in the context of this book, but it certainly establishes relevant foundations to sustain the importance of eHealth to deliver fundamental human rights: both health care, and also the right to receive equal access to public services. eHealth is a key element for the successful delivery of these fundamental rights.

Health care also embraces different organizations and services to promote health, either by curing, preventing or by way of palliative interventions for individuals or groups of population (World Health Organisation, 2009).

A Healthcare system refers to those structures, processes, people and other resources such as financial and information which are involved in the delivery of health care to specific groups within the population. Better performance is focused on three main areas: health, satisfaction of population expectations and finance, particularly funding and savings (World Health Organisation, 2009).

There are different models of healthcare systems across the world, and the variations are determined by the groups of the population

Figure 1. Relation between fundamental concepts involved in eHealth

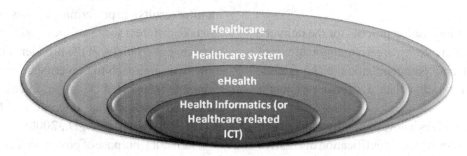

targeted and the funding methods involved by combining private and public resources, such as taxes, insurance, donations, volunteer effort and direct payment.

ICT

For most people ICT or Information and Communication Technologies are related to electronic equipment, like computers or routers, which are used to manage data. This is far from the actual depth of the concept. The most controversial aspect involves the understanding of what "technology" means. It is an innovation process by application of knowledge, both new and existent, both scientific and non-scientific, to practical scenarios (Goodman, C., 2004). It may include tools and products, but also intangibles like processes, methods, techniques, systems or any other organisational structure.

By developing this concept is it possible to prepare a definition of ICT that approaches the concept from the innovation point of view, as an application of knowledge into the information and communications field. In this sense ICT involves related tools and products; like hardware or software, processes like extract, transform, and load (ETL), architecture design, software development, systems design or service oriented architecture (SOA) implementations, between other processes, methods and related techniques involved in any of the information, communication and related technologies fields.

Health Informatics

Health Informatics is a mix of sciences: information, telecommunication, computing and health. It involves tools usually associated with ICT but also a wider spectrum of related sciences that influence the new ICTs. Examples include radiology ICT enabled tools that are influenced by sciences related with digital images, and laboratory ICT enabled tools that are influenced by applications of chemistry. There are multiple links between other sciences and Health Informatics.

Health Informatics is regulated by different organisations in different regions of the world, such as the IMIA (International Medical Informatics Association) which has existed since the 1970s. More recently, newer bodies are taking an important role in regulating this field like the European Federation for Medical Informatics, the Office of the U.S. National Coordinator for Health Information Technology (ONCHIT), the U.S. Certification Commission for Healthcare Information Technology (CCHIT), the Asia Pacific Association for Medical Informatics (APAMI) and the Australian College of Health Informatics (ACHI), between many others.

eHealth

eHealth is an innovation process for the delivery of better healthcare by creative applications of information and communication technologies. It is a process rather than a structure or just a technology.

eHealth involves innovation and organisational change, as it requires the identification of creative ways to adapt technologies and methods already available and applied in other arenas for use within the healthcare field. Many technologies are well-understood and are available for multiple applications; it is a matter of applying what already exists to improve the healthcare value chain. Samples of these innovations are the applications of wireless, internet or laptops to get more mobility not only for practitioners but also patients, carers, executives, etc. These innovations are broadly implemented across health care organisations, but there are other, more specific examples. Such as scanning applied to electronic documents for patient records, integration middleware for integrated patient history, teleconferencing or GPS for remote diagnoses, or virtual worlds to replicate experiences and learn from healthcare virtual networks. These innovations, together with the practice of effective delivery of these innovations into actual healthcare organisations, is eHealth.

eHealth subsumes a number of other concepts like mHealth (mobile devices applied to telemedicine), teleconferencing (remote conferencing ICT enabled), KmHealth (knowledge management), TeleHealth or TeleMedicine, eCare, PAS (Patient Administration Systems), PACS, SCI, EPR (Electronic Patient Records). The number of such examples increases more innovations are designed and implemented within the eHealth process.

IT AND EHEALTH GOVERNANCE

Governance is the set of management or leadership processes used by people structures to take decisions, grant power to make decisions happen and monitor results and performance. These structures can take different forms of socio-political or economical *government,* in the broader sense of this term. This approach to Governance as a concept is broadly supported (Dignam, 2006) including the World Bank and the International Monetory Fund (IMF) (Kaufmann, D., 2000).

The natural purpose of governance is to provide assurance to all stakeholders that things will go as expected, in other words: that the results achieved will be in line with the decisions taken.

In the wider sense, governance implies a macro management or leadership process to make socio-political and economical decisions followed by the government structures put in place to achieve those decisions. From the healthcare perspective it implies the whole range of decisions taken by societies to deal with the healthcare issues of different collectives.

By analogy, using the above definitions related with Healthcare and Healthcare System, we can explain what Governance means within the context of the health care system: a process to ensure results are achieved in line with a set of taken decisions related with the direction, fundamental rules and structures established by each HCO or healthcare Board to move the healthcare system as a Corporations in that direction.

This analogy can be applied to develop the IT and eHealth Governance concepts. The difference strives on the scope of the decisions taken within the spheres of influence and accountability of each of these sub-structures of the healthcare system.

eHealth deals with innovation and organisational change to ensure creative ways to get the most of information and related technologies and methods within the healthcare field. In this sense, eHealth Governance is the process to ensure this happens in line with the healthcare Board strategy in place. eHealth can involve Information Governance, IT Governance and Project Governance between others.

Figure 2. Relation between governance and healthcare concepts

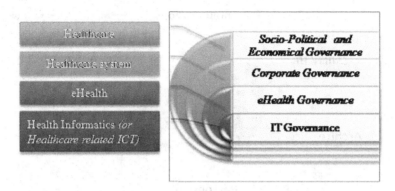

Throughout this chapter, we have adopted the approach presented by Mårten Simonsson and Pontus Johnson in their effort to consolidate a vast literature available around this concept (Simonsson, M., 2006). They suggest that IT governance is about taking IT related decisions and implementing them by using Governance practices and resources.

In terms of frameworks for IT Governance implementations, we considered CobIT® as a reference throughout the study presented in this chapter. CobIT® was developed by ITGI, the IT Governance Institute which promotes original research and case studies that executives can refer to in their IT Governance duties (ITGI, 2009).

The CobIT© framework presents the elements involved on IT Governance in terms of "dimensions": goals, processes, people, information (data), applications, technology and facilities (infrastructure).

CobIT present specific reference models for each relevant IT Governance process describing the following aspects of Governance maturity (Hardy, G., 2006):

- Awareness and communication
- Policies, standards and procedures
- Tools and automation
- Skills and expertise
- Responsibility and accountability
- Goal setting and measurement

EHEALTH AND HEALTH SERVICE ORGANISATION STRATEGIC ALIGNMENT

As Prof. Luftman outlined in a recent interview, there is no one thing IT can do for the business, there is a bunch of things IT can do (Kontzer, T., 2009).

In this section we share the lessons learned from a project implementing IT Governance in the Health Sector in Scotland, and the activities indicated that allow us to succeed in getting better alignment of ICT within HCOs, in other words, to improve eHealth.

Studies conducted over the last decade coincide in identifying the lack of alignment between IT and the business strategy as a common issue for most of the organisations consulted.

Since 2000, surveys like the HIMSS (Health Information and Management Systems Society) on information technology (Tschida, 2000) show this misalignment as one of the most important concerns of executives. This finding has been reinforced by later studies such as Silvius' business & IT alignment theory (Silvius, 2007), the most recent HIMSS 2008 survey (Hiner, 2008), the "IT Governance Global Status Report 2008" (PriceWaterhouseCoopers, 2008) and finally the CIO Insight and SIM surveys (Kontzer, 2009).

Although the ITGI report shows some positive figures regarding the actual level of IT-Business

Figure 3. Dimension of eHealth - HCO alignment. Based on the six criteria proposed by Luftman.

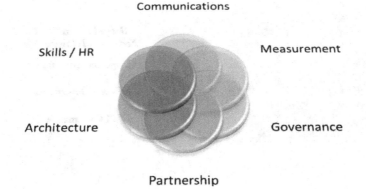

alignment, it concludes that there is still room for improvement. According to this report, 62% of the organisations consulted world-wide consider their actual level of alignment to be at least good, and 19% consider it to be very good. These are not isolated results. Along with these recent surveys, there are also multiple references in other formal studies and conference proceedings reflecting the need to improve the alignment of ICT with the business. The reason why CIOs and CEOs are concerned about aligning IT with the business is because "good alignment translates into increased innovation and revenue" as Prof. Luftman recently stated in relation with the latest SIM survey results (Hoboken, 2008).

Healthcare organizations have similar concerns. This has been broadly expressed during the last few years in studies from the UK (Muir, 2007), New Zealand (Bolevich, 2009), Australia (Eysenbach, 2008), India (Khandelwal, 2006), and Canada (Causi, 2009).

This view has been corroborated by a survey we conducted within the NHS Scotland eHealth Demonstrator Project for IT Governance implementation (Scottish Government, eHealth Programme, 2009). As part of this project a series of workshops were held to discuss lessons learned, strategic alignment and perceived benefits with the main stakeholders involved in the implementation of IT Governance in three National Health Service Boards in Scotland selected for this demonstrator exercise. Boards participating were close geographically and culturally, but have different structures, goals and priorities; also are different in terms of processes in place and resources. In this way we obtained an insight from three different but related case studies.

People involved in the workshops came from the relevant eHealth departments of the three Boards involved.

We employed a reduced version of the Luftman survey to drive the discussion within the workshops exploring the following areas:

These are the same areas defined by Luftman in previous studies (Luftman, J., 2000); but we adapted a subset of the original statements provided for each area in order to adjust the survey instrument to the workshop format.

The adapted instrument is shown in Figure 4.

The responders provided a level of agreement with each statement from strongly disagree (1) to strongly agree (5). Responses were obtained both from individuals and from groups of individuals who were providing a collective view as an outcome of the workshop discussions. Moreover, the responses were classified by the following groups of interest representing different perspectives within the organisations involved:

Figure 4. Aspects included for an abbreviated format of the Luftman instrument assessing perceptions of strategic alignment.

Area of alignment : Communications
1. Business and ICT speak the same language
2. Business and ICT management have a shared vision of the role of ICT in enabling business strategies
3. Business management has a good understanding of the impact of ICT on the business
Area of alignment : Partnership
4. Business and ICT planning and management processes are tightly connected and integrated
5. Innovations in ICT are taken into account when determining the business strategy
6. Your organisation fosters a clear business ownership for ICT projects
Area of alignment : Architecture
7. Strategic business/ICT alignment processes at a centralised level are in line with strategic business/ICT alignment processes at a decentralised level
8. Business processes are adequately supported by ICT
9. Your organisation systematically determines the impact of new ICT investments on existing business processes, systems and infrastructure
Area of alignment : Value Measurement
10. Your organisation is able to clearly demonstrate the value for its ICT investments
11. New ICT investment and enhancement spend is prioritised against business strategy
12. The performance of new ICT investment projects is regularly monitored and benchmarked against strategic objectives
Area of alignment : Governance
13. ICT performance management impacts budget allocation
14. There is transparency in the levels of authority and responsibilities for making decisions with respect to ICT projects
15. There is transparency in the levels of accountability for outcomes for ICT projects
Area of alignment : Human Resource
16. Your organisation is able to minimise the resistance to change that comes with new ICT projects
17. Your organisation fosters a clear stakeholder management for ICT projects
18. In your organisation key-Users participate in the design and development of new ICT systems

- **Business perspective**, involving the perception of the HCO side, not only from the clinical or patient-related services point of view, but also from administration and other corporate services.
- **eHealth perspective**, involving the point of view of the senior management level of eHealth related departments
- **Independent perspective**, usually provided by the external consultant(s) and the local facilitators or project coordinators with a global picture of the project and

the organisation, after reviewing the IT Governance maturity across the Board.
- **Process owners,** either eHealth related managers or eHealth process owners. The processes owners invited to participate on each workshop depended on the scope each Board implemented their own IT Governance initiative. In any case, the assessment was based on the processes suggested by CobIT©.

The results presented in the following section are a comparison between the collective and individual views expressed by these informed interest groups. This analysis will show who within the NHS Boards recognise the benefits and the need to improve IT/eHealth Governance, and also which of this groups can see IT Governance and CobIT as a potential solution to achieve the expected benefits, including better alignment IT-HCO. Finally we'll contrast and compare the level of adoption of CobIT within the HCOs involved.

PERCEPTION OF BUSINESS-IT ALIGNMENT

Adapted and Abbreviated Version of the Luftman Survey Instrument

Overall Perception of Alignment

The analysis is based on the maturity level adapted by Luftman from the CMM model (Luftman, J., 2000) presenting five levels of alignment maturity as follows, starting from a previous Level 0 for those scenarios where nothing in place to manage the process:

The results of the alignment assessment conducted as part of an eHealth Demonstrator Project, shown the overall perception was that eHealth and the NHS Boards are in the earlier stages of the alignment process, which is consistent with the outcome of the IT Governance assessment conducted in these Boards as part of the implementation of the CobIT© framework. This result is interesting as demonstrates in some degree that both instruments, the Luftman survey and CobIT©, using different approaches arrive to similar conclusions, at least at a higher level. As these instruments work with different sets of questions, statements and controls, at a lower level, the conclusion are difficult to compare in later stages of the assessment, but at least the results are consistent if we are looking for a view at a glance of the overall maturity of the IT Governance (CobIT© assessment) in the organisation or the level of alignment between eHealth/IT and the HCOs/Business (Luftman SAM Survey).

This corroborative result also indicates that the instrument worked even when applied within the relatively small groups of participant in the eHealth Demonstrator workshops.

In general terms the NHS Boards consulted perceived the level of alignment is at some point between a "Committed" (Level 2) and an "Established" (Level 3), but seems to lay closer to Level 2 than 3 (Figure 5), mainly because to be considered in a specific level all the relevant aspects of compliance need to be achieved. The only area in which a large variation in perceptions was found was "governance" (Figure 6) indicating the wide differences in the degrees of awareness of governance issues and standards across the boards.

When we consider the perceptions of groups of interest (Figure 7 and Figure 8) we see repeated evidence of a trend for those who are responsible for – rather than observers of, or workers within an area, to have a higher perception of alignment levels. Moreover, this higher level is still, for the most part, between levels 2 and 3, indicating that no role-group has a perception of highest alignment levels, and that those who work within eHealth on a day-to-day basis perceive a lower alignment, between 1 and 2 in most of the dimensions. In general, independents' perspective is stricter, setting the lowest levels of perceived alignment with the exception of the skills dimension, where despite of coinciding with other groups regarding lack of consistency across functions are more optimistic identifying emerging skills across the Boards, as required by eHealth departments nowadays as value service providers

The areas where alignment is better perceived, in general, are Governance, Communications and Architecture. The areas considered more mis-aligned are measurement, partnership and skills.

As mentioned before, the business/eHealth perspective tend to be more optimistic in terms of alignment than process owners or independents;

Figure 5. Perceived level of eHealth-HCO alignment

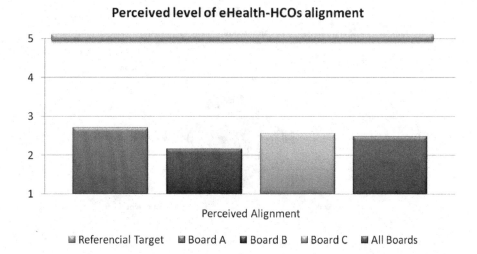

Figure 6. Alignment perceptions detected within some NHS Boards in Scotland. 2009

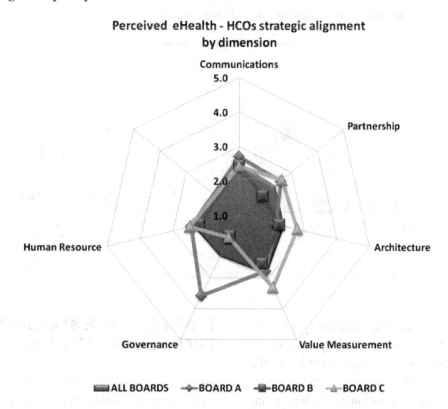

these ones are more rigorous and severe in their perception, perhaps because it was influenced by the outcome of detailed assessments conducted using CobIT© throughout the Boards.

Nevertheless, the overall perception across the Boards and groups of interest remains between level 2 and 3; the higher the level of management

Figure 7. Perceived alignment by groups of interest (radar view)

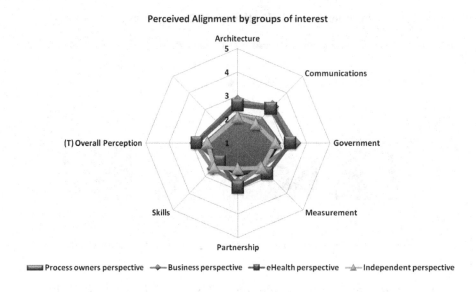

Figure 8. Perceived alignment by groups of interest (bars view)

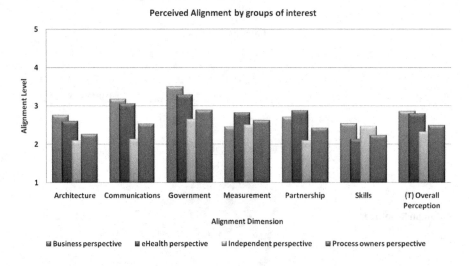

the better perception of alignment but, in any case, no quite distant from other groups perceptions.

The transition from level 2 to level 3 from the six dimension reviewed progress as shown in Figure 9, giving explicit definitions of the limitations and differences between the two levels.

IT GOVERNANCE STANDARDS, FRAMEWORKS AND TOOLS

Now that we have motivated a link between the perceptions of misalignment and low levels of governance, we present a more detailed exposition of different standards, frameworks and related tools suitable for IT and eHealth Governance. We compare their scope and benefits, with emphasis on their possible application in the health sector.

Figure 9. Example of some characteristics of the level of alignment perceived within the NHS based on the Luftman proposed dimensions of alignment

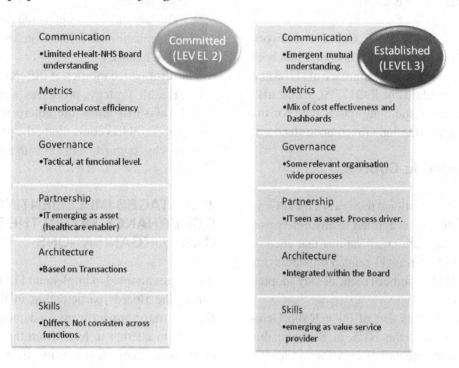

There are many IT-related management frameworks, methodologies and standards in use today. None of them, on their own, forms a complete IT governance framework and there are significant overlaps between and across them, but they all have a useful role to play in assisting enterprises to manage and govern their information and related technologies more effectively. The international standard for IT governance is the recent ISO/IEC 38500 which has only been available since 2008. There are several widely-recognised, vendor-neutral, third party frameworks that are often described as 'IT governance frameworks'. Important examples include:

- ITIL®, or IT Infrastructure Library®, was developed by the UK's Office of Government Commerce as a library of best practice processes for IT service management. Widely adopted around the world, ITIL is supported by ISO/IEC 20000:2005, against which independent certification can be achieved.

- CobIT®, or Control Objectives for Information and related Technology, now in version 4.1, was developed by the United States' IT Governance Institute. CobIT is increasingly accepted as good practice for control over information, IT and related risks. Its guidance helps organizations implement effective governance over enterprise-wide IT. In particular, CobIT's Management Guidelines component contains a framework for the control and measurability of IT by providing tools to assess and measure the enterprise's IT capability for the 34 identified CobIT processes.

- ISO17799, now embedded within ISO27002 and supported by ISO27001, (both issued by the International Standards Organization in Geneva), is the global best practice standard for information security management in enterprises.

We have employed the CobIT framework throughout this study, since it encompasses both the continual improvement approach of ITIL3 and the security standards of ISO17799, whilst also providing support and compliance with for the UK National Information Governance standard.

The Framework: CobIT®

CobIT® is an international framework for IT Governance which can be applied to any enterprise, including health care organisations that encompasses the most relevant IT related standards (i.e. ISO/IEC and ITIL), some of them already adopted across the HCO.

It was selected as part of the eHealth Demonstrator project at the NHS in Scotland due to its wide implementation over the world, but also because it is supported by comprehensive automated tools and the availability of certified professionals to help with its implementation. There are multiple successful previous experiences all over the world, some of them documented and available for reference.

In the particular case of the eHealth Demonstrator project, some Boards are internally and externally audited using CobIT framework as well, and also at further monitoring and improvement stages.

CobIT presents good practices across all areas of eHealth services including the management of the eHealth programme, information services and IT, and provides a set of recommendations to comply with best practices in terms of:

- Which processes need to be improved
- How mature each process is (5 levels presented in a maturity model)
- What's required to achieve the desired level of maturity filling the gap

- What activities need to be performed on each process
- Who should be responsible for/accountable/consulted/informed on each process (RACI charts)
- Performance metrics at different levels (at eHealth strategy, processes and activities levels) that allow the enterprise to know how far it has come along the path towards process maturity and eHealth alignment.

THE STAGES IMPLEMENTING IT GOVERNANCE WITHIN THE HEALTH CARE ORGANISATIONS

The stages adopted to implement IT Governance across the Boards participating in the eHealth Demonstrator project were fundamentally identical in an attempt to learn from the experience and make recommendations in the event of future roll out across other healthcare Boards. Figure 11 shows the basic stages adopted, following a common improvement cycle approach.

The eHealth Governance Momentum

We now describe what motivated the adoption of formal approaches to eHealth Governance in different HCOs in order to set conclusions and recommendations that can be applicable to other health organisations.

In particular, we explore the drivers, expectations and assumptions involved in this process at NHS Scotland as part of the eHealth Demonstrator Project.

Drivers

The Boards involved identified the following main drivers when deciding to implement formal eHealth Governance frameworks:

Figure 10. IT Governance model based on CobIT® applied to eHealth at NHS

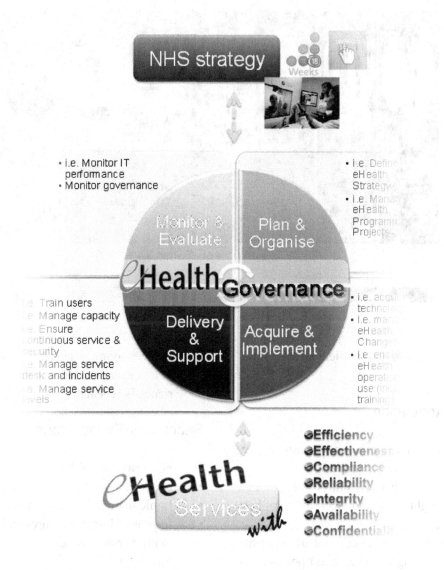

- Perception of limited alignment between eHealth service and Health Care needs along with organisational pressures to achieve more and quicker alignment.
- More demanding health care.
- Limited contribution of eHealth at Health Board level and vice versa, usually eHealth not being seen as part of the NHS value chain but as a health care support instrument.

- Boards often play a passive role in ensuring the organisation gets the most of eHealth.
- Audit recommendations to improve documentation and formal processes in some areas.

Expectations

These factors were perceived to be the benefits delivered by eHealth Governance by the involved

Figure 11. Stages implementing IT Governance in the NHS based on CobIT®

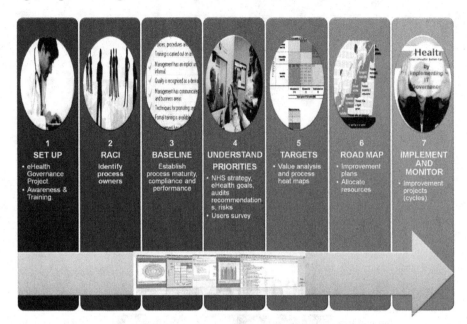

stakeholders, before the implementation took place.

Primary Expectations

- To become more efficient, as funding restrictions are commonplace
- Demonstrate that eHealth is doing things in the right way and according to best practices.
- Ensure (by governance) and demonstrate (by measuring achievements) positive returns on eHealth investment.
- Improve audit outcomes, both internal and external.
- Improve customer satisfaction and communicate it throughout the Board. By customers we mean all actors or stakeholders involved in health care who benefit directly or indirectly from eHealth.
- Set the required systems and processes in place to improve the customer experience.

- Deliver common and standardised services in a consistent manner, ensuring the experience is repeatable.

Secondary Expectations

- Formalise eHealth processes.
- Achieve agreed service levels (SLAs)
- Implement audit recommendations.
- Improve Human resource utilisation within the Service Desk.
- Manage IT Risks.
- Measure where HCOs are compared to industry standards and IT best practices.
- Help specific areas to operate in a standardised way, mainly after a series of changes in the evolution of the NHS Trust.
- Standardisation of practices across the Department. Repeatable processes in place.
- Improve quality and service performance (demonstrate).

Adverse Assumptions

We detected established assumptions about eHealth and eHealth Governance held within the NHS, but frequently shared across other HCOs. Many of these preconceived ideas are obsolete and act as barriers to the successful matching of the high expectations for a modern healthcare system. Important examples include:

- eHealth (IT) supports health care but is not a clear part of the value chain. It is not perceived as an element that is transforming but supporting healthcare.
- The health service has to be provided with or without eHealth; healthcare is the priority and eHealth is less important, is secondary.
- Rigour inhibits the creativity and skills required by eHealth innovations.
- Best practices are bureaucratic and time and resources consuming. NHS Boards therefore cannot afford it.
- Collaboration between Boards: using synergy to achieve better or quicker results is idealistic; each Board has to look after itself, move forward and quickly react to satisfy a highly demanding and unpredictable healthcare; there is no time or resources for other approaches even if they are interesting. Collaboration is time and resources consuming, thus NHS Boards cannot afford.
- NHS (or our Board) is different; these approaches don't apply to us.
- We know what we have to do; it's just that we don't have time and resources to do it.

Lessons Learned

Based on analysis of the NHS Scotland eHealth Demonstrator project, we monitored the changes in expectations throughout the IT Governance implementation, identifying what worked and what didn't work in these three different health care boards. This forms the basis for our suite of recommendations for successful eHealth Governance at the health board level and governmental levels.

The key factors for successful outcomes are shown in Figure 12.

The exact balance of these factors to give the best outcome depends on variables such as board structure, scope of services under consideration, existing and planned infrastructure and personnel capabilities. However, there are a number of common observations and findings that are recommended for any future implementation of eHealth Governance in Scotland. Since these recommendations are independent of funding model and political environment, we present them as global recommendations for governments and health care organisations in any modern democracy.

Ready-Steady-Go

In the following, we use the term HCO to signify any health care organisation (local, regional, or national; public or private) but this term can be replaced throughout by any organisation providing centralised services related to eHealth and/or eHealth Governance, such as local, regional and national government departments. For these latter organisations, each recommendation should be taken as a facilitator for helping HCOs implement eHealth Governance; the recommendation is therefore external rather than internal.

Top 10 Recommendations for eHealth Governance

1. Investigate what other HCOs are achieving and check what eHealth Governance can do for your HCO. eHealth Governance can make a difference.
2. Sell it across your HCO: eHealth Governance can help to improve eHealth. Remember that better eHealth is designed to lead to

Figure 12. Key success factors to implement eHealth governance

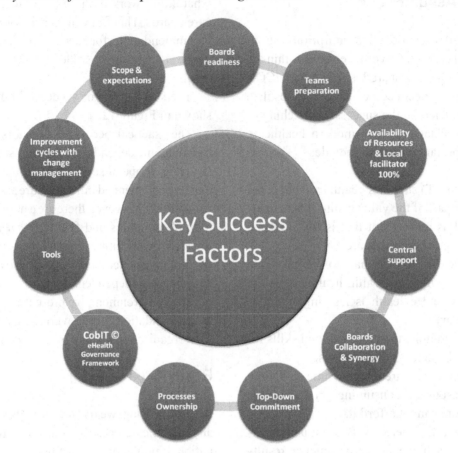

better care. Design and deliver a campaign to raise awareness and readiness of your HCO. Remember that eHealth Governance is not only about technologies but how to get the most of the Information and related IT by adding value to patient care. It involves the whole organisation and implies an organisational change. It is more complex to deal with organisational change than pure technology, so sell it before anything else, the more the organisation buys it the easier to implement. In this context, organisation means people who have to be convinced of the benefits or at least in a position to support the transition towards better eHealth Governance.

3. Adopt a framework for IT (eHealth) Governance. Select a framework widely implemented across the world and supported by professionals and tools. Our experience at NHS in Scotland suggests CobIT but there are other frameworks and standards that can be applicable. ITIL is progressing in an interesting and wider approach more aligned with new approaches to service oriented architectures applied to Healthcare than previous versions. Ensure the skills, knowledge and tools to support the implementation of the selected framework are easily available in your HCO environment. Check the framework selected is not focussed only in a particular dimension of Governance, for example security or a specific part of

the service, but that encompasses all the processes involved in eHealth. Moreover, the central aim of the framework should be alignment of IT with eHealth strategies and eHealth with the Healthcare business.

4. Adopt automated tools to support eHealth Governance. Particularly tools with an embedded knowledge base so the implementation can produce quicker results, demonstrate the benefits and re-enforce the transition towards better eHealth Governance. Nowadays, tools tend to offer a platform from which to develop what the organisation requires. It is good in terms adaptation to the HCO preferences but is time and resource consuming. There are tools in the market offered with a knowledge base that collects other organisations expertise so it is easier and quicker to start with and get results. The availability of this embedded knowledge can make a difference to succeed implementing eHealth Governance. Check tools assessed by professional bodies. For example, but is not the only one, the ISACA is specialised in IT Governance and offers links and assessments of different tools supporting CobIT© and other related standards, frameworks and guidelines.

5. Provide local support and advice on eHealth Governance to help process owners, particularly but not exclusively, in the earlier stages.

6. Get the benefits of synergy and collaboration. Use central expertise and participate actively within opportunities for sharing the experience with other HCOs.

7. Be creative to encourage continual internal collaboration and synergy to learn from your own experience and tune your new way of working as a team, as an organisation. Involve all stakeholders from the outset.

8. Do not underestimate the amount time and resources required at the earlier stages. Run a pilot to better understand how eHealth Governance works and the organisational change implications for your HCO.

9. Show the results. Monitor the progress in your HCO and create opportunities to show it across the HCO.

10. Try to get a certification (i.e. ISO/IEC 38500) or at least show your audit result prior to and after any process improvement cycle implemented in your HCO.

We believe that it is vital for governmental agencies and funding bodies to provide support, central external advice, central training facilities, and a central knowledge repository at the earliest possible stage. This is because successful implementation at the HCO level is greatly assisted by expert assistance with the concepts, techniques and organisational changes involved: readiness is key. There is an obvious synergy in this situation: early support from the centre leads to quicker and more cost-effective eHealth improvements, giving both financial and health care benefits to the entire community.

We also concur with earlier findings of Luftman from similar studies that management commitment and project buy-in are also vital. This hardly needs to be stated, since eHealth Governance involves planned organisational change in all cases, and all best management practices for these changes apply. In fact, the main complexities of eHealth Government involve the organisational transitions, with the ICT aspects playing a secondary part. Hence any effort spent in improving the readiness of the HCO, getting commitment at all levels, preparing a detailed project plan and managing expectations is worthwhile. This can be best achieved, in our opinion, by initially focussing on a small number or core processes, rather than attempting an implementation over multiple, broad areas.

In summary, our findings are motivated by an initial study of perceptions of alignment levels, followed by a demonstrator project involving three HCOs; they coincide with, and extend, the findings of previous studies of this type, including that of Luftman. Our recommendations apply in most political and socio-economic models and describe the key enablers of eHealth Governance implementation.

REFERENCES

Bolevich, Z., & Mules, C. (2009). *A coherent future: Aligning health service and ICT trends*. NZ Ministry of Health. Retrieved from http://www.slideshare.net/HINZ/aligning-health-service-and-ict-trends

Causi, S. P. (2009). *Healthcare by 2015*. Canada GHBN. Retrieved from http://www.slideshare.net/GHBN/healthcare-by-2015-mar-2009

Datasec & NHS Fife. (2009). *eHealth demonstrator project for IT governance*. Edinburgh: Scottish Executive.

Dignam, A. J., & Lowry, J. P. (2006). *Company law* (Dignam, A. J., Ed.). 3rd ed.). Oxford: Oxford University Press.

Goodman, C. S. (2004). *HTA 101: Introduction to health technology assessment.*

Hardy, G. (2006). Using IT governance and CO-BIT to deliver value with IT and respond to legal, regulatory and compliance challenges. *Information Security Technical Report, 11*(1), 55–61. doi:10.1016/j.istr.2005.12.004

Hiner, J. (2008). SIM survey: Top 10 IT management concerns of 2008. *Techrepublic*. Retrieved from http://blogs.techrepublic.com.com/hiner/?p=882

Hoboken, N. J. (2008). *National survey finds information technology and business alignment a struggle for American companies*. Retrieved Sep 9, 2009, from http://www.stevens.edu/press/pr/pr1206

Kaufmann, D., Kraay, A., & Zoido-Lobatón, P. (2000). Governance matters: From measurement to action. *Finance & Development, 37*(2).

Khandelwal, A. (2006). E-health governance model and strategy in India. *Journal of Health Management, 8*(1), 145–155. doi:10.1177/097206340500800111

Kontzer, T. (2009). Why IT and business can't get in sync. *CIO Insight*. Retrieved from http://www.cioinsight.com/index2.php?option=content&task=view&id=882683&pop=1&hide_ads=1&page=0&hide_js=1

Luftman, J. (2000). Assessing business-IT alignment maturity. *Communications of AIS, 4*(14).

Muir, R. (2007). *eHealth governance, security and privacy. the UK perspective*. UK: slideshare.net. Retrieved from http://www.slideshare.net/HINZ/ehealthgovernance-security-and-privacya-uk-perspective

PriceWaterhouseCooper. (2008). *IT governance global status report 2008*. USA: IT Governance Institute. Retrieved from http://tais3.cc.upv.es/V/BEA6QVG8VHQPKT7UM-V26BICX9F7VFJXNB5GINHXXF77Y2N-LQUP-00908?func=quick-1

Scottish Government. E. P. (2009). *eHealth demonstrator project of IT governance at NHS in Scotland*. Scotland, UK: NHS Scotland annual conference 2009. Retrieved from http://www.nhsslearning2009.scot.nhs.uk/poster-gallery.aspx

Silvius, A. J. G. (2007). *Business & IT alignment in theory and practice*. Paper presented at the 40th Hawaii International Conference on Systems Science (HICSS-40 2007).

Simonsson, M., & Johnson, P. (2006). Defining IT governance-a consolidation of literature. *18th Conference on Advanced Information Systems Engineering CAiSE'06,* Luxembourg.

Tschida, M. (2000). Prior-IT-ies (health information and management systems society survey on information technology). *Modern Physician.* Retrieved from http://www.accessmylibrary. com/article-1G1-62408652/prior-ies-health-information.html

World Health Organisation. (2009). *eHealth for health care delivery.*

Section 2
Security in the Healthcare Industry

Chapter 7
Business Continuity and Disaster Recovery Considerations for Healthcare Technology

Edward M. Goldberg
Capella University, USA

ABSTRACT

As the healthcare industry moves towards adoption of electronic collection and storage of health data it becomes increasingly dependent on the successful functioning of these technologies in order to ensure access to this important information. This chapter explores the technical, ethical and legal issues associated with the importance of careful planning and implementation of robust disaster recovery procedures as well as the importance of business continuity activities in assuring that this data is available following a system failure or other event that may introduce risk of data loss.

INTRODUCTION

The Rationale for Contingency Planning to Protect Healthcare Technology

Traditional emphasis for protecting healthcare technology systems and the data they serve is focused on preventing data corruption, mis-

appropriation and misuse of the information (Bandyopadhyay & Iyer, 2000). Due to resource constraints, the potential for the loss and/or unavailability of these systems is often overlooked and/or neglected. The past decade provided ample rationale for seeking to protect society's critical infrastructure from acts of terror, hurricanes, tsunamis, floods, etc. Healthcare technology is now an inextricable element in that infrastructure and preparing for such eventuality is arguably an ethical responsibility of those responsible.

DOI: 10.4018/978-1-60960-174-4.ch007

Given the substantial reliance upon and critical nature of electronic health records, the focus on the security and ethical use of such information is appropriate (Ahlfeldt et al, 2009). The unit cost of storage and the systems which process and make that information useful generally decreases over time as for most such technology. The amount of storage needed has been growing exponentially for several years and will likely continue to do so for the foreseeable future. Similarly, the need for increased processing power to handle all of that information, periodic technology refreshes to keep pace with the computing environment in which the information exists as well as increased bandwidth and network capacity contribute to a substantial and ongoing cost. That cost and shrinking budgets in healthcare create a barrier to creating a resilient computing environment, thereby leaving these systems vulnerable to disasters and other major business interruptions.

Business Continuity and Disaster Recovery Defined

Business Continuity (BC) plans provide for the logistics, resources, infrastructure and strategies that allow an organization to perform its critical business processes during and after a disaster or other event that would otherwise cause the interruption or cessation of those processes (Goldberg, 2008; DRII, n.d.). These are plans that an organization uses to maintain the processes that it considers most important and necessary for its continued existence and ongoing viability. Typically, BC plans are designed to account for the loss of facilities, people and/or systems (any one of these or any combination of them). The details of the processes an organization must continue and how it does so vary widely, as do the risks and scenarios that could challenge its ability to perform effectively.

Disaster Recovery (DR) plans provide for the continuance or timely recovery of Information Technology (IT) systems. DR plans prioritize the work required to recovery computer systems, telecommunications systems, networks, data, etc., during and after a disaster or other disruptive event (Goldberg, 2008; DRII, n.d.). *DR plans are based upon BC plans.* Recall that BC plans account for loss of facilities, people and/or systems. The pervasive use of technology has embedded IT systems into many business processes. BC plans typically include *Recovery Time Objectives (RTO)* and *Recovery Point Objectives (RPO)* which define the timing and order by which the organization needs IT systems restored to be able to fulfill its BC planning objectives.

Specifying DR Needs: Recovery Time Objectives and Recovery Point Objectives

RTO is the time from when a disaster or other disruption disables an IT system until it is restored to service (Disaster Recovery Institute, n.d.). Faster recovery times generally require more expensive solutions than longer recovery times, so RTO is generally set to the longest time that the organization can practically continue without the system.

RPO is the point in time to which data restoration is made following a disaster or disruption (Disaster Recovery Institute, n.d.). While a 24 hour RTO means that a system will be available for use within 24 hours, a 24 hour RPO means that the data will be 24 hours old when the system is restored, and data after that point is not available. The criteria for establishing RPO for various IT systems varies by organization, and is typically a risk/cost/benefit analysis. For example, financial institutions typically have RPO of zero for their systems which are transaction-based because the loss of even one transaction could be very costly, disruptive and perhaps prohibited by regulation.

It is conceivable to have no data loss (RPO = 0) but still have an RTO that is not zero. Email systems are often so configured – when the system becomes available, all of the email from before the event as well as email that came in during the outage are all buffered and made available. Similarly, there are systems where RTO is low or zero (meaning the system is essentially always available during and after a disaster or disruptive event) but where the RPO is not zero. Utility companies, for safety, liability and regulatory reasons, always maintain the ability to take customer calls and dispatch crews, but customer billing data may not be available for some time afterwards. In such an instance, the utility has determined that some of their system data need not be available because it is less critical than safety-related information (Goldberg, 2008).

HEALTHCARE TECHNOLOGY CONSIDERATIONS

The use of technology in healthcare processes requires a higher degree of rigor than many less critical processes (Bandyopadhyay and Iyer, 2000). Specifically, the loss, delay, unavailability or corruption of healthcare data can have catastrophic results. Besides the costs associated with traditional business continuity and disaster recovery infrastructure, health care technology presents both special needs and special opportunities that warrant commensurate attention. Regulations such as Health Insurance Portability and Accountability Act (HIPAA) and other health information privacy requirements require close scrutiny. Even records relating to the use of sensitive information warrant such enhanced attention. Traditionally, the transfer of records from paper to electronic form required an infrastructure that provided for the same level of protection against misuse of information as was present previously for the paper forms. Protection and tracking of records in electronic form is often still analogous to those processes implemented for paper records. However, the availability and transportability of electronic health records makes possible and facilitates the use of the health information for a wide variety of purposes not feasible in paper form.

Such ease of use and movement also facilitates misappropriation of that same data, hence the need to carefully consider the right level of contingency planning in concert with continuance of systems that protect data in electronic form.

Current and future use of existing information should be considered with respect to DR as it is for any other infrastructure/resource consideration (Bandyopadhyay & Iyer, 2000). For example, performing research on existing records, both current and archived, will likely prove to be fertile ground for new knowledge in healthcare. Applying a rigorous approach to the infrastructure that supports such activities will require a unique approach to both disaster recovery and business continuity. In fact, the pervasive nature of technology in healthcare coupled with the subsequent value of research will likely warrant a higher level of availability than is now justified, with shorter recovery times and substantial commitment to preventing loss of data, etc.

The process for specifying RTO for healthcare technology is not different from the process used for any other use of information technology (Disaster Recovery Institute, n.d.). It is both typical and logical for people to consider the work they do to be important. In many organizations, technology users routinely describe the critical nature of their work and the work processes they perform. With the pervasive nature of technology in so many such work processes, it is often no longer possible to perform those processes manually i.e. without the process-embedded technology upon which those processes rely. This common scenario often results in overly rigorous specification of RTO. For example, end users most affected by a computer system outage may request a very short or zero RTO, meaning that the loss of that system due to a disaster would be very short-lived or otherwise unnoticed, respectively, by the end user. Short RTO's typically require more expensive infrastructure than longer RTO's, and so a business analyst or other IT-business interface must translate the requested RTO into business terms such as cost/benefit analysis, etc. The cost of implementing a short or zero RTO is often prohibitive or excessive, and the nature of the work is better considered with respect to a disaster to arrive at a reasonable compromise. Some healthcare technology systems are indeed often part of life or death processes, but not all have such implications.

It is important to classify all of the organization's technology systems in terms of RTO and RPO to ensure the ability to effectively recover from a disaster without undue burden on the organization (Disaster Recovery Institute, n.d.). Doing this properly involves taking inventory of all of the organization's business processes and ranking them based on their criticality. It is not always a straightforward or intuitive assessment. Background functions such as payroll can be determined to be critical while seemingly crucial major processes may be deferred. The process of determining business process needs and establishing recovery time and point objectives is often referred to as a *business impact analysis (BIA)*.

A PROJECT APPROACH TO HEALTHCARE TECHNOLOGY BC/DR PLANNING

Once the BIA is complete, the DR planning process can be started (Goldberg, 2008). The first time this process is performed, it is essentially a project and should be treated as such. It is very important to note that treating planning as a project is an effective approach only for the initial creation of plans for the healthcare organization. DR plans need to be living documents given the fluid nature of people, organizations, systems, and the business processes these entities support. Supporting such ongoing change requires an ongoing and sustained effort. Projects are effective for unique, time-limited activities. That mindset carries over into the business, and often prioritizes urgency over long-term effect. Creating DR plans and a

DR planning process fits with the definition of a project, but maintaining and testing such plans is a post-project process.

The DR planning process (recall that DR plans support and are therefore driven by a BC plan) depends upon the active engagement of the relevant business process owners (Goldberg, 2008). Absent their engagement, plans become stale and irrelevant in terms of both the business processes and their stakeholders. Any number of changes to the organization, the regulatory environment, personnel contact information, and to the business process itself can cause a BC plan and supporting DR plans to be worse than useless, often providing a false sense of security and causing missteps during a disaster.

Healthcare Technology Resiliency: A Cultural Perspective

Healthcare organizations have cultural traits unique to healthcare as well as traits that distinguish each such culture from those in other healthcare organizations. The success of DR plans relies upon a culture that supports preparedness (Goldberg, 2008). Absent a mindset that preparedness is important and is affected by people in the organization, plans will rapidly drift out of date and grow less useful with the passage of time. On a technical level, the rapid rate of change in systems due to security patches, software and hardware upgrades, technology refreshes, configuration management and change management issues contributes to the likelihood that even the most rigorous DR environments will face challenges when needed.

Creating an organizational culture that supports DR does not imply that the entire organizational culture needs to change for DR planning to be effective (Schein, 1992). Rather, those implementing DR planning should be aware of the organization's culture, seeking to change only that which is within leadership's sphere of influence. Simply knowing what the existing culture is serves to facilitate successful DR planning and maintenance activities. Culture determines the degree to which resistance to change affects the rollout of any program. Culture also determines degrees of accountability and ownership of business processes. Similarly, the organization's tolerance for risk, a cultural outcome, helps to determine DR strategy. Lastly, the ability to get things accomplished within the organization is a characteristic of culture. The organization needs to be aware of DR and BC in all of its activities because contingency plans can be affected by those activities. Another way of describing the inextricable nature of BC and DR with culture is a logical chain: Executive sponsorship begets ownership, ownership begets accountability, accountability instantiates a process into people's consciousness, consciousness creates routine everyday behavior, and routine everyday behaviors reflect the culture. In the end, culture is sustainable, albeit fragile. BC and DR need to be a conscious part of an organization's everyday behavior – part of the culture.

Changing Culture for DR: Change Management

Discussing culture as it affects DR and BC planning is a purely academic exercise unless there is something actionable about it. Edgar Schein (1992) of Massachusetts Institute of Technology (MIT), a renowned expert on modern organizations and change management, describes a three-step change management process: demonstrating what is wrong with the current state, vividly describing the desired future state, and creating a safe means for all involved to move from current state to future state. This proven process is supported in both practical and academic circles. It is simple to design for any organization, is relatively easy to measure (progress), and is repeatable. The change process serves a higher purpose beyond simply creating a robust DR-supportive culture. Kurt Lewin, the classic and germinal source of change management theory, proved that one can-

not know and understand an organization without trying to change it (Schein, n.d.). Logically, that would imply that BC and DR planners would need to change their organization just to learn about their organization. While this might seem absurd – an expensive and potentially disruptive education – once the process begins, it immediately reveals what needs to change and why. The least it can do is establish healthy communications and instantiate a DR planning processes such as developing and testing plans and keeping them current, etc. With proper attention, the change process can make DR planning a conscious part of ongoing business dialogue, and a priority for the organization. (Contemporary literature includes many substantial discussions of the influence of leaders on culture, the use of change management, the value of pervasive communications and numerous cultural traits, but the topic is broad and can be researched separately from this focused discussion.)

MANAGING A DR ENVIRONMENT AND A BC CULTURE IN A HEALTHCARE SETTING

As one might conclude from the preceding discussions, managing a disaster recovery environment is a complex and challenging undertaking. In this limited discussion, it is not possible to cover the extent and depth of the topics and subtopics that comprise the state of the art/science of disaster recovery and business continuity planning. There is a widely accepted body of knowledge within the field of contingency planning provided and kept current by the Disaster Recovery Institute () ("professional practices", n.d.). Within that tome are ten subject areas of practice relevant to any setting and certainly to the healthcare/technology environment. Much of that body of knowledge is geared specifically towards the business continuity aspects of preparedness, but from prior discussion it was shown that disaster recovery – the information technology piece of the puzzle – supports and is integral to business continuity. Within a healthcare setting, that thought process serves to explain the inextricable nature of pervasive IT within healthcare and, therefore, the need for rigorous infrastructure and processes.

Healthcare Technology Disaster Recovery Implementation

Disaster recovery, at the lowest level, involves making copies of important data, storing it safely and providing an infrastructure to be able to use it during and after a disaster (Read, 2007). Consideration must be given to the nature of the organization and its resiliency so that the DR environment can be appropriately designed and implemented. There are a myriad of technology solutions for storage and recovery, all with benefits and costs that must be considered.

For a simple but telling example, a small hospital with a robust medical records system needs to maintain access to those records no matter what happens to the computer systems. Copies of records on tape shipped to an offsite location would be sufficient to protect the data from loss due to the destruction of the datacenter. Tape is relatively inexpensive, and making copies on tape is a viable solution with available technology. Further, tape backup stored offsite is a common legacy configuration for disaster recovery, but it is fraught with issues that have caused organizations to switch to solutions that are more robust.

Tape stored offsite raises many questions that need to be addressed to determine if the configuration is adequate for the organization's needs (Read, 2007). Consider recovery time objective – RTO. If the organization has a four hour RTO for the data on the tape, it is not likely that the datacenter could be restored to functionality after a destructive disaster (i.e. fire) in four hours. Therefore, to meet the four hour RTO, a second datacenter is needed, one that has enough equipment to begin operations within the four hour window. Such

an alternate location could be owned, leased or shared with others. There are many vendors who provide such facilities as a service.

Other considerations for meeting the healthcare provider's RTO include the volume of data on tape and the ability to restore that data within the time allotted (Read, 2007). Tape is a relatively slow media compared to solid state, disk or optical storage. Further, given its serial nature, it is difficult to restore files selectively. Rather than tape, many organizations use other storage facilities at remote locations – disk storage, for example. Need and cost determine the nature of that storage – whether it is connected and copied synchronously or asynchronously.

Synchronous copies are often limited by distance due to the time lag for the communications link (Read, 2007). Synchronous storage is expensive and relies on robust communications over short distances to have live copies of data in two places. Such configurations are very effective in fast restoration, and since the data simply exists in two places, the restoration time relies mainly upon how quickly the second location can be started to replace the primary location. It is often not possible to operate both locations simultaneously due to address and other configuration conflicts, so a failover mechanism (automated or manual) must generally be employed. Additional considerations include the vulnerability of data copied – in other words, the backup location's mirrored storage will make a perfect copy of the primary site's data, even if it is corrupt and/or infected.

The vulnerability of the data itself is of great concern in a healthcare setting, with life and death consequences (Bandyopadhyay and Iyer, 2000). In addition to the RTO restoration considerations discussed above, recovery *point* objectives must be met. In other words, it is necessary that any restoration include recovery of data to the last time the data was valid. That may mean the loss of some data that became corrupt, and it also requires that the organization specify its RPO. That RPO may be zero, meaning that it can afford no loss of data, and there are technology solutions to accommodate such needs. Logically, shorter RPO and RTO times require more expensive disaster recovery solutions.

Assuring Appropriate DR Solutions Based on the BC Plan

DR solutions can be very expensive (Read, 2007). Alternate datacenters, robust communications links, offsite storage, vendor-supported implementations or in-house staffing of alternate work locations, transportation of equipment and data and the maintenance of the equipment and a ready workforce can be staggering in terms of cost. Having inadequate DR solutions can be even more expensive because of the likelihood that data will be lost, healthcare operations severely and adversely affected and the organization's viability threatened. Unlike other organizations with less critical charters, an inadequate DR solution in a healthcare setting can cause harm and/or death.

For the aforementioned reasons, the DR solutions employed in a healthcare setting must meet or exceed the organization's needs without being wastefully onerous. To return to the example used previously, a small hospital may not even need an alternate datacenter. The loss of the facility may mean the cessation of all operations, not just IT. If the hospital's BC plan is to transfer patients to a nearby hospital and cease operations, it makes no sense to restore IT functionality elsewhere. Loss of facilities would not be a DR consideration in such a scenario. Loss of systems in that scenario, however, would be a valid concern, and for that local redundancy and storage would likely be adequate.

CONCLUSION

Healthcare environments require special consideration in the design and implementation of disaster recovery for their technology (Bandyopadhyay &

Iyer, 2000). Such systems are so pervasive and integrated into basic processes that the reliance on IT to provide healthcare requires robust planning to ensure continuity of operations. DR plans cannot be designed and implemented in a vacuum. It is necessary to first determine BC needs. BC needs are driven off the organization's culture as is the maintenance of plans, environment and infrastructure. DR plans are driven by BC plans. In the end, culture must be modified to support all forms of contingency planning and a high state of readiness.

The field of healthcare technology and disaster recovery within that field warrant ongoing study. Both IT and healthcare are rapidly evolving technological settings, and the intersection of these sciences is a rich place for study. Such investigation needs to find innovative ways to meet ever-increasing needs which include reducing costs. The information being stored and used today and since the inception of pervasive technology in healthcare will provide substantial data for studies within healthcare. The need to store, manipulate, access and process enormous amounts of data is being driven by the advancement of medicine. Disaster recovery of the systems that support such activity will be evermore critical with that advancement.

REFERENCES

Ahlfeldt, R., Erikson, N., & Soderstrom, E. (2009). Standards for information security and processes in healthcare. *Journal of Systems and Information Technology, 11*(3), 295–308. doi:10.1108/13287260910983650

Bandyopadhyay, K., & Iyer, R. (2000). Managing technology risks in the healthcare sector: Disaster recovery and business continuity planning. *Disaster Prevention and Management Journal, 9*(4), 257–270. doi:10.1108/09653560010351899

Goldberg, E. (2008). Sustainable utility business continuity planning: A primer, an overview and a proven, culture-based approach. *The Electricity Journal, 21*(10), 67–74. doi:10.1016/j.tej.2008.10.016

Professional Practices. (n.d.). Disaster Recovery Institute (n.d.). *Professional practices*. Retrieved September 8, 2009 from https://www.drii.org/professionalprac/prof_prac_details.php

Read, T. (2007). *Architecting availability and disaster recovery solutions: Sun blueprints online*. Retrieved September 8, 2009, from http://www.sun.com/blueprints/0406/819-5783.pdf

Schein, E. (1992). *Organizational culture and leadership*. San Francisco: Jossey-Bass, Inc.

Schein, E. (n.d.). *Kurt Lewin's change theory in the field and in the classroom: Notes toward a model of managed learning*. Retrieved September 8, 2009, from http://www.a2zpsychology.com/articles/kurt_lewin's_change_theory.htm

Chapter 8
E–Discovery and Health Care IT:
An Investigation

Vasupradha Vasudevan
Management Sciences and System, USA

H.R. Rao
Management Sciences and System, USA

ABSTRACT

The increase in electronic health records has introduced an increase risk of litigation related to collection, storage and exchange of health information. This chapter explores the issues associated with activities involving legal discovery that can result from failure to properly manage this stored data. It offers insights into strategies that organizations can use to protect against litigation resulting from failure to properly consider and mitigate against unexpected outcomes involving legal discovery involving stored health data.

INTRODUCTION

The computer revolution has increasingly improved firm productivity. Communications and archival systems to electronic documents help firms cut costs and quickly respond to everyday challenges. Storage of information in the electronic format helps organizations transfer confidential patient information safely and securely, save time in searching for files and helps gain better control over information. However, hidden costs may also exist in the form of high litigation risks. The risk of litigation can also impose heavy costs in terms of archiving and preservation of electronic documents. (Thru-Group, nd)

DOI: 10.4018/978-1-60960-174-4.ch008

E-discovery is a concept that health care organizations need to keep in mind, as it can greatly affect their daily operations. Many firms and organizations adopt E-discovery to save their organizations from incurring huge monetary losses in litigations.

E-Discovery

Discovery is the process by which one party to a lawsuit exchanges information with the other party. This exchange of information is vital to proving the claim or defense of a party. The scope of discovery is extremely broad.

E-discovery is the process of accessing, using and preserving information, data and records created or maintained in electronic format. It refers to discovery of information in civil litigations in which information is stored in electronic format and is also referred to as Electronically Stored Information (ESI).

The electronic format prevents spoliation of information as it also contains Metadata of the information preserved in the records. Examples of information sources that are most often used for e-discovery include instant messaging, e-mail, accounting databases, files etc. It is possible to generate large volumes of data at very low costs with the replication of ESI.. Furthermore, electronic content can be easily edited and can be backed up. Special software may, however, be required to access electronic information. (Dirking and Kodali, 2008)

Any information pertaining to a patient that is kept in the possession of a hospital or a healthcare provider whether on paper, or stored in electronic format, can be subject to disclosure in lawsuit. "E-discovery" however deals only with electronically stored information. In today's world, more than 99% of business information is stored in electronic format. In a lawsuit, any physician or CEO of a large healthcare organization will be called upon to produce ESI. E-discovery therefore requires the production of electronically stored information or ESI.

In 2004, President George W. Bush called for an electronic health records system to be maintained and preserved for all the Americans by 2014. Thus, a new office was established within US Department of Health and Human Services (Office of the National Coordinator for Health Information Technology).

On December 1 2006, amendments to the federal rules took effect that will henceforth have an impact on how ESI is created and stored. Healthcare providers are required to establish procedures to comply with these rules and communicate about the same to their staff.

Electronic Health Records are believed to contain a wealth of information about a patient. These records provide a critical source of evidence in all kinds of legal proceedings, such as medical malpractice cases and workers' compensation cases. Two other types of records that are maintained and preserved electronically by a healthcare organization are Business records and Employee records. (Brouillard, 2008) and (Miller and Tucker, 2009)

Associated Roles

The information technology (IT) specialists, keeper of medical records, health information management (HIM) personnel, financial officers, risk managers and corporate officers should understand the rules related to ESI to protect their organization from litigation.

HIM personnel should work in agreement with the IT staff and with the organization's attorneys to address the privacy issues of sensitive information like HIV, mental health, substance abuse and employee records as all of these are impacted by the new amendments in the federal rules. HIM personnel should be prepared to handle any issue relating to the organization's information management systems, including the location, preservation, retention and accessibility of electronic healthcare information.

The in-house counsel should also be conversant with the new rules in order to work in cooperation with outside counsel to establish, implement and enforce policies and procedures internally in the organization to ensure compliance.

Information to be Produced

Information about patients is either stored as on paper as patient records or stored on disks. These records are further linked to medication records. Computerized medical charts are used in some cases like labor and delivery, and during other emergency and critical conditions. In case of a lawsuit all these information must be produced in the ESI format.

Under the new rules, the requesting party may suggest a form in which this information has to be produced for which there may be objections from the other party. If the two parties are unable to resolve the differences and come to a consensus, a court will balance the burden of providing the ESI against its potential benefits to the lawsuit by weighing factors such as cost of production etc. HIM personnel will have to provide all these details to their counsel in order to resolve the differences.

Steps to be Taken

Certain steps have to be taken immediately in the event of a lawsuit to save your organization from foul play. Identification of the most knowledge-able IT and HIM people in the organization is a must and they should be brought in to review all record management and retention policies of the organization. A protocol has to be developed for an immediate and complete preservation of ESI. Constant working with the outside counsel is required to develop compliance.

The healthcare provider should properly handle ESI in order to protect themselves and the organization during a lawsuit. A very knowl-edgeable attorney is required to help you handle and manage ESI effectively. In case of lawsuit, key personnel within the organization should be trained to preserve all the ESI pertaining to that suit. (Callahan, 2007)

Preparing for E-Discovery

All HIM professionals will have to process an e-discovery request at some point in their career. It is not enough if they just know how to process a request. They also need to know the ins and outs of the electronic record management of their organization.

GET TO KNOW THE SYSTEM BETTER

Organizations will have to consider the ways in which they release information from multiple sources. HIM professionals need to learn their electronic systems thoroughly. Knowing how to access the electronic system's information is required to help both the inside and outside counsel during a lawsuit.

An understanding of where the records are stored, what is stored in the records, how to access the information in the records, what information is accessible and what information is not accessible, how to operate these systems and who is the owner of these systems is required.

Have a plan:

An overall records management plan is required for every organization to be prepared for litigation. An e-discovery request will require information to be obtained from multiple systems.

Specific guidelines and policies should be followed by organizations for the retention and preservation of the electronic data they handle. Enacting strict deletion policies would help an organization during litigation. Establishment of good-faith procedures is necessary

Talk it over:

In preparing for e-discovery, an organization's key personnel must know what is contained in the system and what could potentially be requested during a trial. Organizations must also decide on how to obtain the data the attorneys ask for during litigation.

Many healthcare organizations develop task forces aimed at preparing for e-discovery requests. An ideal task force would develop policies and procedures, build compliance models and work out retention schedules for its records management throughout the organization.

HIM professionals will also need to know where all the information comes from, how they are all organized and how to access the organized information. Designation of an e-discovery liaison is also required.

Storing only important information:

HIM professionals suggest that only those records that are routinely used are the ones that are to be included in a preset records management plan. This information would have either a business use or legal use. (Dimik, 2007)

LAWS RELATING TO THE HEALTHCARE INDUSTRY

An Outline of the Federal Rules of Civil Procedure

The FRCP governs all legal proceedings for civil lawsuit in the US district courts. These are propagated by the United States Supreme Court and approved by the United States Congress. These are comprised of 11 different categories and 86 different rule sets. The 11 categories are:

- Scope (purpose of the rules)
- Commencement of civil suits (rules that provide for the commencement of civil suits),
- Pleadings and Motions (civil suit pleadings, motions and defenses and counterclaims),
- Parties (capacities in which a party or parties can be sued),

- Discovery (contains rules governing discovery)
- Trial (provides for the plaintiff's right to a trial by a jury or court)
- Judgment (provisions containing legal judgments and costs)
- Provisional and final remedies and special proceedings (series of rules that provide for the final provision or remedy of a case)
- Special proceedings (rules governing special civil action proceedings)
- District courts and clerks (provides direction containing the business and the operations of civil courts)
- General provisions (explanation of which proceedings the rules apply to)

The US district judge has the ultimate authority in courtroom legal procedure and a very important role in courtroom legal procedure. Magistrate judges or special masters can also resolve E-discovery disputes. However, using judges and special agents for e-discovery disputes can achieve significant litigation cost and time savings. Each state will have, or adopt, its own rules for e-discovery. Most of the rules pertaining to a state will be adopted based on the FRCP, and the landmark case. HIM professionals must further be very cognizant of their state laws regarding discovery, and seek the advice of their legal counsel as a must when responding to e-discovery requests. (Baldwin-Stried, 2006)

Aspects of the New Rules Applicable to Health Information Management

Several of the new rules are directly relevant to Health Information Management. Especially rules discussed above (Rules numbered, 16, 26, 33, 34 and 37) have component parts relevant to Health Information Management. (Rebelo, 2007).

Discovery and disclosure: Under the new set of rules, any organization is required to establish processes in order to address scheduling and pretrial conferences and the agreements that parties reach for the preservation, disclosure and format of electronic records. Health Information Management and IT professionals must coordinate with inside and outside counsel prior to pretrial conferences. In addition, the HIM professionals should work with legal counsel and IT professionals to ensure that added privileges be added for sensitive information such as HIV, mental health, substance abuse and employee records. HIM professionals should be cognizant of the location, retention and accessibility of the health information records. Most importantly, under the new rules the parties in a lawsuit must prepare for and schedule a conference to address the organization's e-discovery and production policies within 120 days of filing the lawsuit.

Retention and destruction: These are critical concepts in e-discovery. Organizations must always know where all information important to the organization is stored and establish a routine policy and practice both for retention and destruction, which specifically details on when certain information's useful life is over in order to destroy it. The new Rules provide a safe harbor wherein certain information that has been destroyed using a routine policy and cannot be produced again is exempt. Sanctions can however be imposed on information for improper destruction.

Litigation hold or preservation order: In the context of e-discovery, a litigation hold or preservation order is the same concept as that applied to a paper-based medical record. Organizations must establish a policy and procedure that especially addresses the suspension of the usual record retention and destruction policy, in the event a litigation hold or preservation order is issued. This policy should specify who would have the authority to suspend the usual policy, who would be responsible for communicating the litigation hold or preservation order within the organization, who would be responsible for implementing the hold and who would have the authority to lift the hold.

Spoliation: This is the legal term for intentional destruction, alteration or concealment of evidence critical to a lawsuit. An organization's records must be reasonably protected from spoliation. The efforts to prevent spoliation of records must be closely tied to an organization's policies and procedures for record retention and destruction and for a litigation hold or preservation order.

Disaster Recovery: A plan for Disaster Recovery should be a part of any organization's record retention policy. This plan is composed of two parts: (1) Preservation of patients' medical records in the event of a disaster and (2) Return of the organizations normal flow of functions as quickly as possible with as little disruption as possible. Back-up processes are critical to an organization's resumption of operations after a disaster. However, old back-up tapes are also considered a legal liability. Consideration of the destruction of these back-up tapes should also be a part of the retention policy of an organization. (Christie, 2009).

IMPLEMENTATION OF A POLICY TO ADDRESS THE NEW E-DISCOVERY RULES

Establishing policies and procedures prior to lawsuits allows organizations to respond to e-discovery challenges in an appropriate and cost-effective manner. Before responding to any challenge, Health Information Management professionals must discuss and understand the retention and preservation policies of electronic records with inside and outside counsel. Senior management should be informed of, and involved in, the organizational development of e-discovery policies and procedures. Once the policies and procedures have been developed, they must be communicated to all the appropriate personnel within the organization as well as the outsiders who conduct business with the organization or have access to the organization's business records.

Continuous monitoring of compliance with the policies and procedures is crucial to ensure a systematic approach to electronic records management that is in accordance with the state and federal requirements. (Rebelo, 2007)

The Sedona Guidelines

- An organization should have reasonable policies and procedures for managing its information and records.
- An organization's information and records management policies and procedures should be realistic, practical, and tailored to the circumstances of the organization.
- An organization need not retain all electronic information ever generated or received.
- An organization adopting an information and records management policy should also develop procedures that address the creation, identification, retention, retrieval, and ultimate disposition or destruction of information and records.
- An organization's policies and procedures must mandate the suspension of ordinary destruction practices and procedures as necessary to comply with preservation obligations related to actual or reasonably anticipated litigation, government investigation, or audit. (Baldwin-Stried, 2006)

OVERVIEW OF THE NEW ELECTRONIC DISCOVERY RULES

The various discovery rules govern the process by which two parties to a lawsuit exchange information between them. Amendments to the rules were approved on April 13, 2006 and the new rules went into effect on December 1, 2006. ([Shorter, 2008) and (Cornell University Law School, 2009).

In order to cope with this growth in electronic communication, message management techniques and archiving systems are being adopted by many organizations. Well-defined processes for preserving and retrieving email messages are the essential parts of a message management system. Most organizations do not have proper storage systems. It is also a must that most organizations need to comply with the requirements of the Health Information Portability and Accountability Act, but they do not.

To overcome the challenges posed by privacy and security issues and the changing requirements in the rules made by regulatory bodies, organizations often follow either the "save everything" or "save nothing", which still is not adequate. It has also been mistakenly believed that backup and disaster recovery policies are sufficient for organizations. Locating the required information on backup tapes is difficult. A proper message archive that is indexed, available and searchable only meets the real needs of organizations.

BEST PRACTICES FOR MESSAGE MANAGEMENT

An established policy is required for retaining, retrieving and destroying email and other electronically stored information. This forms the starting point of implementing a message management system. The management program should also cover the important aspects of retention and recovery capability of instant messages and shared documents.

An email management system should provide secure access for corporate email and web-based program that allows access for auditors and other authorized users. An effective mail management system should also minimize the risk of leakage of confidential personal health information of patients, and help providers defend against internal litigation or human resources complaints. A complete message management and archiving system reduce storage requirements.

Table 1. An overview of the FRCP

Rule	Description	Impact
Rule 16	This describes the litigation and the discovery process the attorneys follow even before the case begins. It creates a framework for the parties and the court. It includes the provisions for electronic discovery.	HIM and IT professionals must work with the healthcare organization's attorney to discuss the need of electronic information available and provide additional security to sensitive data prior to trials.
Rule 26 (a)(1)(B)	This rule makes the "electronically stored information" explicitly subject to discovery The term "electronically stored information" is meant to denote the information created, manipulated, communicated, stored and best utilized in digital form requiring the use of hardware and software The term encompasses a wide range of data including metadata	HIM and IT professionals must work with counsel to identify what all information pertaining to an organization is "electronically stored information". These professionals must be aware that electronic data is exponentially greater in volume.
Rule 26(b) (1)	This rule describes the parties' legal duty to maintain and disclose records to claim or defense of any of the parties	HIM professionals must work with legal counsel to get to know what documents have been requested and whether they are relevant to claim or defense
Rule 26(b) (2) (B)	Addresses the issues raised by difficulties in locating, retrieving and providing discovery of some ESI Grants the judge authority to request production on information even if good case has been shown	HIM and IT professionals must be able to explain why certain information is not reasonably accessible
Rule 26(b) (5) (B)	This rule establishes a procedure for parties that the information that has been involuntarily produced is protected by the attorney-client privilege or work-product doctrine	HIM and IT professionals must work with legal counsel to ensure that such an information is not disclosed. Avoid inadvertent loss of such privileges
Rule 33(d)	This rule allows a party to respond to an interrogatory by producing the ESI that contains the answer the interrogatory is requesting only if the response would incur the same burden for both the parties	HIM and IT professionals must be able to verify the authenticity of that retrieved ESI and thy must ensure that that ESI can be located and identified by the interrogatory party and can give a reasonable opportunity for the interrogatory to examine, audit or inspect
Rule 34	This rules provides that electronically stored information is as discoverable as paper documents Specifically applies to the documents that are stored by healthcare organizations in the usual course of the business	HIM and IT must establish policies and procedures for the retention, storage, destruction and production of data (to ensure that the produced documents were kept in the usual course of the business)
Rule 37(f)	This rule describes what sanctions will be imposed for failing to provide the agreed upon documents Provides a safe harbor for information that has been lost because of a routine good-faith operation. Courts will not hesitate to impose sanctions for violation of e-discovery rules Safe harbor: good-faith Party believes that the information is reasonable re-discoverable Party is subjected to an obligation to preserve the information Party's intervention to modify or suspend certain features Party may not exploit the opportunity Litigation hold: Suspend an organization's normal practice Create a duty to preserve	HIM and IT professionals must work with the legal counsel of the organization to understand what the organization's discovery obligations are and how they are met HIM and IT professionals must understand how its electronic information storage system operates and they must be able to describe the routine losses of information

Figure 1. Designing and implementing a message management and archiving program

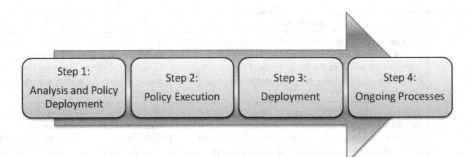

A well-designed message management system provides hierarchical storage management. As instant messages and shared documents become more prevalent, a comprehensive message management system is required to include intelligent archiving these types of data.

In addition to all these capabilities, tools to simplify e-discovery requirements must also be incorporated into the message management and archiving systems. These tools must also be able to initiate a litigation hold program. An effective litigation hold program should show that a healthcare provider is making a good faith effort to comply with the e-discovery issues.

Steps for Developing and Implementing a Message Management and E-Discovery Program

The first step in this is to identify the threats of not having a proper message management system. Without a proper management program, an organization faces increased financial risks and greater susceptibility to public penetration.

- Document Retention and Policy Deployment for the development of a system
  Step 2:
    a. Email, Instant Message and Collaborative Document Archiving

    b. File Archiving

    c. Database Archiving

Step 3:

    a. Message Management and File Archive

    b. Structured Data

Document Retention, Employee Training and Auditing

Message Management System Attributes

1. **Automatic, secure and scalable message management:** a high-quality archiving solution with intelligent filtering, retention and review policies should be implemented

2. **Efficient archiving:** hierarchical storage management technology should be adopted.

3. **Improved content control:** providers are restricted from releasing personal health information. A robust message management system also allows the IT administrators to frame policies to clock archive access for some users. A completely integrated message management system can protect a provider against inbound and outbound security threats from messages.

4. **Elimination of personal storage and incorporation of legacy data:** a high-quality email management program converts personal message stores to indexed files. This

Figure 2. The e-discovery process

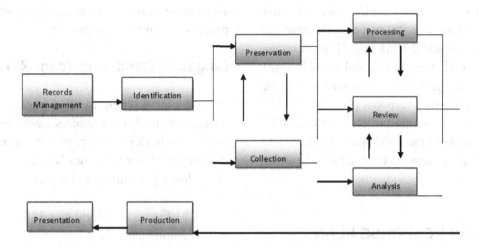

program would also convert legacy data into usable indexed files.

5. **Message recovery in native formats:** electronic communications is presented in the native format of the original message. The same is true for instant messaging and document-sharing applications.

An Approach to E-Discovery

E-discovery is a complicated process that often involves multiple internal and external stakeholders. These parties to the e-discovery process typically require access to these archives. An archiving solution must be able to support automated data transfer with chain-of-custody tracking from the archive. This is a reactive and proactive approach to e-discovery. (Kazeon, 2008)

CAPABILITY TO ENFORCE A LITIGATION HOLD

When an organization receives a discovery order, it will immediately initiate and enforce a hold on all of its electronic documents. The normal policy of the organization regarding the destruction of records must be suspended until notice. The

e-discovery program must be capable of accommodating multiple holds at the same time.

Message Management and E-Discovery Program Benefits

Ample amounts of money can be saved by the organization in three basic areas: archival storage, administration and response to discovery or regulatory inquiries. The management system can significantly alleviate the demand for storage. Administrative costs also decline because a high-quality email management system reduces the need for new servers. Finally, a comprehensive message management system that includes an e-discovery component makes retrieving of documents simple in response to an e-discovery request. (Symantec, 2007)

Litigation Response Planning and Policies for E-Discovery

The legal discovery process in healthcare is taking a radical turn with the enactment of changes and recent additions to the Federal Rules of Civil Procedure (FRCP). These rules vary from state to state, district to district depending on the court jurisdiction.

In order to comply with these rules, Heath care organizations must develop a well-defined structure and process to successfully manage e-discovery requests. HIM and IT professionals should work with inside and outside legal counsel to manage electronic discovery process, implement a litigation response plan and develop or update organizational policies. HIM and IT professionals should seek the opinion of the organization's legal counsel in the final development of the policies.

LITIGATION RESPONSE PLAN

Conduct an Evaluation of Applicable Rules

The organization's legal counsel plays a crucial role in e-discovery preparation. It should educate all the governing body members, HIM and IT professionals within the organization about the process. Within the organization the actual process followed for the discovery of electronic documents will depend on the court's jurisdiction, and the type and complexity of the case to be litigated.

Identify a Litigation Response Team

Fundamental to the management and administration of an e-discovery process, is the group of interdisciplinary professionals who are on the organization's litigation response team.

This team should conduct an assessment of the organization's current policies and procedures that are applicable to the organization and jurisdiction. It should then implement new policies and procedures necessary to successfully manage the e-discovery process. It should also govern the identification, preservation, search, retrieval and production of responsive electronic and other information pertaining to pending and current litigation.

The team should also govern the ongoing review, monitoring and evaluation of e-discovery process within the organization.

Litigation Response Team Roles

This team should comprise of representatives from the legal counsel or risk management, HIM and IT professionals. Depending on the type, structure and complexity, the organization's team will contain the following members and more:

*   Chief medical information officer
*   Compliance officer
*   Executive management (chief operating officer, chief information officer)
*   Executive nursing management (vice president of nursing)
*   Financial officer
*   Other designated department or business process manager

The governing board must take the ultimate responsibility to look after the organization's e-discovery management process. It should also approve the plan for e-discovery.

The CEO or the other designee should work in close collaboration with the legal counsel or risk management team. That status of the e-discovery litigation should be reported to the governing board on a regular basis.

The legal counsel and risk management may operate as a single department depending on the size and the structure of the organization. Legal counsel plays an important role in overseeing the e-discovery process while working collaboratively with the IT and HIM personnel.

The IT department provides the needed technical support for the organization. The IT department will be a valuable resource for the legal counsel.

The HIM department would provide the authoritative and technical knowledge about the management of health information within the organization. The HIM department has been traditionally considered as the custodian of the patient's medical records. The HIM personnel should work closely with the IT professionals and be involved in the organization's information management plan.

The organization is also required to define the role of the medical staff on an e-discovery team and the response to e-discovery requests. Many healthcare organizations designate one of its medical staff with extensive clinical background as the chief medical information officer. Depending on the size and structure of the organization, a compliance officer may or may not be designated.

Analyzing Issues, Risks and Tasks

Before developing organizational policies and procedures, the litigation response team must analyze the issues, risks and challenges resulting from e-discovery. In addition, the gaps in the organization must be identified. Here the team must take into consideration issues like ESI (electronically stored information), where it is located and what will be the policies and procedures the organization will follow to identify and disclose relevant ESI. One of the greatest costs associated with the e-discovery process is the potential waiver of privilege for ESI that could result in inadvertent costs. Thus, the team has to take into consideration the organization's policies and procedures with regard to the screening for access privileges.

Meet and Confer Sessions

A special master, judge or magistrate will oversee the litigation between two parties. Prior to the trial, the parties will meet and confer with the judge or any other special master. One or more such confer sessions must be conducted.

Some of the issues that have to be taken into consideration:

- How an organization would search, index, classify to produce all potentially responsive information for an e-discovery request
- How an organization will determine its true cost to carry out the above mentioned activities
- The benefits that an organization would get by implementing an enterprise content and records management system
- The organizational description of a good-faith operation
- Identification of all the record custodians
- Is the legal counsel having current copies of the organization's information management plan and information technology operating procedures

Four Levels of Custodianship

Level 1: Primary or Direct Custodians

People who work with the data or information directly or have direct knowledge or involvement of the events of the case belong to this level

Level 2: Data Owners or Stewards

Individuals who have the responsibility to oversee the business processes and operations belong to this category.

Level 3: Business Associates and Third Parties

Contractors and other third parties; who serve a variety of functions involving the information of the parties to litigation but who do not have direct contact with the litigation.

Level 4: Official Record and System Custodians

The HIM department has always been designated as the overall custodian of the health information and the medical records of the organization.

In this regard, some of the issues that have to be taken into consideration are:

- How exactly does an organization define and designate the official custodians of business and health records
- Identification of the data owners, stewards and the respective records they manage
- Communication of the requirement for such identifications to the respective stake holders in the organization.

Preservation and Legal Holds

The organization has the legal duty to preserve all the information responsive to e-discovery requests in the face of threatened or impending litigation.

Some of the issues to be taken into consideration in this regard are:

- The organization's comprehensive retention and destruction schedule, to identify all enterprise and medical records as well as the owners
- The trigger to initiate a potential litigation hold
- The person within the organization responsible for the litigation hold
- Protection of all evidence in the event
- When, how and who will lift the hold

Accessibility of Information

The FRCP provides provisions for a two-tier approach to discovery: reasonably accessible information and not reasonably accessible information discovery.

ESI that can be easily located with the help of technology is considered "accessible" and if not, is considered as "not reasonably accessible".

Some issues to be taken into consideration in this regard are:

- Cost considerations for accessing "accessible information" versus "inaccessible information"
- Production of ESI from the Electronic Health Records system

Legacy Data Systems

The retrieval and retention of the ESI contained on legacy systems is subjected to warrants in certain cases. In the case of legacy systems, the issues to be taken into consideration are the organization's provisions to provide for the efficient and effective migration of legacy data, the need for legacy data and the mechanism of destruction of legacy data.

Back-Up Media

ESI are being constantly replicated by organizations wholesale on mirror image as a precautionary act to prevent loss of information. This poses serious problems to organizations. Here the issues that are to be taken into consideration are the policies and procedures that organizations must follow with regard to the disposition and processing of these back-ups and the retention and destruction schedules of all back-up tapes.

Develop an Organizational Policy and Procedure

The next step is updating the organization's policies and procedures related to e-discovery.

Preparation for a pretrial conference: This policy outlines the steps to be completed before the legal counsel attends a pretrial conference. The goal is to make an organization to be adequately prepared for the conference.

Preservation and legal holds for health records and information: This policy outlines the process for preservation of records and information.

Retention, storage and destruction of electronic health information and records: This policy establishes the time-periods and conditions for the retention, storage and destruction of the records and information.

Production and disclosure of electronic health information and records: This policy outlines the steps in the production and disclosure process.

Develop a System for Ongoing Monitoring and Evaluation

The response team's responsibilities also extend to the evaluation of the efficacy of the organization's policies and procedures after implementation of the new ones. This includes regular reviewing of staff, auditing and monitoring activities, including audits of business process areas as well as random audits of human resources. The litigation response team should work with the compliance office to establish triggers and monitors.

CONCLUSION

E-discovery is the process of accessing, using and preserving information, data and records created or maintained in electronic format. The electronic format prevents spoliation of information as it also contains Metadata of the information preserved in the records. Any information pertaining to a patient that is kept in the possession of a hospital or a healthcare provider whether on paper, or stored in electronic format, can be subject to disclosure in lawsuit.

In the event of a lawsuit, the aspects that are important to an organization are the people associated with information critical to an organization, the information to be produced by the organization in a lawsuit, the process of e-discovery and the steps to be taken in the organization.

The Federal Rules of Civil Procedure govern all legal proceedings for civil lawsuit in the US district courts. These are comprised of 11 different categories which define the Scope, Commencement of civil suits, Pleadings and Motions, Parties, Discovery, Trial, Judgment, Provisional and final remedies and special proceedings, District courts and clerks and the General provisions. The FRCP contains 86 rule sets in addition.

In any organization, e-mail is the primary means of communication and all exchange of important data and information take place through e-mail. Thus establishing a proper message management system in organizations is critical. The steps for establishing a proper message management and e-discovery program include analysis and deployment of an appropriate policy, execution of the policy, policy deployment and executing all the other ongoing processes. Among the many benefits, an organization has in implementing a proper system is that the system can help an organization save ample amounts of money.

The legal discovery process in healthcare is taking a radical turn with the enactment of changes and recent additions to the Federal Rules of Civil Procedure (FRCP). In order to comply with these rules, Heath care organizations must develop a well-defined structure and process to successfully manage e-discovery request.

The development of a well-planned litigation response system, a well-informed and reliable litigation response team, well-established organizational policies for e-discovery and a strong message management and e-discovery system are critical to an organization as seen in the above sections. These make an organization highly proactive and respond to e-discovery challenges better making it get a clear advantage at the time of lawsuit.

REFERENCES

Anonymous. (2008). *Kazeon eDiscovery solution*. Retrieved June 17, 2010, from http://www.zeh.com/pdf/kazeon_brochure.pdf

Baldwin-Stried, K. (2006). E-discovery and HIM: How amendments to the federal rules of civil procedure will affect HIM professionals. *Journal of American Health Information Management Association, 77*(9), 58–60.

Brouillard, C. P. (2008). *Emergency liability issues specific to healthcare technology.* Retrieved June 17, 2010, from http://www.slidefinder.net/B/Brouillard/13847638

Callahan, J. (2007). *What health care providers need to know about e-discovery. Central New York M.D.* News.

Christie, J. S. J. (2009). *Electronic discovery for healthcare providers.* Birmingham, AL: Bradley Arant Rose & White LLP.

Cornell University Law School. (2010). *Federal rules of civil procedure.* Retrieved June 17, 2010, from http://www.law.cornell.edu/rules/frcp/

Dimik, C. (2007). E-discovery: Preparing for the coming rise in electronic discovery requests. *Journal of American Health Information Management Association, 78*(5), 24–29.

Dirking, B., & Kodali, R. R. (2008). *Strategies for preparing for e-discovery.* Information Management Journal.

Miller, A. R., & Tucker, C. E. (2009). *Electronic discovery and electronic medical records: Does the threat of litigation affect firm decisions to adopt technology?* Retrieved June 17, 2010, from http://www.ftc.gov/be/seminardocs/090430amiller.pdf

Rebelo, M. J. (2007). *E-discovery in health care litigation.* Physician's News Digest.

Roberts, J. G. J. (2006). *Federal rules of civil procedure.* Retrieved June 17, 2010, from www.supremecourt.gov/orders/courtorders/frcv10.pdf

Symantec Corporation. (2007). *Managing electronicmessaging and E-discovery for healthcare providers.* Retrieved June 17, 2010, from http://eval.symantec.com/mktginfo/enterprise/white_papers/ent-whitepaper_managing_messaging_healthcare_11-2007.en-us.pdf

Thru-group. Managing sensitive records in health care: Industry solution profile.

Chapter 9
The Nationwide Health Information Network:
A Biometric Approach to Prevent Medical Identity Theft

Omotunde Adeyemo
TEKsystems, USA

ABSTRACT

The Nationwide Health Information Network (NHIN) promises many benefits, but may be prone to a new phenomenon in healthcare fraud now rapidly drawing attention and commonly referred to as medical identity theft. As the medical industry continues down the path towards overall infrastructure digitization, it is anticipated that associated electronic records will become more portable hence facilitating efficient exchange. Problem however is, the enhanced transferability may also open a new vista of advantages to fraudsters. To address this risk, the NHIN implementers must implement stringent access control measures. One such solution is using a biometric cryptosystem-based solution. For defense-in-depth, a security strategy suggesting successive layers of controls, the PKI cryptographic scheme is recommended to intrinsically protect medical records when in use, storage or even in the event they are successfully stolen.

INTRODUCTION

In 2004, former US president George Bush, signed an executive order to implement an interoperable

Health Information Technology (HIT) framework. The directive, expected to be fulfilled within ten years of the order, birthed the design and continued implementation of the Nationwide Health Information Network (NHIN) (Lafferty, 2007, p.15). NHIN, a "network of networks"

DOI: 10.4018/978-1-60960-174-4.ch009

(Rishel, Riehl and Blanton, 2007, p.7) is planned to interconnect major healthcare establishments designated as Electronic Health Records (EHR). There is however one impending problem with this initiative: it may present new opportunities to cyber criminals perpetrating medical identity theft. The medical industry has experienced a traumatic rise of cases in recent times, of this new trend in healthcare fraud. This chapter discusses the planned healthcare information highway, NHIN and the potential dangers medical identity theft poses to the project. A strong authentication mechanism that leverages cryptography and biometrics is prescribed for the problem.

Medical records are largely characterized by personal health information held at healthcare institutions. The act of stealing or the misuse of an individual's medical record in any manner including illicit submission for claims is a derivative of healthcare fraud (Lafferty, 2007) but now more commonly referred to as medical identity theft.

BACKGROUND

Healthcare fraud continues to be a huge expense for the United States (US) government. According to Hoffman and Podgurski (2007), it has been projected that total health expenditures in the United States (US) will rise to over $4 trillion by 2015, and fraud will account for about 10 percent of that expenditure (p. 12). The statistic accentuates the gravity of the problem and suggests an area government can turn for huge savings.

The problem is observed to be taking an upward trend and it appears economic gains is a leading motivator and attraction for perpetrators. Conn (2006), citing the executive director of the World Privacy Forum (WPF), Pam Dixon, claims medical data is currently being peddled at $50 a record in the black market. To the fraudster, it seems truer now than ever, healthcare is now "where the money is" (Conn, 2006, p.27; Lafferty, 2007, p. 12).

The returns promise to be huge and an enticing incentive for criminals to make larger gains perhaps even easier since more records can potentially be handled in electronic formats given the advent of newer technologies. It is now possible to store relatively larger amounts of data on increasingly smaller and cheaper devices which require very minimal technical expertise.

Central to the problem therefore is, as medical data become more accessible in electronic format across the NHIN, so will it become more portable. This ease of portability, according to Lafferty (2007), is on the one hand, for the good of the initiative, but on the other hand, a risk since it may potentially grant criminals similar ease of access to individuals' records. McGraw, Dempsey, Harris and Goldman (2009) share the same view. They expressed concerns about the privacy issues and potential implications of any single breach of electronically held medical records.

Medical identity theft, as is later shown always involves unauthorized or wrongful access to the victims' personal health records. Those accesses are made either at the point of initial record theft, to falsely obtain medical services, or later when updates are being made to the victim's records by unsuspecting medical officials. While specific laws targeting the crime as a separate issue than the classic financially-driven identity theft are still awaited, other measures must be taken to mitigate the problem. Strong security and privacy strategies with access control measures, rising to the severity of the risk, must be planned. A strong multifactor authentication method is later discussed in later sections as one such compensating control, to address the problem. It is further suggested that all electronic personal records on the NHIN must be encrypted at all times, whether at rest or in transit.

The Nationwide Health Information Network

According to the U.S. Department of Health & Human Services (HHS), in a News Release

(2005, November 10), HHS Secretary Mike Leavitt, claimed major advancements towards accomplishing a secure, portable health information for consumers have been made. According to the Secretary, contracts have been awarded to four Health-IT consortia to develop conceptual models of the proposed Nationwide Health Information Network. The secretary expressed hope that the contracts will bring together technology developers and stakeholders within the healthcare industry to develop a secure and interoperable state-of-the-art network. He argued the initiative will result in a healthcare system that will offer higher quality, lower costs, less hassle, and better care for US consumers. In his article, McDonald (2009) also agrees that sharing healthcare information in this manner will improve the quality of medical services and reduce costs.

According to HHS, the firms selected to lead the four consortia are, Accenture, Computer Science Corporation (CSC), International Business Machines (IBM), and Northrop Grumman. All four were charged with the same requirement; that each must develop a prototype for sharing information among hospitals, pharmacies, laboratories and physicians within three selected communities. The consortia will test their prototypes for secure patient identification and information location; as well as for authentication and access control. All four consortia are further required, according to the HHS secretary, to collaborate and ensure information can move seamlessly within and across all four network prototypes. This seamlessness in movement of health information opens new doors and vistas of opportunities to the US healthcare industry, as the NHIN concept comes to fruition and reality.

The Office of the National Coordinator (ONC) for Health IT (2008), in a synopsis of their four-year plan for the scheme, suggested that the full NHIN, a "network of networks" (Rishel, Riehl and Blanton, 2007, p.7), would eventually evolve, but only at a gradual pace. According to the report, as information increasingly move among EHRs and PHRs, (definitions in the next section) "individuals will connect with their clinicians, clinicians will connect with other care providers, and health-related communities will connect with each other" (p. 8).

The ONC asserts EHRs and PHRs will play a key role in the coming years to enable the expected transformation of healthcare services. The primary outcome anticipated with this change is incorporating requirements for "authorized access to … individual health information for patient care [and] consumer self-management of health" (Rishel, Riehl & Blanton, 2007, p. 9). With such sprawling national network infrastructure and plans to make consumers' personal health information (PHI) available across its length and breadth, proper attention must be paid to security and privacy concerns.

Definition and Description of Key Terms

The incursion of IT into healthcare, otherwise referred to as Health Information Technology (HIT), has led to the introduction of new terms that better define the new operating domain. For the most part, the basic roles of the various components are not changing, rather what has changed is the manner information management and services are being delivered. This has led to new definitions and terminologies. To help understand other sections within this chapter, some of the most salient components of the NHIN are defined in the following paragraphs.

Personal Health Record (PHR): The National Alliance for Health Information Technology (2008) defined PHR as an individual's electronic record of health-related information. According to Kahn, Aulakh and Bosworth (2009) medical records for individuals may originate from disparate sources including employers, health plans, family members, and other providers. The PHR places control and access to medical records into the hands of the individuals that own them.

Electronic Medical Records (EMR): The EMR holds electronic records of an individual's health-related information. Medical records will be created, collected, managed, and consulted by authorized clinicians and staff within one health care organization.

Electronic Health Record (EHR): This refers to "an electronic record of health-related information on an individual that conforms to nationally recognized interoperability standards and that can be created, managed, and consulted by authorized clinicians and staff across more than one health care organization" (National Alliance for Health Information Technology, 2008)

EMR vs. her: According to the National Alliance for Health Information Technology (NAHIT), the principal difference between an EMR and an EHR is the ability of an EHR to exchange information according to a predetermined standard. The expectation is, following widespread adoption of the standardized information exchange systems for interoperability, EMRs will become irrelevant. According to the National Alliance for Health Information Technology (2008), "EMRs and EHRs are tools for providers, while PHRs are the means to engage individuals in their health and well-being" (p. 14).

EHR vs. PHR: To be a PHR, access to the record must be managed and controlled by individuals. When control over medical record shifts to the individual, then from the individuals perspective, there is a shift in meaning from EHR to PHR. The health care provider operating the EHR system typically exposes a web-accessible portal. Individuals leverage these systems to manage their PHR. The source of control for the records is vital in determining whether a system is a PHR or remains within the meaning of an EHR. This suggests that as medical data arrive from disparate sources to a health institution for an individual, the records remain EHR-defined until the owning individual assumes control over the records. The PHR concept has been likened to the library system, with the intent that individu-

als will have control over who has access to the records, who can "check out" records, how much information to include, record maintenance, and ordering (National Alliance for Health Information Technology, 2008)

Health Information Exchange (HIE): These are systems designed to interconnect EHRs and PHRs. An HIE may also connect with other HIEs. Rishel et al (2007) suggested that HIEs would typically participate in the movement of data at the state and regional levels. The National Alliance for Health Information Technology (2008) defined HIE within the meaning of its application, as the electronic movement of health-related information among organizations. The term has been employed interchangeably both in the sense of its basic use for electronic data transmission, and as an infrastructure for data exchange.

Health Information Organization (HIO): The term describes organizations that oversee and govern the exchange of electronic health records amongst institutions. This is the basic and most generic description of these entities to represent institutions that facilitate the exchange of electronic medical data without regard to geography, community or a specific agenda. (National Alliance for Health Information Technology, 2008).

Regional Health Information Organization (RHIO): A health information organization that brings together health care stakeholders within a defined geographic area and governs health information exchange among them for the purpose of improving health and care in that community (McDonald, 2009; National Alliance for Health Information Technology, 2008; Thielst, 2007).

NHIN Architectural Components

Rishel, Riehl and Blanton (2007) presented a summary report of the NHIN prototype architectures submitted by the four consortia. The 4 organizations reported on the progress they had made so far. Rishel et al. analyzed the various approaches the four consortia adopted in developing their initial prototypes. The prototypes were demonstrated live at the "NHIN Prototype Architecture Project Third NHIN Stakeholder Forum on 25–26 January 2007" (p. 3).

According to Rishel, the intent is for the network to securely connect consumers, providers, and other persons wishing to use health information and services, without compromising confidentiality of records. Several of the critical components planned to provide connectivity at the local and national levels were discusses. Though the four consortia differed in their choice of certain definitions, the prototypes generically included EHRs and PHRs at the local levels.

EHRs and PHRs will be owned by hospitals or other healthcare practices. They will be interconnected by Health Information Exchanges (HIEs). An HIE will then connect with other HIEs. Rishel et al. however did not indicate how HIEs operating at the local levels differ from those at the regional levels, but McDonald (2009) offers some perspectives in this regard in his discussions about Regional Health Information Organizations (RHIOs). According to McDonald, "[RHIOs] focus on the care organizations in a region" (p. 447), hence they could be pictured at one geographical level higher than an HIE or HIO. HIEs opting to make the required investments may elect to be setup at the National level and designated as a NHIN Health Information Exchanges (NHIE) (Rishel et al, 2007, p. 31). NHIEs will ultimately implement the NHIN architecture at the highest level to include all network services, standards, requirements, process, and procedures. A NHIE will connect to HIEs and other NHIEs to form the full NHIN infrastructure. As shown in Figure 1, a NHIE could also choose to provide all the operational services a regular HIE would, in addition to fulfilling the requirements at the national level.

Figure 2, illustrates how NHIEs will interconnect using the Internet as the backbone to implement the network of networks.

Typical User Path through NHIN

To connect with, and traverse the NHIN, consumers will rely on their designated PHR; a local EHR holding their personal medical records. The PHR may connect to an HIE which in turn provides the needed access to NHIN (Rishel, Riehl and Blanton, 2007, p. 9). There may be a need for an HIE to connect to another NHIE if the HIE is not one so designated, in order to deliver a national service. Customers who do not have access to a PHR may still have the option of connecting directly to an HIE through their web portal.

Customers' medical records will primarily sit within the PHR. Since the NHIN scheme is not designed to host data or any centralized systems at the national level, (Rishel et al., 2007), PHRs will therefore play an important role safekeeping medical records. Senior Management of those operations must therefore understand the security ramifications and significance of their facilities within the overall scheme.

Medical Identity Theft

Medical identity theft is a subset of both healthcare fraud and identity theft (Lafferty, 2007, p.12). According to Lafferty, the phenomenon is characterized by a combination of medical privacy violations, identity theft, and healthcare fraud. In terms of healthcare fraud, the major issue is the "intentional submission of false claims" by criminals (Lafferty, 2007, p. 13). Though the crime is similar to the classical financial identity theft, in that for both, the victim's identity is compromised, and both may result in financial impacts, there are still several distinctions between the two. Medical identity theft goes beyond classical identity theft (Tomes, 2009) in that wrong medical treatments may be administered due to inaccurate information entered into the victim's records. The crime is therefore one that introduces threat to victims' lives.

Figure 1. Components of NHIN (as illustrated by Rishel et al. (2007))

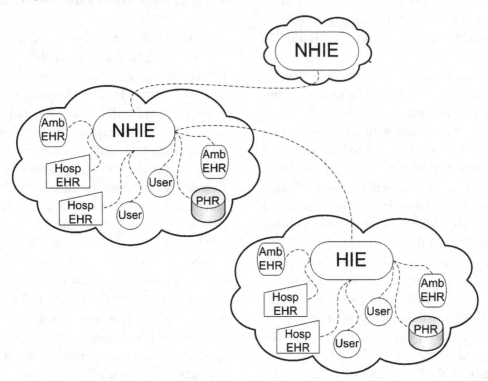

Figure 2. HIEs and NHIEs Implementing the Network of Networks

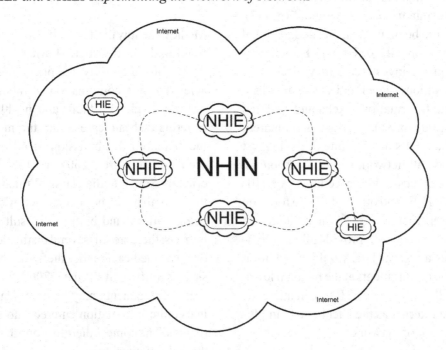

Medical identity theft may be plotted in various ways. One common example is when perpetrators use their victims' information to obtain treatment resulting in wrong entries and updates made to the victims' records (Lafferty, 2007, p.13). A second category according to Lafferty is the falsification of patients' records by medical practitioners either for cover-up or for financial gains. Another class may be categorized as organized crime; to pull this off, perpetrators lure Medicare patients into clinics staffed with either legitimate or illegitimate physicians. The perpetrators make illegal money by billing the government while the patients are oblivious of the crime. A fourth kind of the crime is when insiders of a healthcare organization, for example an EHR, literarily steal customers' heath records from their companies' systems. They then offer the records for sale in the black-market. With health data now being sold for about $50 per record (Lafferty, 2007, p.17) profits from the crime can quickly add-up to large sums considering the volume of records that can be stolen in electronic formats.

Hoffman and Podgurski (2007) also discussed other categories of the theft related to privacy; including blackmail, where a criminal could potentially demand money from individuals, such as politicians, whose public images could be damaged when their personal health histories are disclosed. Other privacy related examples include discriminations when making applications with various organizations for health insurance, mortgages, employments, or college admissions. Victims of the crime may be disqualified from gaining employment opportunities due to poor health conditions reported in their records as a result of the crime (Tomes, 2009).

According to Tomes (2009), physicians may also be at risks of lawsuits when perpetrators of the crime make wrongful updates to medical records in a manner that incriminates them. Such lawsuits may have far-reaching implications on doctors if the case is lost. Consequences may involve huge fines and impacts on their professional practices.

In all the categories of the crime discussed above, one common observation is, in each case, access to the victim's medical records is required. The records are accessed either at the point of theft, or when the victim's information is presented by the impostor for services at a hospital, or when the victim's record is falsely updated. Another point of access is when claim submissions are made under the victim's identity, for example, to Medicaid or Medicare. This finding suggests, access to data is an important, if not the most significant factor for the scheme to succeed.

It therefore makes sense to give individuals ultimate control over who accesses their medical information. Granting control to customers may also protect healthcare organizations and medical practitioners by providing a means of retaining undeniable proof of access authorization, an access control factor known as non-repudiation. One proven solution offering these functionalities and many more is the Public Key Infrastructure (PKI) cryptographic scheme.

The Risks of Digitization and Portability

It is believed that as the NHIN continues to work its way through national adoption, one adverse spin-off to its anticipated boost to medical data portability, will be a commensurate amplification in the occurrence of theft (Lafferty, 2007). The network will also boost exchangeability of records which criminals can further leverage to illegally steal records nationwide. It is imperative that proportionate levels of safeguards, robust enough to address these risks, be explored.

As reported by Rishel et al. (2007), stewards of the NHIN effort identified several security requirements including the following:

- **Data integrity checking:** To prevent unauthorized changes to data and to ensure data is free of errors prior to processing.

- **Non-repudiation:** To prevent the sender of a message from denying that it was the source of the message. Also prevents the receiver from denying receiving the message.
- **Secure transport:** To ensure secure data transmission and delivery between systems.
- **Authorization:** Granting rights and accesses based on permissions. Authorization is dependent on good identity and authentication controls.
- **Authentication:** Authentication of users prior to NHIN access. Acceptable authentication strengths are still being determined.

Access control is a critical pedestal for authentication and identification. And since it could be the most significant concern in the battle against medical identity theft, a case is being made that strong authentication be considered for the proposed digital facilities. *Strong Authentication* is a stringent access control method typically based on multifactor authentication techniques. To guarantee data is intrinsically protected even when stolen, it is further recommended that medical records be encrypted at all instances of storage, exchange, or use. This strategy is referred to, in security parlance, as defense-in-depth. Later in this chapter, a cryptosystem-based, biometric access control model is discussed as one solution offering such level of control.

Healthcare Legislations

To address security related consumer risks arising from healthcare digitization, the government moved to legislate the Health Insurance Portability and Accountability Act of 1996 (HIPAA). HIPAA was passed as a federal law to protect the privacy and security of consumers' electronic protected health information (EPHI) (Hoffman and Podgurski, 2007, p. 6). According to Hoffman and Podgurski, the Security Rule of HIPAA is contained within an associated Privacy Rule, provided by the legislation. The security rule is enforced by the Centers for Medicare & Medicaid Services (CMS), an agency within HHS. The security rule, pursuant to HIPAA, was signed into law on April 20, 2005. The enhancements within the rule mandated new administrative, physical, and technical measures for safeguarding consumers' medical records.

Under HIPAA, Covered Entities, that is, health care clearing houses, health plans, and health care providers, who transmit EPHI as part of their business are mandated to protect the confidentiality, integrity, and availability of consumer data. Covered organizations are mandated to employ "reasonable and appropriate" levels of safeguards to control access to EPHI. The safeguards are categorized into two areas namely; "required" and "addressable". While the required specifications are mandatory, the addressable specifications can be handled using discretionary approaches. Some examples of required safeguards organizations must implement include having a disaster recovery plan and having an emergency-mode operations plan. While password management and log-in monitoring are examples of addressable specifications of the law.

Some experts have however found gaps with HIPAA. For example, in its definition of the term "covered entities", McGraw, Dempsey, Harris and Goldman (2009) and Hoffman and Podgurski (2007) observed the law may exempt many EHRs, PHRs, HIEs, and other NHIN components from its requirements. This is a huge gap that places responsibilities on security and privacy practitioners within Healthcare related institutions, especially those within the definition and meaning of the terms EHRs and PHRs, to demonstrate due diligence in their practices, regardless of their coverage status under HIPAA.

Current government efforts are however underway to address several of HIPAA's weaknesses. In February 2009, as part of the American Recovery and Reinvestment Act (ARRA), more commonly known as the stimulus package of the Obama Administration, the Health Information Technology for Economic and Clinical Health (HITECH) Act was signed into law (Waldren Kibbe & Mitchell, 2009; Anonymous, 2009). HITECH is expected to make changes to HIPAA's security and privacy rules (Anonymous, 2009). Aimed primarily at encouraging the adoption of HIT and the proliferation of EHRs, the law is expected to mandate operators to report disclosures of unprotected data. With HITECH, fines for data breaches have been reviewed from the current $100 per violation under current HIPAA provisions, to new fines as high as $1.5M "per calendar year for all violations of an identical requirement or prohibition" (Waldren Kibbe & Mitchell, 2009, p. 23). The new law is expected to go into effect for current EHRs, January 1, 2014.

While it is still early to determine the overall effectiveness of HITECH and how well it improves on the gaps and weaknesses presented by HIPAA, one immediate observation is its inclusion of any medical operation, adopting the national HIT initiative, and operating as an EHR. This development addresses the gap in HIPAA's definition of covered entities, which limits its coverage to include only specific healthcare institutions.

SOLUTIONS AND RECOMMENDATIONS

This section prescribes a solution to the issues discussed in this chapter. The approach involves a combination of biometrics and the public key infrastructure (PKI) encryption techniques.

The Public Key Infrastructure

The public key infrastructure allows the use of public networks such as the Internet to securely exchange sensitive data. The technique leverages a public/private cryptographic key pair (SearchSecurity, n.d.) to protect data storage and

exchange. For classic implementations, keys are obtained and shared through a trusted certificate authority (CA). The CA issues and validates all digital certificates for participating entities within a scheme. The PKI is also commonly referred to as asymmetric cryptography and is opposed to symmetric cryptography that utilizes a single key approach in its implementation. With PKI, the key pair is created simultaneously from the same algorithm (SearchSecurity, n.d.). The private key is kept secret by the owner, while the public key is made available to the public. The private key is used to decrypt data initially encrypted using the corresponding public key. PKI offers personal and institutional authentication, identification, confidentiality, and non-repudiation

PKI and Access Control

Encryption of data over the Internet in not a new concept, what this chapter however proposes is a solution to leverage a combination of biometric and PKI techniques. The uniqueness of the solution is the inclusion of an individual's biometric data in the cryptographic key algorithm.

Biometric Authentication Based on CryptoKeys Containing Biometric Signatures

Biometrics is the use of human characteristics for authentication and identification in an access control system. Kay (2005) defined biometric authentication as the "verification of user's identity by means of a physical trait or behavioral characteristics that can't easily be changed" (p. 26). According to Bhargav-Spantzel, Squicciarini, Modi, Young, Bertino, and Elliot (2007), the technique adds a new paradigm to user authentication by using the characteristics of the subject itself. Biometric authentication grants automated access by using one of the following characteristics; fingerprint verification, iris recognition, retina analysis, face recognition, hand outlines patterns, ear shape recognition, detection of body odor, voice verification, patterns of DNA, and sweat pores (Zorkadis and Donos, 2004, p. 128).

Biometric authentication technologies are characterized by their use of the multifactor authentication concept that verifies *who you are*; physiological characteristics, or *what you do*; behavioral patterns. This is contrasted to the concepts of *what you know*; as is the case in systems relying on the subject's "knowledge of a password or other secrets ... and/or *what you [have]* (such as ... an ID card)" (Zorkadis and Donos, 2004, p. 125). The biometric solution proposed here suggests a multifactor approach that employs the use cryptographic keys

Biometric authentication solutions are not without problems. Zorkadis and Donos (2004) for example noted that the technology is vulnerable to replay attacks because biometric characteristics are not really secret information, arguing "we leave our fingerprints everywhere" (p. 130). and many of our other physiological characteristics can be forged. This is one reason the approach proposed here is based on a multifactor scheme that does not only rely on the - *who you are* factor.

Privacy concerns with biometrics have their roots in the need to collect and store data in order to implement the solution. Since the information being collected is essentially personal data, the risks of violating users' privacies is evident. One way to address the issue, and remain compliant with privacy laws, is to adopt a biometric system that processes "anonymized data" (Zorkadis and Donos, 2004, p, 130). In such application, the biometric data rather than being collected and held on a central server remains with the subject, stored on a handy device such as a smartcard. If such is adopted at a PHR, in addition to the elimination of privacy concerns, those facilities will also be freed of the extra burden of managing a central server.

Yet, biometrics has several benefits. Some of its advantages according to Tillmann (2007), include:

- Strong authentication and identification through multifactor techniques.
- Significant cost savings compared to the high costs of password management systems.
- Mitigates the risks associated with lost passwords, PINs or badges.
- Can be used to proof compliance with HIPAA for covered organizations.
- Helps preserve privacy and protect against identity theft.
- Biometric characteristics are permanent.
- Biometric characteristics are not transferable.
- Biometric characteristics cannot be lost or forgotten.

The advantages of biometric technology, listed above, can bring lots of value to the NHIN scheme if adopted.

According to Itakura and Tsuji (2005), there already is today, a solution developed to control "biometric personal identification by unlocking digital signatures or cryptographic communications using a corresponding secret key" (p. 290). Those solutions also utilize the conventional personal authentication controls typically designed into biometric technologies for the initial phase of an authentication request. Once the initial check on the biological information is successful, the system then activates the secret crypto-key, stored on a smartcard for example. The key would later be used to make calculations for the cryptographic signature.

Itakura and Tsuji's (2005) proposal builds upon the approach just described. They proposed a multifactor authentication method that utilizes two kinds of data; (1) the biometric information of the subject and (2) cryptographic data which is also derived from the subject's biometric information for its creation. The distinguishing factor in their model is the fact that it uses the biological information of a person in creating the secret and public keys. For the former approach, the biological information authentication module is separate from the cryptographic module, and a signal is only sent to the cryptographic module when the biometric authentication is successful. There is no other relationship between the two modules. With Itakura and Tsuji's approach however, the biometric information that is being verified through the authentication process is the same information used in generating the asymmetric keys in the cryptographic module. One benefit of embedding the user's biometric information in the cryptographic keys is "zero knowledge", meaning no biometric information is provided for inspection (p. 291).

The value that Itakura and Tsuji's (2005) approach offers, and the reason their work was selected and recommended for use with the NHIN access control model are as follows:

- The ability to use anonymized data by placing a person's biological information on a smartcard rather than on a central database server. This approach complies with the principles of "purpose and proportionality" (Zorkadis and Donos, 2004, p. 130), thus addressing some of the privacy concerns associated with biometrics today.

- In addition, leaving biological information on users' access cards eliminates the potential database management issues that may arise where the solution is adopted on a large scale effort such as the NHIN. As the number of customers on the network continue to grow, so will the size of the database storing their biological information. This would have otherwise necessitated the use of huge facilities for processing (Itakura and Tsuji, 2005, p. 291). The server may also potentially grow so large and become unmanageable. The approach to leave the information on a smartcard prevents this scenario.

- Support for strong multifactor authentication access control, that utilizes aspects

of: *what you are* (biometric information), what you have (smartcard), and what you know (PIN).

- For even stronger security, the model utilizes cryptographic systems, leveraging keys that contain the user's biometric information. This protects the authentication system even when biological information is stolen.

A Biometric Cryptosystem Authentication Solution for NHIN

As suggested throughout this chapter, the implementation of NHIN is expected to introduce significant level of privacy related risks to consumers. At the heart of this problem, are the opportunities digitization of healthcare records may present to medical identity thieves, as a result of easier portability and ubiquity of records. It was also earlier established that one critical requirement for the success of medical identity theft is access to medical records. Therefore, the need to implement stringent access control measures around consumer electronic medical data cannot be overemphasized. The solution must also be robust enough to continue providing confidentiality and records integrity even in the event of successful data breaches and theft. There should be an avenue for persistent assurance, preventing an assailant from using a victim's stolen information either to illegitimately obtain medical services or make false claims. The solution should also mitigate the risk of introducing wrongful updates to victims' medical records; a hazardous event that may present life threatening circumstances to the affected persons. It was also argued that the avenue provided by law, to protect citizen's electronic medical records, that is HIPAA, is defective. The following recommendations are suggested as an effective approach towards the protection of consumers on the proposed NHIN:

- A cryptosystem based multifactor biometric solution should be adopted such as that proposed by Itakura and Tsuji's (2005) as the base authentication model.
- The proposed multifactor approach should utilize finger print scanning for biometric authentication, for the *who you are* factor; a smartcard for *what you have;* and the smartcard PIN for *what you know*. The finger print option was proposed because it is one of the most common and cost effective biometric techniques. There might be a need to accommodate pre-registered authorized representatives as backup authorizers or co-authorizers, for each consumer, for times he or she is unable to complete the access control process due to poor health conditions. In this case, the finger print approach provides the additional advantage for patient identification. The patient's fingerprint can simply be taken to complete the authentication process, while authorization can be provided by the pre-registered representative.
- The PKI scheme should be adopted for encrypting medical records.
- Users' electronic protected health information (EPHI) must be encrypted at all times, either in storage or when transmitted.
- Medical records must be encrypted using the customers' public keys and decrypted using their associated private keys.
- Itakura and Tsuji's (2005) approach should be enhanced to utilize the same keys used for the authentication mechanism in the PKI scheme for encrypting medical records. Once the authentication phase is successful, the user's key pair should be activated and further employed to decrypt the data.

These proposal fulfills all the identified security requirements presented earlier in the paper, including, Authentication, Data Integrity, Non-repudiation and Secure Transport of records.

Typical Application of the Proposed Model

For the protection model proposed, a biometric solution will be deployed at each organization designated as an EHR or PHR since medical records will primarily reside there. The fingerprint scanner is about the most widely used biometric technique and perhaps one with highest user acceptance. The finger print scanner may therefore be the most ideal for this solution.

With this proposal, hospitals, pharmacies, and other Healthcare organizations designated as PHRs, would have scanners on site to serve patients and other categories of walk-in consumers. The greatest benefits of the model will be realized when the PHRs enable the same level of access control for remote use through the heath provider's web portal. In that case, consumers will have the option of procuring portable finger print scanners, for home computer usage. See Figure 3 for an illustration of this application.

Apart from the strong access control offering of this approach, its enhanced accessibility, flexibility, and convenience affords consumers the opportunity to readily authorize access to their records from almost anywhere across the globe over the Internet. Fingerprint scanners are relatively cheap and most are handy enough for easy transportation. Many fingerprint scanners also come with technologies that allow them to be readily attached and automatically installed on almost any modern personal computer.

The accessibility feature will also come handy in cases where a consumer is incapacitated. In such situations, that individual may need to rely on a relative, or other pre-registered persons, approved for emergency situations, to fulfill the access authorization requirements. With the biometric solution, the authorization may be jointly completed by taking the fingerprint of the patient,

Figure 3. Typical application of the biometric access control model used from home and onsite.

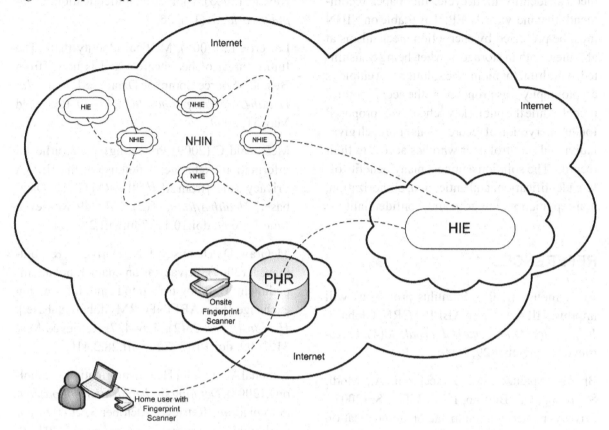

while the authorized person supplies other access information, such as the smartcard PIN. The approved representative can thus be at a remote location to complete the authorization.

The model requires the retention of a Certificate Authority (CA) to manage trusts throughout the network. The CA could be one designated solely to the NHIN scheme or could be any of the reputed organizations serving the larger internet population.

FUTURE RESEARCH DIRECTIONS

Future work can further investigate the implementation of the PKI scheme for the NHIN infrastructure. An inquiry into the integration of certificate

authorities is key to successfully implement the PKI solution discussed.

CONCLUSION

The medical identity theft is a real threat to the healthcare industry. But the risks it presents are about to be amplified as the nation launches the much anticipated healthcare super-highway; the Nationwide Health Information Network. Medical records will be transformed to electronic format as they become ported onto the network. Once in electronic format, the records become much more portable, this offers many benefits to the project, but so does it provide opportunities to perpetrators of healthcare fraud. Since access to medical records is always a required step to complete the medical identity theft cycle, this paper recommends that individuals' EPHI available on NIHN must be protected by encryption mechanisms at all times, both in storage or when being transmitted. A multifactor biometric solution that employs cryptography was proposed as the access control model, while the public key scheme was proposed for the encryption of records. This approach gives individuals control over who has access to their records. The solution amongst many benefits offers identification, authentication, authorization, non-repudiation, integrity and, confidentiality.

REFERENCES

Anonymous,. (2009). Stimulus provisions will improve HIPAA. [from ABI/INFORM Global.]. *Information Management Journal*, *43*(4), 6. Retrieved September 29, 2009.

Bhargav-Spantzel, A., Squicciarini, A., Modi, S., Young, M., Bertino, E., & Elliot, S. (2007). Privacy preserving multi-factor authentication with biometric. *Journal of the Computer Security*, *15*(5), 529–560.

Conn, J. (2006). A real steal. [from ABI/INFORM Global database.]. *Modern Healthcare*, *36*(40), 26–28. Retrieved May 31, 2009.

Hoffman, S. & Podgurski, A. (2007). Securing the HIPPA security rule. *Journal of Internet Law* *10*(8), 1, 6-15.

Itakura, Y., & Tsujii, S. (2005). Proposal on a multifactor biometric authentication method based on cryptosystem keys containing biometric signatures. *International Journal of Information Security*, *4*(4), 288–296. doi:10.1007/s10207-004-0065-5

Kahn, J., Aulakh, V., & Bosworth, A. (2009). What it takes: Characteristics of the ideal personal health record. *Health Affairs*, *28*(2), 369–376. doi:10.1377/hlthaff.28.2.369

Kay, R. (2005). Biometric authentication. *Computerworld*, *39*(14), 26.

Lafferty, L. (2007). Medical identity theft: The future threat of healthcare fraud is now. [from Business Source Complete Database.]. *Journal of Health Care Compliance*, *9*(1), 11–20. Retrieved May 31, 2009.

McDonald, C. (2009). Protecting patients in health information exchange: A defense of the HIPAA Privacy Rule. [from ABI/INFORM Global Database.]. *Health Affairs*, *28*(2), 447–449. Retrieved June 1, 2009. doi:10.1377/hlthaff.28.2.447

McGraw, D., Dempsey, J. X., Harris, L., & Goldman, J. (2009). Privacy as an enabler, not an impediment: Building trust into health information exchange. [from ABI/INFORM Global database.]. *Health Affairs*, *28*(2), 416–427. Retrieved May 31, 2009. doi:10.1377/hlthaff.28.2.416

National Alliance for Health Information Technology. (2008). *Defining key health information technology terms.* Retrieved October 3, 2009 http://healthit.hhs.gov/portal/server.pt/gateway/PTARGS_0_10741_848133_0_0_18/10_2_hit_terms.pdf.

Office of the National Coordinator for Health IT. (2008). *The ONC-coordinated federal health information technology strategic plan: 2008-2012.* Retrieved on June 8, 2009, from http://healthit.hhs.gov/portal/server.pt/gateway/PTARGS_0_10731_848084_0_0_18/HITStrategicPlanSummary508.pdf

Rishel, W., Riehl, V., & Blanton, C. (2007) *Summary of the NHIN prototype architecture contracts.* Gartner, Inc. Retrieved on June 1, 2009 from http://healthit.hhs.gov/portal/server.pt/gateway/PTARGS_0_10731_848093_0_0_18/summary_report_on_nhin_Prototype_architectures.pdf

SearchSecurity. (n.d.) *PKI.* Retrieved on June 12, 2009, from http://searchsecurity.techtarget.com/sDefinition/0,sid14_gci214299,00.html

Tillmann, G. (2007). Will biometric authentication solve corporate security challenges? *Optimized, 6*(2), 24.

Tomes, J. P. (2009). You are not a HIPPA Covered entity–you may be a red flag covered entity as well. *Journal of Health Care Compliance, 11*(1), 5–13.

U.S. Department of Health & Human Services. (2005). *HHS awards contracts to develop nationwide health information network.* Retrieved on June 8, 2009, from http://www.hhs.gov/news/press/2005pres/20051110.html

Waldren, S., Kibbe, D., & Mitchell, J. (2009). Will the feds really buy me an EHR? and other commonly asked questions about the HITECH act. [from ABI/INFORM Global.]. *Family Practice Management, 16*(4), 19–23. Retrieved September 29, 2009.

Zorkadis, V., & Donos, P. (2004). On biometrics-based authentication and identification from a privacy-protection perspective. *Information Management & Computer Security, 12*(1), 125–137. doi:10.1108/09685220410518883

Chapter 10
A Medical Data Trustworthiness Assessment Model

Bandar Alhaqbani
Queensland University of Technology, Australia

Colin J. Fidge
Queensland University of Technology, Australia

ABSTRACT

Electronic Health Record systems are being introduced to overcome the limitations associated with paper-based and isolated Electronic Medical Record systems. This is accomplished by aggregating medical data and consolidating them in one digital repository. Though an EHR system provides obvious functional benefits, there is a growing concern about reliability trust (trustworthiness) of Electronic Health Records. Security requirements such as confidentiality, integrity, and availability can be satisfied by traditional data security mechanisms. However, measuring data trustworthiness is an issue that cannot be solved with traditional mechanisms, especially since degrees of trust change over time. In this chapter, a Medical Data Trustworthiness Assessment model to assist an EHR system to validate the trustworthiness of received/stored medical data based on who entered the data and when is presented. The MDTA model uses a statistical approach that depends on the observed experiences available to the EHR system. In order to provide an accurate trustworthiness estimate for historical medical data, a time scope around the time when the data was entered was used. This scope enables the model to capture the dynamic behavior of the data entry agent's trustworthiness. To conduct this assessment medical metadata is used to extract information about the medical data sources (e.g. timestamps, and the identities of healthcare agents and medical practitioners) and, thereafter, this information is used in a statistical process to derive a trustworthiness value for the medical data. The result can then be expressed in the displayed health record by manipulating the EHR's metadata to alert the medical practitioner to possible trustworthiness problems.

DOI: 10.4018/978-1-60960-174-4.ch010

INTRODUCTION

Electronic Health Records can enable efficient communication of medical information, and thus reduce costs and administrative overheads (Blobel, 2004; Gunter & Terry, 2005). However, to achieve these potential benefits, the healthcare industry needs to overcome several significant obstacles, in particular concerns about the trustworthiness (reliability) of EHR medical data. Trustworthiness is a crucial factor that has a strong effect on how medical practitioners use data (Iakovidis, 1998). This concern is raised because EHR data is typically composed from different healthcare providers' Electronic Medical Record systems, from paper-based medical reports, and from referrals that patients get from those healthcare providers who do not have an EMR system or an electronic connection with the EHR system. Furthermore, by using an EHR system, a medical practitioner will thus be exposed to historical medical data with varying levels of reliability; the data might originate from a healthcare organization that does not satisfy patient safety requirements, e.g. one which is known to habitually enter inaccurate or incomplete data, or be entered by a medical practitioner who fails to satisfy medical guidelines, e.g. someone who is known to violate medical procedures. As a consequence, the trustworthiness of EHR data depends on the trustworthiness of its sources.

In general, in order to measure the trustworthiness of an agent, reputation systems (Xiong & Liu, 2003, 2004) provide an accumulative trustworthiness measure of an agent where all past experiences and/or feedback about the agent are combined. Most reputation systems are built to assess the trustworthiness of an agent at the present time. In other words they predict the expected future behavior of an agent based on its current trustworthiness. However, they do not provide a way to assess an agent's trustworthiness at a particular time in the past. Evaluating the trustworthiness of past data entries is crucial in the healthcare domain because an EHR combines *historical* medical data.

To illustrate this requirement, consider the following example. Assume that in year 2009 EHR system A received two medical reports, Patient Y's diagnosis and Patient Z's prescription, that were created by Dr X in 2000 and 2005 respectively. The EHR system maintains a database where it stores its observed experiences with external agents. It uses an eBay-like (Schneider et al., 2000) reputation system (though this is not an appropriate mechanism as we will see in the following section) in which it records the number of observed positive and negative experiences with an agent per annum and uses this to calculate a cumulative trust measure (Figure 1). In this case, these positive and negative experiences are generated from previously evaluated medical entries that were created by Dr X. Correct diagnoses and accurately following medical procedures are examples of positive experiences whereas misdiagnoses, incomplete or careless data entry, and failure to follow medical procedures are negative events. Figure 2 represents the observed trustworthiness of Dr X that EHR system A maintains over time. Now, let's see how EHR system A will evaluate the trustworthiness of the two received medical reports.

In current reputation systems, the calculated trustworthiness value for Dr X in the year 2009, i.e. 0.48, will be used as the trustworthiness of the two medical records, however this is an inaccurate measure because it represents Dr X's expected *future* behavior instead of his behavior at the time the records were created. From Figure 2, we notice that Patient Y's diagnosis was created at a time period when Dr X was evaluated to be trustworthy, whereas Patient Z's prescription was written during a time period when Dr X was believed to be untrustworthy. Therefore, assigning the trustworthiness value that is calculated in year 2009 to these two medical records is inappropriate due to the fact that trustworthiness is a dynamic attribute and varies according to Dr X's behavior.

Another approach is to consider Dr X's absolute trustworthiness value in 2000 and 2005 for these two records. Although this approach provides a better estimate, it does not consider the dynamic variability of the trustworthiness attribute. For example, between 1999 and 2001, inclusive, Dr X was believed to be providing trustworthy medical data. However in 2002 he was found not to have followed appropriate medical procedures in his diagnosis of a particular case, and this error was detected more than once. Therefore, this dynamic change of Dr X's trustworthiness should have an impact on his immediately preceding data entries, and the same thing can be said about the impact of his previous trustworthiness behavior on following medical data entries. (In general, we would expect the behavior of a medical practitioner or healthcare organization to change gradually over time, so there should be a correlation between successive data entries.)

Figure 1. The EHR system's observed cumulative trustworthiness of Dr X

Time	Number of observed Experiences		Trustworthiness
	Positive	Negative	
1999	1	1	0.5
2000	2	0	0.75
2001	3	0	0.85
2002	1	6	0.5
2003	0	7	0.33
2004	0	7	0.25
2005	0	5	0.21
2006	1	0	0.23
2007	6	0	0.35
2008	5	0	0.42
2009	6	1	0.48

Figure 2. The EHR system's continuous trustworthiness measurement of Dr X

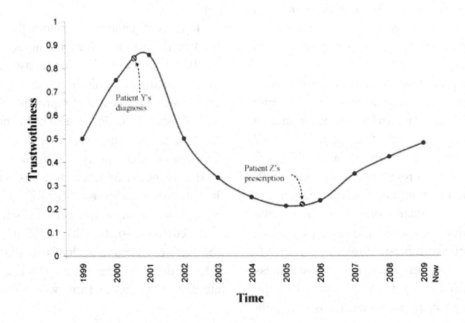

RELATED WORK

Reputation systems represent an important input for assessing the trust (or reliability) of a certain agent or service. These systems provide a reputation score for an agent calculated from the agent's ratings as voted on by others who have experienced a transaction with the agent. For instance, eBay's (www.ebay.com) feedback forum is one of the earliest reputation systems; it collects buyers' feedback (either +1, 0, or —1) and aggregates them equally (Resnick & Zeckhauser, 2002) to produce a global reputation score for the seller. The global score is further processed to provide the percentage of positive feedback that is gained by the seller. However, this additive scheme ignores the personalized nature of reputation measures (Mui et al., 2001). A slightly better approach, the average reputation scheme (Schneider et al., 2000) provides an improved calculation because it computes the reputation score as the average of all ratings. This principle is used in the reputation systems of many commercial web sites, such as Revolution Health (www.revolutionhealth.com) and Amazon (www.amazon.com). Although the average reputation scheme is better than the additive scheme, it still has the same weaknesses.

In the Peer-to-Peer (P2P) research arena, many reputation models have been proposed to assist in assigning reputation scores to those agents within the P2P network. These scores help an agent (service seeker) to make its own decision to trust and connect to the most honest and reliable agents (service providers). EigenTrust (Kamvar et al., 2003) is a reputation-based trust management system that aims to minimize malicious behavior in a peer-to-peer network. It computes the agents' trust scores through repeated and iterative multiplication and aggregation of trust scores along transitive chains until the trust scores for all agent members of the P2P community converge to stable values. PeerTrust (Xiong & Liu, 2003, 2004) is another reputation-based trust management system for P2P eCommerce communities. It

is even more cautious and examines the received ratings for their quality. It uses five factors to do so, namely feedback in terms of the amount of satisfaction, the number of transactions, the transaction's context factor, and the community context factor. These factors are used to discount the agent's trust value. However, our work differs from these two models in two aspects. Firstly, in the healthcare context, it's crucial to have on hand the identity of the agent who created the medical data (i.e. the healthcare provider or medical practitioner) in order to ensure accountability. In this way, the healthcare context differs significantly from the P2P context. Secondly, in our MDTA model we follow a time-variant mathematical approach by using Beta and Dirichlet probability density functions for combining feedback and for expressing reputation ratings, and subjective logic to represent the trust value where we consider agent's uncertainty factor, which makes our model capable of evaluating the trustworthiness of historical data that the former two models fail to achieve.

A Bayesian approach is used in more sophisticated reputation systems (Teacy et al., 2006; Wang et al., 2006) to produce the reputation score. For example, Mui et al. (2001) proposed a reputation model that uses Beta probability functions to represent the distribution of trust values according to an interaction history. This model calculates trust either by considering direct observations, if any, or by taking the recommendation of neighboring agents. However, this model does not distinguish between two trust aspects in its calculation, namely functional trust and referral trust (Jøsang et al., 2007), in which case functional trust values are assigned to neighbors in calculating the transitive trust on a specific agent, while the referral trust supports accurate calculation. TRAVOS (Teacy et al., 2006) is another system that uses the Bayesian approach to calculate a reputation score from binomial ratings and it considers referral trust in its transitive trust calculation. However, in the absence of any evidence, the TRAVOS system will assign an agent a default 0.5 reputation score that results from using the initial settings for the Bayesian parameters α and β. This system does not consider other factors that will have an impact on the default reputation score for these new agents. By contrast, our Medical Data Trustworthiness Assessment model employs a dynamic community base rate that is the average reputation score of the whole community that the agent belongs to. This dynamic community base rate is used in evaluating the reputation of any known or unknown agent, which improves the reliability estimation process since the community base rate dynamically reflects the trustworthiness of the whole community at any one time.

Even more relevant to our approach is Hedaquin (Deursen et al., 2008), a system for measuring the quality of health data that is entered into a patient's health record. Hedaquin is based on a Beta reputation system and uses the credentials of the health data supplier, ratings for the health data supplier, and metadata supplied by measuring devices. Hedaquin's goal is similar to our Medical Data Trustworthiness Assessment model, but instead of assessing the quality of the raw health data, our MDTA model assesses the trustworthiness of the medical data as entered into the patient's Electronic Health Record. Also, Hedaquin uses some ad hoc factors to discount the final quality value and does not provide an accurate trustworthiness estimate of new agents because it follows the same approach as TRAVOS and, in addition, it does not provide a mechanism to assess the trustworthiness of previously entered data. By contrast, our approach for assessing data trustworthiness uses two reputation systems, namely Beta and Dirichlet, which accepts binomial and multinomial ratings and makes our MDTA model capable of expanding and accepting ratings from various trusted agents (Alhaqbani et al., 2009). In addition, the MDTA model assesses new agents by considering their surrounding community's trustworthiness and takes into account the agent's dynamic trustworthiness behavior and is capable

of measuring the trustworthiness of old data (Alhaqbani & Fidge, 2009). In this chapter we combine both of these outcomes in a single model.

A TRUST NOTATION FOR ELECTRONIC HEALTH RECORDS

Manifestations of trust are easy to recognize because we experience and rely on it every day. At the same time trust is quite challenging to define because the term is used with a variety of meanings. Jøsang (2007b) has recognized two types of trust: *reliability trust*, which we call trustworthiness, and *decision trust*.

As the name suggests, reliability trust can be interpreted as the trustworthiness of something or somebody. In Electronic Health Record systems this can be interpreted as the trustworthiness of healthcare providers, medical practitioners, and medical data, assuming that all medical data transmission occurred in a secure and reliable way. A definition by Gambetta (1990) provides an example of how this can be formulated:

Definition 1 (Reliability Trust): Trust is the subjective probability by which an individual, *A*, expects that another individual, *B*, performs a given action on which *A*'s welfare depends.

However, trust can be more complex than Gambetta's definition suggests. For example, Falcone & Castelfranchi (2001) note that having high *reliability trust* in a person is not necessarily sufficient for deciding to enter into a situation of dependence on that person and they suggest to introduce some saturation-based mechanisms to influence the decision trust.

Definition 2 (Decision Trust): Trust is the extent to which a given party is willing to depend on something or somebody in a given situation with a feeling of relative security, even though negative consequences are possible.

In an EHR system, healthcare workers, including medical practitioners, are those who make the decision on whether or not to trust a given patient's medical data because they are legally accountable for any decision or action they made. However, there are several factors beside data trustworthiness that might influence the medical practitioner's decision trust, namely: utility (e.g. possible outcomes), risk attitude (e.g. risk taking, risk averse), and situation context (e.g. emergency).

PREVIOUS WORK: REPUTATION SYSTEMS

Reputation systems collect ratings about users or service providers from members of a community. The reputation system is then able to compute and publish reputation scores about those users and services. Reputation systems use different rating levels, which might be binomial or multinomial. These reputation scores are used to assist in measuring or evaluating the trustworthiness of a certain agent. In this section, we review the reputation systems that are used in our model, namely Beta and Dirichlet reputation systems, and the Subjective Logic trust model we employ.

BETA REPUTATION SYSTEM

Binomial reputation systems are based on a Beta probability function (Ismail & Jøsang, 2002), which can be used to represent the probability distribution of binary events, and are therefore called Beta reputation systems. In a reputation calculation process, the Beta reputation system updates its two parameters α and β to adjust its statistical Beta Probability Density Function as shown in the following definition.

Definition 3 (Beta Probability Reputation Score): Let r be the number of positive observations, and s be the number of negative observations that an agent X has about agent Y. By using the Beta reputation system, the *a posteriori* reputa-

tion score that X has about Y is computed as the expected probability, $E(p)$.

$$E(p) = \frac{\alpha}{\alpha + \beta},$$

where

$$\alpha = r + Wa, \quad \beta = s + W(1-a),$$

where a expresses the the base rate, and W is the weight of the non-informative prior, and normally $W = 2$.

As an example, let an agent A have 8 positive and 2 negative observations about agent B. Further assume that the base rate a is set to be 0.5. By using Definition 3, the probability expectation value is equal to 0.8. This can be interpreted as saying that the relative frequency of a positive observation in the future is somewhat uncertain, and that the most likely value is 0.8.

DIRICHLET REPUTATION SYSTEM

Multinomial Bayesian systems are based on computing reputation scores by statistical updating of Dirichlet Probability Density Functions, which therefore are called Dirichlet reputation systems (Jøsang, 2007b; Jøsang, Luo et al., 2008). The *a posteriori* (i.e. the updated) reputation score is computed by combining the *a priori* (i.e. previous) reputation score with new ratings.

In Dirichlet reputation systems agents are allowed to rate other agents or services with any value from a set of predefined rating levels, and the reputation scores are not static but will gradually change with time as a function of the received ratings. Initially, each agent's reputation is defined by the base rate reputation. Following the receipt of ratings about a particular agent, that agent's reputation will change accordingly.

Let there be k different discrete rating levels L. This translates into having a state space of cardinality k for the Dirichlet distribution. Let the rating level be indexed by i. The aggregate ratings for a particular agent are stored as a cumulative vector, expressed as:

$$\vec{R} = (\vec{R}(L_i) \mid i = 1 \ldots k).$$

This vector can be computed recursively and can take factors such as longevity and the community base rate into account (Jøsang, 2007b). The most direct way of representing a reputation score for an agent y is to simply aggregate the rating vector $\vec{R}_y$ which represents all relevant previous ratings. The aggregate rating of a particular level i for agent y is denoted by $\vec{R}_y(L_i)$.

For visualization of reputation scores, the most natural approach is to define the reputation score as a function of the probability expectation values of each rating level. Before any ratings about a particular agent y have been received, its reputation is defined by the common base rate vector $\vec{a}$. As ratings about a particular agent are collected, the aggregate ratings can be computed recursively (Jøsang, 2007b; Jøsang, Luo et al., 2008) and the derived reputation scores will change accordingly.

Definition 4 (Dirichlet Probability Reputation Scores): Let agent A have ratings $\vec{R}_B$, with k different discrete rating levels L, to represent A's ratings of an agent B. By using the Dirichlet reputation system, The corresponding Dirichlet probability reputation scores, $\vec{S}_B$, is defined as follows:

$$\vec{S}_B : \left(\vec{S}_B(L_i) = \left. \frac{\vec{R}_B(L_i) + W\vec{a}(L_i)}{W + \sum\limits_{j=1}^{k} \vec{R}_B(L_j)} \right| i = 1 \ldots k \right),$$

where parameter W represents the non-informative prior weight, with = 2 usually the value of choice, although larger values for constant W can be chose if a reduced influence of new evidence over the base rate is required.

The reputation score $\vec{S}$ can be interpreted like a multinomial probability measure, as an indication of how a particular agent is expected to behave in future transactions. It can easily be verified that

$$\sum_{i=1}^{k} \vec{S}(L_i) = 1$$

While informative, the multinomial probability representation can require considerable space on a computer screen because multiple values must be visualized. A more compact form can be used to express the reputation score as a single value in some predefined interval. This can be done by assigning a point value v to each rating level L_i, and computing the normalized weighted point estimate score ε.

Definition 5 (Point Estimate): Let agent X have k different rating levels with point values $v(L_i), 1 \leq i \leq k$, evenly distributed in the range $[0,1]$ according to $v(L_i) = (i-1)/(k-1)$ The point estimate reputation score of a reputation $\vec{R}$ is then:

$$\epsilon = \sum_{i=1}^{k} \nu(L_i)\vec{S}(L_i)$$

Such a point estimate in the interval $[0,1]$ can be scaled to any range, such as 1-5 stars, a percentage or a probability. Bootstrapping a reputation system to a stable and conservative state is important. In the framework described above, the base rate distribution $\vec{a}$ will define the initial default reputation for all agents. The base rate can, for example, be evenly distributed over all rating levels, or biased towards either negative or positive rating levels. This must be defined when

Figure 3. Base rate probability expectation values

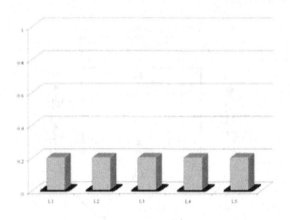

Figure 4. Update probability expectation values

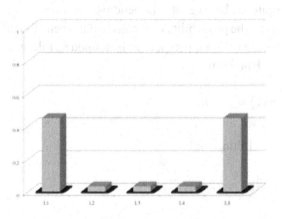

setting up the reputation system in a specific community.

As an example, consider a rating scale with five levels:

L1: Bad
L2: Mediocre
L3: Average
L4: Good
L5: Excellent

We assume a default base rate distribution a = 0.2. Before any ratings have been received, the multinomial probability reputation score will be represented as in Figure 3.

Now assume that 10 ratings are received, where 5 are bad, and 5 are excellent. This translates into the multinomial probability reputation score of Figure 4. The point estimate reputation score is calculated by using Definition 5, and equals 0.5.

SUBJECTIVE LOGIC

Subjective logic (Jøsang, 1997, 2001, 2007a) is a type of probabilistic logic that explicitly takes uncertainty and belief ownership into account. Arguments in subjective logic are subjective opinions about states in a state space. A binomial

opinion applies to a single proposition, and can be represented as a Beta distribution. A multinomial opinion applies to a collection of propositions, and can be represented as a Dirichlet distribution. Subjective logic defines a trust metric called opinion.

Definition 6 (Multinomial Subjective Opinion): Let $X=\{x_i|i=1,\ldots,k\}$ be a set of exhaustive and mutually disjoint states x_i. Let $\vec{b}$ be a belief vector, let u be the corresponding uncertainty mass where $\vec{b}, u \in [0,1]$ and $\sum \vec{b} + u = 1$, and let $\vec{a} \in [0,1]$ be a base rate vector over X, all seen from the viewpoint of agent A. The composite function $\omega_X^A = (\vec{b}, u, \vec{a})$ is then A's subjective opinion (trust) over X.

Definition 7 (Binomial Subjective Opinion): Let $X = \{x, \overline{x}\}$ be a binary partitioned state space. A's binomial opinion about the truth of statement x is the ordered quadruple $\omega_x^A = (b, d, u, a)$ where b is the belief mass in support of x being true, d is the belief mass in support of x being false, u is the uncertainty mass, a is the a *priori* probability in the absence of a committed belief mass.

In Subjective logic, the opinion probability expectation is used to derive the *posteriori* trust score of an agent, that is calculated as per the following definition.

Definition 8 (Subjective Opinion Probability Expectation): Let agent A have a subjective opinion about agent X. Depending on the opinion's state, the probability expectation that agent X is in a state x from A perspective is defined as follows:

Binomial:

$$E(x) = b + au$$

Multinomial:

$$\vec{E}_X(x) = \vec{b}(x) + \vec{a}(x)u$$

Subjective logic defines trust operators (functions) to calculate the subjective opinion in different trust contexts. For example, assume that Alice needs treatment for her knee and asks her GP Bob to recommend a good physiotherapist. When Bob recommends David, Alice would like to get a second opinion, so she asks Claire for her opinion about David. The trust scope in this case can be expressed as *'to be a competent physiotherapist'*. This situation is illustrated in Figure 5 where the indexes on arrows indicate the order in which the opinions are formed.

When trust and referrals are expressed as subjective opinions, each transitive trust path Alice→Bob→David, and Alice→Claire→David can be computed with the transitivity operator, also called the discounting operator, where the idea is that the referrals from Bob and Claire are discounted as a function of Alice's trust in Bob and Claire respectively. Finally the two paths can be combined using the cumulative or averaging fusion operator. These operators form part of Subjective Logic (Jøsang, 2001, 2007a), and semantic constraints must be satisfied in order for the transitive trust derivation to be meaningful (Jøsang & Pope, 2005). Opinions can be uniquely mapped to Beta PDFs, and in this sense the fusion operator is equivalent to Bayesian updating. This model is thus both belief-based and Bayesian. Algebraically, a trust relationship between A

Figure 5. Deriving trust from parallel transitive chains

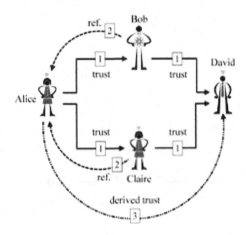

and B is denoted [A, B], transitivity of two arcs is indicated using a binary ":" operator, and the fusion of two parallel paths is indicated with a "◊" operator. The trust network of Figure 6 can then be expressed as:

$$[A,D] = ([A,B]: [B,D]) \lozenge ([A,C]: [C,D])$$

The corresponding transitivity operator for opinions is denoted as "⊗" and the corresponding fusion operator as "⊕". The mathematical expression for combining the opinions about the trust relationships of Figure 6 is then:

$$\omega_D^A = (\omega_B^A \otimes \omega_D^B) \oplus (\omega_C^A \otimes \omega_D^C)$$

MEDICAL DATA TRUSTWORTHINESS NETWORK STRUCTURE

Figure 6 shows our proposed network structure for deriving the EHR system's level of trust in received data fields, via our Medical Data Trustworthiness Assessment model. In this section, we explain the functionality of each component. The protocol by

Figure 6. Medical data trustworthiness network structure

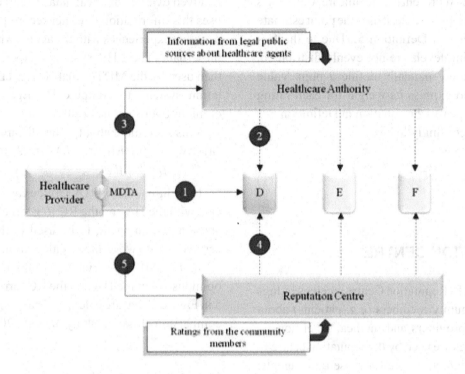

which these components interact is described in MDTA Protocol section below.

HEALTHCARE AUTHORITY

A Healthcare Authority is a legal body that records information gathered from public sources including, but not limited to, reports received from healthcare providers and medical practitioners about incorrect medical data or procedures, and medical misconduct, non-safety, or malpractice cases. The subject of this information is either a healthcare provider, a medical practitioner, or both. The HA uses this information to produce a ratings vector, in which it ranks each reported case according to its severity. This process can be done by applying previously-defined classification rules to each case.

In addition, the HA assigns a base rate for each severity rating level and for the prior behavior of the healthcare agent (either a healthcare provider or medical practitioner). The HA's ratings vector will have k levels representing the severity (danger) levels for reported cases. Here we assume that level 1 denotes the highest level of severity and level $k-1$ the lowest. Level k denotes the special default behavior for the agent's community (in the absence of any other information). In this situation we assume 'perfect' behavior of the community (however the receipt of bad ratings may be used by the HA to lower this value).

From this, the HA provides authorized or registered healthcare providers with its opinion (arrow 2 in Figure 6) about the medical conduct and practice of a certain healthcare provider or medical practitioner. Here, the HA acts as a Dirichlet reputation system and expresses its trust using the Subjective Logic trust metric opinion. For example, $\omega_D^{HA} = (\vec{b}_D^{HA}, u_D^{HA}, \vec{a}_D^{HA})$ is Healthcare Authority *HA*'s trust opinion about healthcare agent *D*. Vector $\vec{a}_C^{HA}$ represents *HA*'s base rate for *D*'s community (C).

In order to represent the Healthcare Authority's opinion as a single value, it uses the point estimate representation in Definition 5.. Due to the fact that the rating levels are not evenly distributed, the HA should manually define a point value vector $\vec{m}$ to express its weight for each rating level. In this case, the equation in Definition 5 is changed accordingly to be:

$$\epsilon_X^{HA} = \sum_{i=1}^{k} \vec{m}(L_i)\, \vec{S}(L_i) \tag{1}$$

REPUTATION CENTRE

In our model a Reputation Centre receives ratings from community members (e.g. patients) about healthcare providers and medical practitioners. These ratings are used by the reputation centre to derive a reputation score for those rated agents; this reputation score represents the RC's subjective opinion (arrow 4 in Figure 6). These opinions are communicated to healthcare providers as needed. The RC acts as a Dirichlet reputation centre and expresses its opinions in the same way that the Healthcare Authority does. For example, $\omega_A^{RC} = (\vec{b}_A^{RC}, u_A^{RC}, \vec{a}_C^{RC})$ is Reputation Centre RC's opinion about healthcare agent A.

MEDICAL DATA TRUSTWORTHINESS ASSESSMENT SERVICE

The Medical Data Trustworthiness Assessment service is employed by the Electronic Health Record system to measure the reliability of medical data sourced from other healthcare agents (e.g. healthcare providers or medical practitioners). The EHR system has a database that records its experiences with other healthcare agents. These experiences are created from the reports that are received from the EHR system's users about those

received external medical data. The EHR system uses this information to either record positive or negative experiences with the agents who created these data. The EHR system's experiences are then used by the MDTA, that acts as a Beta reputation system, to compute the EHR system's opinion about a certain healthcare agent. The EHR systems's opinion about a healthcare agent D (arrow 1 in Figure 6) is denoted as $\omega_D^{EHR^*} = (b_D^{EHR^*}, d_D^{EHR^*}, u_D^{EHR^*}, a_D^{EHR^*})$.

In addition, the MDTA service can communicate with the HA and the RC to get their opinion about a certain agent, to be used in the MDTA service's trustworthiness calculation process. Also, the MDTA service maintains dynamic opinions about the HA and the RC (arrows 3 and 5 in Figure 6) that are calculated based on opinion comparison (Jøsang, Bhuiyan et al., 2008).

MDTA PROTOCOL

In the previous section we introduced the components needed to implement our trustworthiness model. In this section we define the protocol whereby these components interact with one another.

The Medical Data Trustworthiness Assessment service is a supporting service for an Electronic Health Record system. It is responsible for assessing the trustworthiness of given medical data, based on its data entry characteristics, and then communicating this information to the EHR system to update the medical metadata displayed. This process starts by receiving medical data from the EHR system, then the MDTA starts its investigation by consulting the EHR reputation system and seeks, if necessary, opinions from known parties. In this setup, we assume that each entity, including healthcare providers, medical practitioners, the Healthcare Authority, and the Reputation Centre has a well-defined identity that can be verified in a secure context.

Figure 7. Medical data trustworthiness message sequencing

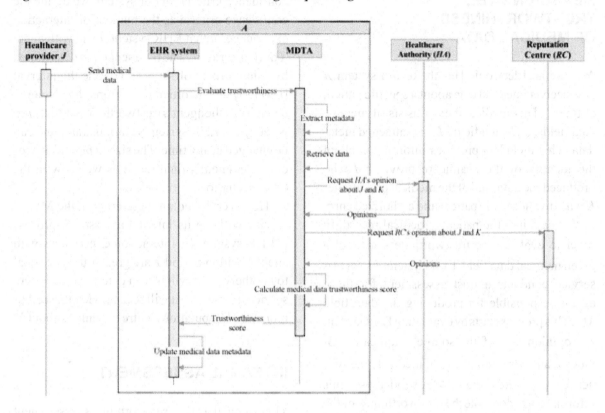

To better understand the functionality of the MDTA service, we use the following steps to depict the messages received and sent by the MDTA service in order to accomplish its task (Figure 7).

1. An EHR system *A* receives medical data for patient *p* from healthcare provider *J*.
2. The EHR system sends this medical data to the MDTA service to evaluate its trustworthiness.
3. The MDTA extracts medical metadata to identify the source healthcare provider, who is *J* in this case, and the identity of the medical practitioner *K* who created this record.
4. The MDTA accesses system *A*'s reputation database to find historical interaction experiences between *A* and *J*, and *A* and *K*.

5. If the recorded experiences do not satisfy *A*'s confidence criteria (see the following section) then:
   a. The MDTA requests opinions about *J* and *K* from Healthcare Authority *HA*; and
   b. The MDTA requests opinions about *J* and *K* from Reputation Centre *RC*.
6. The MDTA service uses the received information to calculate the medical data trustworthiness score.
7. The MDTA service sends the result back to the EHR system *A*.
8. EHR system *A* updates the medical data displayed to reflect the computed reliability score, e.g. by flagging potentially untrustworthy data.

MEASURING THE TRUSTWORTHINESS OF MEDICAL DATA

Assume an Electronic Health Record system A has received medical data about a specific patient at time t. This medical data consists of medical data fields, and each field MF has attached metadata. This metadata provides information about the identity of the healthcare provider J who produced the data, and of the medical practitioner K who diagnosed the patient and authorized entry of this data into the patient's medical record. In order to evaluate the trustworthiness φ_{MF}^A of a given medical data field, EHR system A's MDTA service conducts a trust assessment for those agents responsible for producing the data field MF. This process starts by evaluating EHR system A's opinion ω_J^A of the source healthcare provider J, and A's opinion ω_K^A of medical practitioner K. Afterwards, the MDTA service uses this information to compute the trustworthiness of the medical data by using the fusion operator as in the following equation.

$$\varphi_{MF}^A = \mathrm{E}(\omega_J^A \oplus \omega_K^A) \qquad (2)$$

Electronic Health Record system A uses the resulting reliability score φ_{MF}^A to update medical data field MF's metadata to reflect this score in order to alert the medical practitioner relying on the data if its trustworthiness is low.

In order to compute the trustworthiness of medical data field MF, the MDTA service needs to evaluate the trustworthiness of its sources J and K. However, the MDTA service's approach for calculating these two values is similar; so we will denote the trust target as agent X, which represents either J or K. The MDTA service follows two approaches in calculating the trust of a given agent X and the approach chosen is determined by evaluating certain criteria which we call the confidence criteria. In our system, we define the confidence criteria as the number of interaction experiences n that EHR system A had with agent X during period T. The time scope T is determined by using a fixed offset *per* to define the interval $[t-per, t+per]$ in order to capture the dynamic behavior of the agent's trustworthiness. Offset *per* is set by the EHR system's administrator and can be changed at any time. The size of *per* influences our assessment's final result as we show in the Case Scenario section below.

However, based on these criteria, the MDTA service will use its internal assessment process if EHR system A's interaction experiences with agent X within period T are greater than or equal to n, otherwise it will use an external assessment service from which it will seek the Healthcare Authority and Reputation Centre's opinions about X.

INTERNAL ASSESSMENT

The Medical Data Trustworthiness Assessment service uses EHR system A's reputation database to derive A's opinion ω_X^{A*} about agent X by using the positive, r, and negative, s, observations that A has about X during time scope T. EHR system A's opinion parameters are calculated as per the following definition:

Definition 9 (Binomial Opinion Parameters): Let r_X^B and s_X^B be the number of positive and negative observations respectively that agent B has about agent X. Then B's subjective opinion parameters are calculated as per the following:

$$b_X^B = \frac{r_X^B}{(r_X^B + s_X^B + 2)}$$

$$d_X^B = \frac{s_X^B}{(r_X^B + s_X^B + 2)}$$

$$u_X^B = \frac{2}{(r_X^B + s_X^b + 2)}$$

$a_C^B = B$'s base rate for agent X's community C

The base rate in Definition 9 helps the EHR system to set *a priori* trust about a certain agent in the absence of any interaction experiences. On start-up of the reputation system this value is usually set by the authority who provides the system.

Most previous work treats the base rate as a static value that does not change over time. However, this is inadequate for our purposes because the base rate should reflect the evaluator's belief at a certain time towards its targeted community. Therefore, we use EHR system A's base rate for agent X's community (the relevant healthcare provider's or medical practitioner's community base rate) to represent the base rate in A's opinion as is shown in the following definition.

Definition 10 (Community Base Rate): Let an agent A have positive r_C^A and negative s_C^A observations about a community (group of agents) C. Then B's base rate for C during time period T is given as:

$$a_{C,T}^A = \frac{r_{C,T}^A}{r_{C,T}^A + s_{C,T}^A} \quad \text{where} \quad \begin{cases} r_{C,T}^A = \sum_{M \in C} r_M^A \\ s_{C,T}^A = \sum_{M \in C} s_M^A \end{cases}$$

Once the MDTA service has computed A's opinion about X and A's experiences with X satisfy the confidence criteria, the service publishes A's opinion about X as follows.

$$\omega_X^A = \omega_X^{A^*} \tag{3}$$

Once the MDTA service finishes computing A's opinions about J and K, it substitutes these values into Equation 2 to derive A's subjective trustworthiness measure φ_{MF}^A on the medical data.

EXTERNAL ASSESSMENT

In this approach, EHR system A seeks opinions from external parties to be combined with A's self-computed opinion $\omega_X^{A^*}$ in order to derive A's overall opinion ω_X^A about agent X. There are two sources of information: relevant Healthcare Authority HA and Reputation Centre RC. Each source sends its opinion about X during time scope T to A through a secure communications channel. However, these opinions are discounted by EHR system A's opinion about each source. The following equation uses the Subjective Logic fusion operator to compute A's opinion about X using A's self-computed opinion, HA's opinion, and RC's opinion about X.

$$\omega_X^A = \omega_X^{A^*} \oplus \omega_X^{A:RC} \oplus \omega_X^{A:HA} \tag{4}$$

The computation process for discounted opinions $\omega_X^{A:RC}$ and $\omega_X^{A:HA}$ is the same. Therefore, in the following, we show how to compute $\omega_X^{A:RC}$, and the same process can be applied to produce $\omega_X^{A:HA}$.

Firstly, the MDTA service needs to compute A's opinion about RC. Since A does not record any observations about RC, the MDTA service uses an opinion comparison approach via the operator "$\downarrow$" (Jøsang, Bhuiyan et al., 2008) as defined in the following.

Definition 11 (Opinion Derivation Based on Opinion Comparison): Let ω_Z^A and ω_Z^B be opinions that are made on agent Z by agents A and B respectively. A's opinion about B is calculated based on the similarity between their opinions as defined below:

$$\omega_B^A = \omega_Z^A \downarrow \omega_Z^B \quad \text{where} \quad \begin{cases} d_B^A = \left| \left(\dfrac{r_Z^A + 1}{r_Z^A + s_Z^A + 2} \right) - \epsilon(\vec{R}_Z^B) \right| \\ u_B^A = \max\left[u_Z^A, u_Z^B \right] \\ b_B^A = 1 - d_B^A - u_B^A \end{cases}$$

To follow Definition 11, the MDTA service selects an agent Z from A's database, calculates A's opinion $\omega_Z^{A^*}$ about Z, and compares it to RC's opinion ω_Z^{RC} about Z to derive A's opinion about RC.

Secondly, the Reputation Centre RC needs to convert its multinomial aggregate ratings $\vec{R}_X^{RC}$ into a binomial opinion. Reputation Centre RC uses the following definition to derive its binomial rating parameters r and s.

Definition 12 (Multinomial to Binomial Rating Conversion): Let agent A employ a multinomial reputation model that has k rating levels, where $\vec{R}(x_i)$ represents the ratings on each level x_i, and let ε represent the point estimate reputation score. Let the binomial reputation model have positive and negative ratings r and s respectively. The derived converted binomial rating parameters (r, s) are given by:

$$r = \epsilon_X^A \sum_{i=1}^{k} \vec{R}_X^A(x_i)$$

$$s = \sum_{i=1}^{k} \vec{R}_X^A(x_i) - r$$

Afterwards, RC uses Definition 9 to derive its binomial parameters b, d, and u. The base rate a parameter is computed as in the following equation.

$$a_X^{RC} = \frac{\epsilon_X^{RC} - b_X^{RC}}{u_X^{RC}} \tag{5}$$

Finally, the MDTA uses ω_{RC}^A, ω_X^{RC}, and A's base rate a_{RC}^A to derive A's transitive opinion on X, which is version discounted version of RC's opinion on X. To carry out this task, the MDTA service uses the base rate sensitive transitive approach in Definition 13 to calculate A's transitive opinion on X.

Definition 13 (Base Rate Sensitive Transitive Approach): Let $\omega_B^A = (b_B^A, d_B^A, u_B^A, a_B^A)$ be A's subjective binomial opinion about B and $\omega_X^B = (b_X^B, d_X^B, u_X^B, a_X^B)$ be B's subjective binomial opinion about X. Then A's transitive opinion on X is derived from the discounted version of B's opinion on X where B's belief and disbelief on X is discounted by A's opinion probability expectation on B as shown below:

$$\omega_X^{A:B} = \omega_B^A \otimes \omega_X^B \quad \text{where} \quad \begin{cases} b_X^{A:B} = \left(b_B^A + a_B^A u_B^A \right) b_X^B \\ d_X^{A:B} = \left(b_B^A + a_B^A u_B^A \right) d_X^B \\ u_X^{A:B} = 1 - b_X^{A:B} - d_X^{A:B} \\ a_X^{A:B} = a_X^B \end{cases}$$

Once the MDTA service has computed discounted opinions $\omega_X^{A:HA}$ and $\omega_X^{A:RC}$, it uses these values in Equation 4 to derive A's opinion about X, which is either healthcare provider J or medical practitioner K, by using the subjective fusion operator. The fusion operator has two computational approaches depending on the agents' observations time collection. As per the subjective logic calculus, if the observations are collected in disjoint time periods then the cumulative fusion rule is the appropriate approach, where observations are added together. However, if the observations are collected within the same time period, as in our case, the average fusion operator rule is selected where observations are averaged. The following definition shows how the average fusion operator is calculated for two subjective binomial opinions.

Definition 14 (Average Fusion Operator):
Let $\omega_X^A = (b_X^A, d_X^A, u_X^A, a_X^A)$ be A's subjective binomial opinion about X and $\omega_X^B = (b_X^B, d_X^B, u_X^B, a_X^B)$ be B's subjective binomial opinion about X, and assume these two opinions both resulted from observations that has been captured within time period T. The combination of A's opinion and B's opinion is defined as follows:

Case I: For $u_X^A \neq 0 \vee u_X^B \neq 0$:

$$\omega_X^{A\Diamond B} = \omega_X^A \oplus \omega_X^B \quad \text{where} \begin{cases} b_X^{A\Diamond B} = \dfrac{b_X^A u_X^B + b_X^B u_X^A}{u_X^A + u_X^B} \\ u_X^{A\Diamond B} = \dfrac{2u_X^A u_X^B}{u_X^A + u_X^B} \\ d_X^{A\Diamond B} = 1 - (b_X^{A\Diamond B} + u_X^{A\Diamond B}) \end{cases}$$

Case II: For $u_X^A = 0 \wedge u_X^B = 0$:

$$\omega_X^{A\Diamond B} = \omega_X^A \oplus \omega_X^B \quad \text{where} \begin{cases} b_X^{A\Diamond B} = \displaystyle\sum_{C \in \{A,B\}} b_X^C \lim_{\substack{u_X^A \to 0 \\ u_X^B \to 0}} \dfrac{u_X^C}{u_X^A + u_X^B} \\ u_X^{A\Diamond B} = 0 \\ d_X^{A\Diamond B} = 1 - b_X^{A\Diamond B} \end{cases}$$

Finally, the MDTA substitutes A's computed opinion ω_J^A of J and ω_K^A of K into Equation 2 to derive A's subjective trustworthiness measure φ_{MF}^A of medical data field MF.

CASE SCENARIO

We use the following case scenario to demonstrate the functionality of our MDTA model and discuss how the chosen time period *per* can influence our final trustworthiness result. Let us assume that EHR system A received in 2009 a patient's medical diagnosis m that was created in 2005. The medical data was entered by Intern K at Hospital J. Assume that EHR system A, the nationwide healthcare authority HA, and the government-run reputation centre RC have observations about K and J in a time-ordered. Authority HA's reputation system maintains rating $\vec{R}$ about an agent (Table 1) that has five elements, four represent severity rating levels (extreme, high, medium, low) and the fifth element represents 'perfect' behavior. For the sake of simplicity, the base rate vector $\vec{a}$ that represents the *a priori* base rate for those elements in $\vec{R}$ is assumed to be $\vec{a} = (0.002, 0.004, 0.008, 0.01, 0.976)$. Reputation centre RC maintains ratings vector $\vec{R}$ (Table 2) which has five rating levels (bad, mediocre, average, good, excellent), and the base rate $\vec{a}$ that represents the *a priori* base rate for elements in $\vec{R}$ is assumed to be $\vec{a} = (0.1, 0.2, 0.3, 0.2, 0.2)$. EHR system A's reputation system (Table 3) has two values, positive observations r and negative observations s.

When A receives medical diagnosis m, A's MDTA service evaluates the trustworthiness of m. Let us assume that the confidence criteria $n = 8$ and *per* = 1 which means one year, so the time scope is defined as $T = [2004, 2006]$. The MDTA service starts by checking A's reputation system, but finds there are insufficient experience entries recorded either with K or J. Therefore, the MDTA service requests HA's and RC's opinion about K and J. Healthcare authority HA uses Definition 4 to compute its multinomial (Dirichlet) reputation scores $\vec{S}$. Next, it uses its point values $\vec{m} = (0, 0.2, 0.43, 0.67, 1)$ with $\vec{S}$ in Equation 1 to compute its singleton reputation scores $\epsilon_K^{HA} = 0.657$ and $\epsilon_J^{HA} = 0.66$.

The Healthcare Authority HA needs to convert its multinomial reputation scores to binomial opinions in order to pass it to EHR system A's MDTA

Table 1. HA's reputation system

Time	$\vec{R}$		
	K	**J**	**Z**
2002	(0,0,0,0,0)	(0,0,0,1,0)	(0,0,0,0,0)
2003	(0,1,0,0,0)	(1,1,0,0,0)	(0,0,0,1,0)
2004	(0,1,0,0,0)	(0,1,0,1,0)	(0,0,1,0,0)
2005	(0,0,0,1,0)	(0,0,1,1,0)	(0,0,0,0,0)
2006	(0,0,1,1,0)	(0,0,0,1,0)	(0,0,0,0,0)
2007	(1,1,0,0,0)	(0,1,0,0,0)	(0,0,0,0,0)
2008	(0,0,0,1,0)	(0,0,0,0,0)	(0,0,0,0,0)
2009	(0,0,0,2,0)	(0,0,0,1,0)	(0,0,0,1,0)

Table 2. RC's reputation system

Time	$\vec{R}$		
	K	**J**	**Z**
2002	(0,0,1,1,2)	(0,0,0,0,1)	(0,0,0,0,0)
2003	(0,1,0,0,0)	(1,0,0,0,0)	(0,0,0,1,0)
2004	(0,1,0,0,1)	(0,1,1,0,1)	(0,0,1,0,0)
2005	(0,0,1,1,1)	(0,1,0,0,1)	(0,0,0,1,1)
2006	(0,1,1,0,0)	(0,0,1,1,0)	(0,0,0,1,1)
2007	(1,2,0,0,0)	(0,0,0,0,0)	(0,0,0,0,2)
2008	(0,0,0,2,1)	(0,0,0,1,1)	(0,0,0,1,0)
2009	(0,0,2,0,0)	(0,0,3,0,0)	(0,0,0,0,2)

Table 3. EHR system A's reputation system

Time	(r,s)		
	K	**J**	**Z**
2002	(2,0)	(0,0)	(0,0)
2003	(0,1)	(0,2)	(0,1)
2004	(0,1)	(0,1)	(0,1)
2005	(0,0)	(1,0)	(2,0)
2006	(0,0)	(1,0)	(1,0)
2007	(0,1)	(0,1)	(2,0)
2008	(0,0)	(1,0)	(0,2)
2009	(0,0)	(1,1)	(1,0)

service. *HA* uses Definition 12, Definition 9, and Equation 5 to compute its binomial opinions.

$$\omega_K^{HA} = (0.44, 0.23, 0.33, 0.66)$$
$$\omega_J^{HA} = (0.47, 0.24, 0.29, 0.66)$$

Afterwards, the MDTA service uses Definition 11 to compute its opinion about *HA*, with *Z* as the subject of this process. The resulting opinion is $\omega_{HA}^A = (0.53, 0.14, 0.33, 0.8)$, where the base rate trust has been set to $a_{HA}^A = 0.8$. The MDTA service uses Definition 14 with its opinion about *HA*, to compute the service's discounted opinion that *A* holds about *K* and *J*.

$$\omega_K^{A:HA} = (0.35, 0.18, 0.47, 0.66)$$
$$\omega_J^{A:HA} = (0.37, 0.2, 0.43, 0.66)$$

The MDTA service follows the previous approach to compute the discounted opinion held by *RC* about *K* and *J*. However, the only difference in this process is the way that *RC* computes its reputation score. Since *RC*'s rating levels are evenly distributed, it uses Definition 5 to compute its reputation score ε. As a result, the MDTA service's discounted opinions for *RC* about *K* and *J* are:

$$\omega_K^{A:RC} = (0.43, 0.23, 0.34, 0.65) \text{ and}$$
$$\omega_J^{A:RC} = (0.39, 0.27, 0.34, 0.59).$$

In the next step, the MDTA service substitutes its internal opinions:

$$\omega_K^{A\star} = (0, 0.33, 0.67, 0.5) \text{ and}$$
$$\omega_J^{A\star} = (0.4, 0.2, 0.4, 0.5),$$

and its calculated discounted opinions into Equation 4 to compute *A*'s opinion about *K* and *J*.

$$\omega_K^A = (0.35, 0.24, 0.42, 0.61)$$
$$\omega_J^A = (0.39, 0.24, 0.37, 0.59)$$

Finally, the MDTA service computes *A*'s reliability measure φ about medical entry *m* by substituting ω_K^A and ω_J^A into Equation 2 which results in $\varphi_m^A = 61\%$ which shows that the medical diagnosis *m* has a acceptable trustworthiness score.

Now let us set the time period *per* to be 2 years, and follow the aforementioned approach to compute the trustworthiness of medical diagnosis *m*. We find that *A*'s trustworthiness of *m* gets decreased and is equal to 46% which implies the medical data is slightly untrustworthy. This is because *K* and *J* in 2003 and 2007 have received bad reports and ratings at the Healthcare Authority and Reputation Centre, respectively. Let us further change the time period and make *per* equal 3 years. By following the same approach, we find that *A*'s trust on *m* has changed and is now equal to 51% which is higher than the second computed value. This slight increase in the trustworthiness score is due to the fact that *K* and *J* in 2002 and 2008 have shown good behavior as demonstrated by *RC*'s captured ratings and EHR system *A*'s stored observations.

This demonstrates that determining the appropriate size of time period is difficult. If an agent *X*'s trustworthiness is largely stable over time then the size of the time period would not make a big difference in *X*'s trustworthiness evaluation. However, if agent *X*'s trustworthiness is unstable and keeps changing, the time period's size may have a high impact on our trustworthiness calculation. Ideally, the time period should be chosen to be broad enough to encompass the time of interest plus a period of stable behavior sufficient to provide an 'accurate' trustworthiness measure. The degree of accuracy can be calibrated for a particular EHR system based on the percentage

Figure 8. MDTA service application

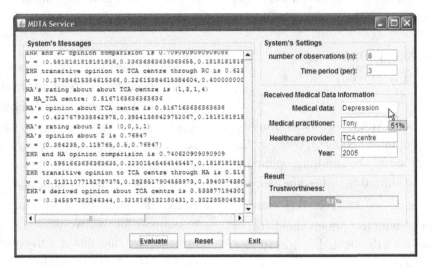

IMPLEMENTATION

To demonstrate the functionality of our model, we have developed a Java application that does the relevant calculations that are introduced in our MDTA model. Also, we have configured a MySQL database server which the MTDA service uses to get the agent's data required in the trustworthiness calculation process. Each agent's database is represented as a database table in our MySQL server. Also, we built a user interface panel which we use to load the incoming medical data and its metadata (Figure 8).

To run our application we set the confidence criteria *n* and time period *per* that the MDTA service will use in its trustworthiness evaluation. Upon receiving incoming medical data, which we simulate by entering manually in the prototype, an evaluation request is sent to the MDTA service which uses the metadata and gets the required internal and, if necessary, external data for trustworthiness calculation process as presented in the aforementioned section. Once the MDTA service has finished the calculation, the trustworthiness value is then used by the application to update the medical data's metadata, e.g. assign the resulted value to the data's field tooltip to indicate the trustworthiness value of the medical data.

CONCLUSION

An Electronic Health Record system overcomes the problems and limitations that are associated with paper based and isolated Electronic Medical Record systems; however, its adoption is hindered by concerns over reliability (trust). Medical data trustworthiness is a vital requirement which has a high impact on how medical data will be utilized. In the current situation, all medical data are usually assumed trustworthy *a priori* so, in the absence of a trustworthiness evaluation, all data will be valued equally; however, this should not be the case.

In this chapter, we presented a dynamic Medical Data Trustworthiness Assessment model that follows a statistical approach to conduct trustworthiness evaluations. Our model uses the metadata attached to incoming medical data, namely the healthcare organization's identity, medical practitioner's identity, and the event timestamp. The trustworthiness evaluation is then conducted by considering the encountered source agent's trustworthiness prior to and after the time at which the medical data was recorded, in order to produce a context-dependent estimate, rather than relying on the agent's perceived trustworthiness at the current time. Thereafter, the resulting trustworthiness value can be communicated to the EHR displayed on a medical practitioner's computer to alert the medical practitioner to any reliability problems.

REFERENCES

Alhaqbani, B., & Fidge, C. J. (2009). *A time-variant medical data trustworthiness assessment model.* Paper presented at the 11th IEEE International Conference on e-Health Networking, Applications and Services (IEEE HealthCom 2009), 16-18 Dec 2009, Sydney.

Alhaqbani, B., Jøsang, A., & Fidge, C. J. (2009). A medical data reliability assessment model. *Journal of Theoretical and Applied Electronic Commerce Research, 4*(3), 64–78.

Blobel, B. (2004). Authorisation and access control for electronic Health Record Systems. *International Journal of Medical Informatics, 73*(3), 251–257. doi:10.1016/j.ijmedinf.2003.11.018

Deursen, T., Koster, P., & Petkovic, M. (2008). *Hedaquin: A reputation-based health data quality indicator.* Paper presented at the 3rd International Workshop on Security and Trust Management (STM 2007), 27 Feb 2008, Dresden, Germany.

Falcone, R., & Castelfranchi, C. (2001). Social trust: A cognitive approach. In Castelfranchi, C., & Tan, Y.-H. (Eds.), *Trust and deception in virtual settings* (pp. 55–99). Kluwer.

Gambetta, D. (1990). *Trust: Making and breaking cooperative relations* (pp. 213–238). Basil Blackwell.

Gunter, T. D., & Terry, N. P. (2005). The emergence of national electronic health record architectures in the United States and Australia: Models, costs, and questions. *Journal of Medical Internet Research, 7*(1), e3. doi:10.2196/jmir.7.1.e3

Iakovidis, I. (1998). Towards personal health record: Current situation, obstacles and trends in implementation of electronic healthcare record in Europe. *International Journal of Medical Informatics, 52*(1-3), 105–115. doi:10.1016/S1386-5056(98)00129-4

Ismail, R., & Jøsang, A. (2002). *The Beta reputation.* Paper presented at the 15th Electronic Commerce Conference, 17-19 June 2002, Bled, Slovenia.

Jøsang, A. (1997). *Artificial reasoning with subjective logic.* Paper presented at the 2nd Australian Workshop on Commonsense Reasoning, Dec 1997, Perth, Australia.

Jøsang, A. (2001). A logic for uncertain probabilities. *International Journal of Uncertainty. Fuzziness and Knowledge-Based Systems, 9*(3), 279–212. doi:10.1142/S0218488501000831

Jøsang, A. (2007a). *Probabilistic logic under uncertainty.* Paper presented at The 13th Computing: The Australasian Theory Symposium (CATS2007), 30 Jan-2 Feb 2007, Ballarat, Australia.

Jøsang, A. (2007b). Trust and reputation systems. In Aldini, A., & Gorrieri, R. (Eds.), *Foundations of security analysis and design, IV* (pp. 209–245). Springer. doi:10.1007/978-3-540-74810-6_8

Jøsang, A., AlZomai, M., & Suriadi, S. (2007). *Usability and privacy in identity management architectures.* Paper presented at the the Australasian Information Security Workshop: Privacy Enhancing Technologies (AISW 2007), 31 Jan 2007, Ballarat, Australia.

Jøsang, A., Bhuiyan, T., & Cox, C. (2008). *Combining trust and reputation management for Web-based services*. Paper presented at the 5th International Conference on Trust, Privacy and Security in Digital Business (TrustBus2008), 4-5 Sept 2008, Turin, Italy.

Jøsang, A., Luo, X., & Chen, X. (2008). *Continuous ratings in discrete Bayesian reputation systems*. Paper presented at the the Joint iTrust and PST Conferences on Privacy, Trust Management and Security (IFIPTM 2008),18-20 June 2008, Trondheim, Norway.

Jøsang, A., & Pope, S. (2005). *Semantic constraints for trust transitivity*. Paper presented at the the Asia-Pacific Conference of Conceptual Modeling (APCCM), Feb 2005, Newcastle, Australia.

Kamvar, S., Schlosser, M., & Garcia-Molina, H. (2003). *The Eigentrust algorithm for reputation management in P2P networks*. Paper presented at the 12th International Conference on World Wide Web (WWW '03), 20-24 May 2003, Budapest, Hungary.

Mui, L., Mohtashemi, M., Ang, C., Szolovits, P., & Halberstadt, A. (2001). *Rating in distributed systems: A Bayesian approach*. Paper presented at the Workshop on Information Technologies and Systems (WITS), 15-16 Dec 2001, New Orleans.

Resnick, P., & Zeckhauser, R. (2002). Trust among strangers in Internet transactions: Empirical analysis of eBay's reputation system. In Baye, M. R. (Ed.), *The Economics of the Internet and E-commerce* (pp. 127–157). Elsevier. doi:10.1016/S0278-0984(02)11030-3

Schneider, J., Kortuem, G., Jager, J., Fickas, S., & Segall, Z. (2000). Disseminating trust information in wearable communities. *Personal and Ubiquitous Computing*, *4*(4), 245–248. doi:10.1007/BF02391568

Teacy, W., Patel, J., Jennings, N., & Luck, M. (2006). TRAVOS: Trust and Reputation in the Context of Inaccurate Information Sources. *Autonomous Agents and Multi-Agent Systems*, *12*(2), 183–198. doi:10.1007/s10458-006-5952-x

Wang, Y., Cahill, V., Gray, E., Harris, C., & Liao, L. (2006). *Bayesian network based trust management*. Paper presented at the 3rd International Conference in Autonomic and Trusted Computing (ATC), 3-6 Sept 2006, Wuhan, China.

Xiong, L., & Liu, L. (2003). *A reputation-based trust model for Peer-to-Peer eCommerce communication*. Paper presented at the IEEE International Conference on E-Commerce (CEC '03), 24-27 June 2003, Newport Beach, USA.

Xiong, L., & Liu, L. (2004). PeerTrust: Supporting Reputation-based Trust for Peer-to-Peer Electronic Communities. *IEEE Transactions on Knowledge and Data Engineering*, *16*(7), 843–857. doi:10.1109/TKDE.2004.1318566

Chapter 11
Using Biometrics to Secure Patient Health Information

Dennis Backherms
Capella University, USA

ABSTRACT

The crime of identity theft has proven to be one of the most costly crimes in American history. Identity theft has become so prevalent in our society today that many laws have been passed, and new bills introduced, to try and combat these troublesome issues. However, recently, a new trend in identity theft has been occurring, individuals are now experiencing medical identity theft. One way to help protect a patient's medical information is through biometric authentication for records access. The technology of biometrics, while thought a novelty at first, has proven to be both a reliable and efficient method for securing patient health records. Biometric technology helps to provide a multi-tiered approach to medical record access and also helps create an audit trail for discovery of unauthorized medical record access. Implementing biometric technology in patient health record security will help substantially reduce the likelihood that medical identity theft will occur.

INTRODUCTION

Organizations and individuals concern themselves everyday with identity theft. Some businesses today have even developed seemingly simplistic products to help prevent thieves from ever get-

DOI: 10.4018/978-1-60960-174-4.ch011

ting an individual's identity for use in fraudulent activity. Stories of identity theft vary from victims who patronize organizations that lose clientele information to children whose parents use their names to procure credit cards and other forms of credit without that child's knowledge. Employer related risks associated with identity theft have also risen in recent years. The reasons for elevated employer risks are because more consumer transactions are occurring online and more employees are in custody of sensitive clientele data.

News stories and print media are notifying consumers how an organization's employees are losing laptops or getting laptops stolen with sensitive clientele data almost all the time. The kinds of sensitive clientele data stored on these lost or stolen laptops include social security numbers, driver's license numbers, and bank account numbers, just to name a few. Identity theft is used, primarily, to defraud businesses and individuals out of billions of dollars annually in the United States alone. Identity theft allows criminals to max out credit cards, open bank accounts or various other financially binding accounts, and grants access to retirement accounts or other long term types of financial nest eggs.

Medical identity theft is equally, if not more, devastating to an individual than identity theft alone. Criminals on the edge of a new frontier, many view medical identity theft as the next step in evolution from identity theft. Medical identity theft has exponential potential to defraud businesses and individuals at levels of financial loss unheard of in years past. Unlike identity theft, medical identity theft has the potential to cause more damage to a victim because of the superfluous information garnered from an individual's medical record. Medical identity theft ranges from opportunists, viewing medical information for personal insight, to people wanting medical attention but do not have their own, or sufficient, medical insurance to cover costs.

The following chapter provides a synopsis on the description of identity theft, actual stories of identity theft, and laws created to help prevent identity theft. The chapter will also describe medical identity theft, actual stories of medical identity theft, and laws created to help prevent medical identity theft. Next, the chapter will focus on biometrics in regards to the history of biometrics, the industry in general, trends in the industry, and how biometrics offers a secure method for authentication. The chapter will also explain how integration of biometric technology into the health industry will provide better security and help to prevent medical identity theft. Finally, the chapter will conclude with ideas for future research directions and how trends in biometric technology will help shape future industry focus.

BACKGROUND

Identity Theft

Criminals, for many years, have been innovating their ways to defraud individuals. Reading studies of criminal activity since the beginning of human times will easily describe criminal mind progression. The progression warrants changes in defrauding tactics used by criminals. One reason criminals change tactics is to overcome newer technological challenges; enter the age of information. The dawn of information has provided individuals with opportunities that may have appeared too futuristic just ten years prior. Organizations can store all types of personal data on wallet-sized cards, some cards are small enough to fit on a key chain, for use in many aspects of everyday life. Digitizing an individual's information, credit cards for example, present an even greater opportunity for the criminal to defraud. Today, identity theft costs the American taxpayers billions of dollars every year and cause problems for an estimated 10 million victims annually (Deybach, 2007).

Identity theft happens more than many people realize and can occur in many different ways. Identity theft is described as a crime in which someone wrongfully obtains someone else's personal data to deceive or commit fraud; typically for economic gain. Identity theft causes hundreds of hours of work to resolve just a single incident and also causes workplace productivity losses because of employees taking the time off needed to resolve issues concerning identity theft. The common story people hear involves someone bringing sensitive data home on a laptop and then the laptop gets stolen. Another common story people hear involves Internet transactions when purchasing online. There are several interesting and groundbreaking cases of identity theft that helped pave the way to legislation regarding the crime of identity theft.

One of the best known cases of identity theft was reported by the US Department of Veterans Affairs. One of the employees had taken a laptop home with over 26 million records stored on it. The laptop had been stolen from the home and recovered sometime later. The largest theft of social security numbers to date, the laptop also contained other personal information of veterans and their wives. Another case of identity theft involved a criminal that stole an individual's personal information and created years of havoc that caused the victim to spend $15,000 and four years of time to rectify the problems. The problems created by the criminal included $100,000 of credit card debt, obtaining a federal home loan, purchases of homes and vehicles, purchases of handguns, and filing for bankruptcy. The criminal also took the time to call and taunt the victim since identity theft, at that particular time, was not a federal crime.

Organizations have also become liable and culpable for the actions and misappropriations of employees. One of the most famous cases involved a Michigan labor union employee. The labor union employee took home many documents containing the personal information of union members. The information in those documents included the names and social security numbers of the union members. The labor union employee's daughter then stole the information to commit fraud. The union was found liable for the action and misappropriation of its employee. Identity theft has become so prevalent in our society today that actions have been prompted at the state and federal level to combat these issues.

Identity Theft Laws

California was the first state to pass any law concerning identity theft. The first law passed required notification to be sent to all affected parties involved in an incident where personal data was breached; other states soon followed suit. In 2006, 31 other states had introduced legislation regarding identity theft; passing into law in at least 12 states (Deybach, 2007). For example, the 2009 Florida Statue described identity theft as "any person who willfully and without authorization fraudulently uses personal identification information concerning an individual without first obtaining the individual's consent" (Fraudulent Practices, 2009). Florida Statue also covers inclusions of minors, deceased individuals, fictitious individuals, and law enforcement officers. Florida law continued by acknowledging the degree level of the crime, the sentencing structure afforded to the legal system when prosecuting criminals, and limitations of prosecution through time restrictions. In response to the debacle of identity theft, federal agencies have also enacted laws that help discern corporate responsibility for the protection of clientele data.

In 2003 and 2004, the US passed two pieces of legislation dealing directly with identity theft, the Fair and Accurate Credit Transactions Act (FACTA) and the Identity Theft Penalty Enhancement Act (ITPEA). The ITPEA's sole purpose was to establish "penalties for aggravated identity theft" (Holtfreter & Holtfreter, 2006, p. 57) and to help reduce both identity theft and financial loss accompanied by identity theft. ITPEA was divided into seven sections that delineated the proper information concerning the improved protection of all consumers and individuals with identity theft woes. The seven key sections addressed were national fraud alert systems, truncation of credit and debit card receipts, indicators of identity theft on credit reports, shared information between debt collectors and creditors concerning identity theft victims, identity theft account blocking, blocking fraudulent debt from being transferred or reported, and enhanced criminal penalties for identity theft (Federal Trade Commission, 2003).

Fraud Alert Systems

Fraud alert systems inform creditors when a consumer's credit report has been associated with real or possible fraud. The creditor is then required to confirm the identity of the consumer prior to "issuing a duplicate credit/debit card, process a change of address, extending credit, or some other consumer related service" (Holtfreter & Holtfreter, 2006, p. 58). Initially believed to eliminate many identity theft problems before they had a chance to escalate out of control, fraudsters quickly found other ways to verify identity that fraud alert systems may not detect. Potential problems with the system immediately surfaced. Clerical errors, such as name misspellings and name conventions, existed and were sometimes hard to dispel.

Truncation of Credit and Debit Card Receipts

Before the law was passed, disposal of credit/debit card receipts allowed fraudsters to gain access to numbers that were in turn used to purchase from retail markets locally, through mail order, or online. Subsequently, in response to requirements of the law, businesses only print the last five digits of the credit/debit card number and do not print the expiration date. The exception to the rule was in situations where vendors only handwrote receipts or used credit/debit card imprints to complete transactions. The provision's intent was to prune fraudster's attempts to gain unauthorized access to an individual's account.

Indicators of Identity Theft on Credit Reports

Another preemptive strike against fraudsters, financial institutions are required to notify card holders when any account information occurs on their behalf pertaining to the same account. A special provision helped establish the validity of the request, especially on accounts which have been inactive for two or more years. The provision established inactive account validity which provided consumers a means of checks and balances for safeguarding personal account information.

Shared Information Between Debt Collectors and Creditors Concerning Identity Theft Victims

Businesses are now required to provide a copy of an application for credit or business transaction to the identity theft victim per their request no later than 30 days of said request. Businesses are also required to give the same report to a law enforcement agency of the victim's choosing. The theory behind the provision was to eliminate many identity theft issues before the issues had a chance to begin.

Identity Theft Account Blocking

If any fraudulent activity has been found, information pertaining to the activity is not allowed to be reported to the victim's credit report. The onus of innocence is therefore placed on the victim and should be removed within four days after said proof is provided. The provision's theory was to eliminate many of the financial problems associated with identity theft before the consumer's credit was ruined beyond repair. Problems with this provision are concentrated on fraudsters who may have used aliases that include the victim's name resulting in adverse affects on the victim's credit report.

Blocking Fraudulent Debt from Being Transferred or Reported

The provision required notification to be sent to debt collectors of collection of fraudulent debt so as not to create an atmosphere to erode a consumer's credit rating further. Debt collectors were also required to notify creditors of such activity and collection status. The provision was created to "assist victims who conduct their own investigations prior to the involvement of law enforcement agencies" (Holtfreter & Holtfreter, 2006, p. 62). The provision is one of the most important provisions to serve as a consumer's rights advocate.

Enhanced Criminal Penalties for Identity Theft

Providing tougher penalties associated with identity theft, individuals convicted of felony identity theft face a mandatory minimum sentence of no less than two years which cannot be reduced by any court. Identity theft felony violations are described in this section for purposes of prosecution. The provision helped establish the legal definition of identity theft and provided a means by which prosecution can punish fraudsters. The potential problem associated with this provision is whether or not "such harsher penalties will really prevent or decrease identity theft" (Holtfreter & Holtfreter, 2006, p. 62).

With many states enacting laws covering various forms of identity theft, and the federal government equally responding to the issue, the hope is that the attempt to rectify some of these issues will decrease the crime of identity theft. Many people still have mixed feelings about identity theft legislation and how identity theft crime will be circumvented. The identity theft laws will continue to evolve as societal needs change. Unfortunately, criminal's tactics also evolve as means to combat their crime change. Recently, a new trend in identity theft has been occurring, medical identity theft.

Medical Identity Theft

Much worse than simple identity theft, medical identity theft has the potential to cause more damage to the victim because of the extra information gained from an individual's medical record. Similar to the portable storage of personal information found on credit/debit cards, medical organizations are now using magnetic storage methods to keep personal medical information on ID cards and other forms of portable devices for use in the medical industry. Besides health insurance and prescription ID cards with magnetic strips on them, individuals also have other devices about their person for quick access to health related information such as bracelets and pendants on necklaces.

Medical identity theft is cause for concern since the incidents related to medical identity theft are on the rise. Medical identity theft includes both financial and human factors. Lafferty (2007, p. 13) noted,

The "human cost" of medical identity theft includes financial losses, false entries in their medical history, the denial of insurance or the use of all available insurance resulting in benefits being "capped," the loss of reputation to the patient, physician, and health care organization depending on who was victimized, the loss of medical record privacy when records are subpoenaed as part of an investigation, and the loss of the proverbial value of time spent trying to correct the damage.

The problems associated with human factors compound over time simply because many medical decisions about an individual result from medical history. If any part of an individual's medical history is falsified, medical decisions based on those false entries can prove deadly.

Medical identity theft can occur in many different ways. Criminals may obtain someone's medical identity to use for medical treatment. Friends or family may use an individual's medical identity to gain medical treatment. Medical professionals can submit false claims against insurance to commit fraud or gain information about an individual for opportunistic reasons; such as gaining information out of curiosity. Opportunistic reasons can also come from co-workers who try to validate rumors about an individual's medical condition, such as confirming debilitating diseases. Whatever the reason may be, medical identity theft introduces new definitions for irreparable damages.

One well known case for medical identity theft involved an individual named Joe Ryan. In 2004, Joe Ryan received a collections notification in the mail totaling $41,000 for surgery he never had. A criminal had used Joe's name and social security number to receive extensive medical treatment and left Joe with the bill. Trying to clear his name with no luck, Joe managed to barely to keep himself out of bankruptcy fighting the injustice. Another case involved a computer hacker who managed to steal 8.3 million patient records and would return the stolen records for a ransom of $10 million; the case is still being investigated. One last case involved a man, who had AIDS, which used his cousin's medical identity to seek medical attention at a cost of $76,000 over a 15 year time period. The man, who had stolen his cousin's medical identity, did not confess to the various crimes until he was on his deathbed.

The worst cases of medical identity theft, to-date, are within the health care industry and organized crime. A psychiatrist diagnosed one of his patient's children, a child that has never been seen by the doctor, and then billed insurance accordingly. A second case involved a podiatrist that killed one of his patients when the patient refused to lie about fraudulent insurance filings made by the doctor. Organized crime is also getting involved in criminal acts of medical identity theft. Organized crime units have been temporarily constructing patient clinics, collecting patient information, and then disappearing after a few short months. The recent rise in medical identity theft has prompted laws at the federal level to combat these issues.

Medical Identity Theft Laws

The most well known and publicized act is the Health Insurance Portability and Accountability Act (HIPAA). Simple, opportunistic, violations could carry up to a fee of $100,000 with a 5 year prison sentence under HIPAA. More complex and malicious violations, those where information is used to defraud, could carry a fee of $250,000 with a 10 year prison sentence. HIPAA violations are enforced by the US Department of Health and Human Services (HHS) Office of Civil Rights (OCR). Congress appropriated funds for HHS to develop three sets of national standards which addressed standards for electronic transactions, standards for privacy of individual health information, and standards used to protect electronic networks and devices used to transport patient health information. In 2006, the President established a collaborative effort between the US Department of Justice (DOJ) and the Federal Trade Commission (FTC) to combat identity theft called the Identity Theft Task Force (ITTF). The ITTF's purpose was three-fold; to bring violators to justice, to mitigate risks for individuals and organizations, and to assist individuals or organizations recover from effects of the theft. The ITTF includes 17 agencies which charged 432 defendants in 2006 with crimes associated with identity theft.

HIPAA Security Rule

The HIPAA Security Rule, part of the HIPAA Privacy Rule and enforced by the Centers for Medicare and Medicaid Services (CMS), was charged to mandate "administrative, physical, and technical measures to safeguard the confidentiality, integrity, and availability of electronic protected health information (EPHI)" (Hoffman & Podgurski, 2007, p. 6). The Security Rule applies to covered entities only, which is a small segment of organizations in possession of EPHI. Covered entities are defined as health plans, health care clearinghouses, and health care providers, all of which transmit electronic health information. Empirical research concerning the rule's effectiveness has yielded unfavorable results. Out of the 178 providers that responded to surveys, only 56% asserted HIPAA Security Rule compliance. Out of the 42 payers that responded to surveys, only 80% asserted HIPAA Security Rule compliance. Reasons given for non-compliance vary from budgetary to difficulty integrating new technology. Researchers determined, in actuality, that only 39% of providers and 33% of payers truly implemented all required security standards and had experienced security breaches within six months of the survey.

Four requirements are needed to meet the HIPAA Security Rule. The first requirement is to ensure the integrity, confidentiality, and availability of EPHI processes. The second requirement is to safeguard against security threats to data. The third requirement is to safeguard against unauthorized uses and disclosures of data. The fourth requirement is to ensure adherence to the Security Rule throughout the organization. Implementation of these requirements varies but general guidelines are provided. General guidelines include physical access to hardware and buildings, log-in monitoring, data backup, disaster recovery, periodic security reminders, password management, and agreement contracts with personnel to adhere to safeguard measures.

Under administrative safeguards, organizations are applying the Security Rule by ensuring the integrity, confidentiality, and availability of EPHI processes. The technologies needed for this deals with computer software and computer hardware considerations, from security track records to the frequency of password changes. Training, user credentials, and evaluations of technical and non-technical personnel are also listed in this guideline. Under physical safeguards, organizations are applying the Security Rule by limiting and controlling access, for all personnel, to site facilities based on role and function. The technologies needed for this deals with describing the nature of access needed, physical systems such as card systems or biometric systems, associating role risk with validation requirements, and mobile device access control. Under technical safeguards, specifications for the encryption of EPHI is given under the Access Control standard and the Transmission Security standard. Organizations are required to encrypt and decrypt EPHI and to encrypt EPHI whenever appropriate. The technologies needed for this deals with appropriate cryptographic techniques, algorithms, protocols, cryptographic key length, distribution and management of keys, and human factors.

Organizations that do not comply with regulations concerning patient information confidentiality continue to expose themselves to the criminal mind. A laptop without proper security protection measures, encryption and biometric authentication for example, gets stolen and now patient health information is available to commit fraud. One particular example happened when a Maryland state health commission board member, who also was a banker, discovered which bank customers had cancer and canceled their loans (Hoffman & Podgurski, 2007). Organizations that do not comply with federal and state regulations risk facing large fines for non-compliance. Liability for organizations losing health information is enormous and should prompt more secure means of health information protection; biometrics may have the solution the health industry needs.

MAIN FOCUS

Biometrics

Biometric technology is not a new concept; in fact, historians have found that 14th century Chinese merchants often used fingerprints to complete business transactions (Bala, 2008). Another common practice during 14th century China was for the government to use fingerprints to identify children (Joyce, 2008). Today's biometric need stems from positive individual identification and secure information system authentication. While the use of biometric technology can be considered relatively new, the ideas behind using biometrics for identification are not. Understanding the relevance of biometrics will help both the IT industry and the health industry understand the validity of using biometrics as a means of positive identification, as well as, using biometrics to provide higher levels of information security and assurance. Over time, the advantages of biometrics have given the IT industry the momentum needed to morph biometric technology into a more efficient and reliable method of information systems authentication. Recently however, biometric technology has started the next phase of exploration by implementing solutions in the health care industry.

Current Industry Examples

The advantages of biometrics start with a better platform for building an efficient and secure means of safeguarding patient health information. Many industries are recognizing the advantage that biometric authentication brings to their organization. Boatwright and Lou (2007) discussed a few examples where organizations implemented biometric authentication with positive results. One particular example involved implementing biometric terminals to identify individuals by the shape and size of their hand. The system was implemented as a result of employees swiping or punching other employees into work to get compensated for work absentee employees did not do. After the implementation of the biometric terminals occurred, the organization claimed to have saved 22% annually in labor expenses.

Some applications of biometric authentication can be used in novelty items, but still provide the same level of security. One interesting way of using voice recognition helped nefarious individuals from accessing a very private and damaging record, pre-teen/early-teen girls' diaries (Markowitz,

2000). The device stores diaries and other personal items and is protected by voice recognition. Anyone who wishes to access the device needs to say a particular password and in the correct manner, otherwise the device stays locked. Although the last example may seem simplistic, it proves how the use of biometric security could also help individuals in other matters.

Another successful example of data security through biometrics, provided by Markowitz (2000), is with the Illinois Department of Revenue (IDOR). The IDOR is charged with tax auditing Illinois based businesses, as well as, tax auditing any out-of-state organizations that conduct regular business in Illinois. Sensitive information was given to auditors from IDOR databases through data disks that were mailed to them, sometimes getting into the auditors hands almost ten days later. To rectify the problem, the IDOR implemented a voice recognition system that permitted voice verification over the telephone prior to granting data line access to auditors in the field. Since auditors were also working at home, in emergency after-hours or weekend situations, the voice recognition system kept auditors from driving into work, sometimes up to 30 miles one way.

Sukhai (2005) noted another successful implementation of biometric authentication at a casino. The casino implemented a system that uses facial recognition software to identify individuals who cause problems and cheat. Based on the success of the facial recognition software, the casino decided to implement biometric systems for employee time-clock management. Similar to the biometric terminals, the installed time-clocks would require employees to scan their hands in order to clock in and out of work (Boatwright & Lou, 2007). The measure was needed to curtail employees clocking in for one another.

The advantages for implementing biometric solutions are numerous. Users no longer would be required to remember complex passwords, PINs, pass phrases, or answers to identity challenge questions. Users would also not have to worry about losing or misplacing devices used for authentication such as smart cards, key fobs, ID badges, key cards, and USB dongles. Since biometric authentication requires measuring biological characteristics of individuals, the likelihood of falsifying this unique information is virtually impossible. Also, once biometric data has been captured and stored, there would be no need to change the information; negating policies that require periodic authentication changes.

While there are many advantages to argue for biometric authentication implementation, there are disadvantages also. One common disadvantage for biometric implementation is public perception. The perception of biometrics has closely associated the technology with that of criminality. Many individuals believe that submitting an iris scan or palm scan, for example, is too intrusive and lends their relinquishment of privacy. Many individuals also worry about who has access to their biometric data and whether that data is going to be shared with other organizations. The rate of error for biometric authentication increases when individuals experience life debilitating accidents, such as the loss of a limb. Accordingly, if an individual needs to verify identity through voice recognition, the individual may have problems legitimately authenticating to an information system while battling the common cold.

Many different industries can benefit from implementing the use of biometric technology. Any industry that processes large quantities of sensitive documents, wireless providers, Internet security providers, telecommunication providers, and order-by-phone organizations, to name a few, can benefit from biometric technology integration. Recently, the health care industry has been required, under certain laws, to develop ways to protect patient health information. In addition to other secure means of user authentication already in place, biometric technology can help provide a multi-layered approach to securing patient health information and the health care industry.

RECOMMENDATIONS

Biometric authentication and identification methods have progressed and expanded in recent years. New methods of biometric authentication and identification include gait analysis, retinal scans, vein scans, voice recognition, and signature verification, to name a few. Biometric technology has also been emerging as the most foolproof method of automated authentication and identification. Since biometric authentication has typically been associated with protecting highly sensitive information in organizations, implementing the same authentication techniques in the health care industry becomes more advantageous. Biometric technology will also help bring the health care industry into compliance with federal regulations, especially HIPAA.

The health care industry should seriously consider implementing biometric technology for several reasons. Since biometric technology requires the measurement and analysis of an individual's unique physical and behavioral characteristics, falsifying information to gain access to patient health information is almost non-existent. Biometric technology can be used to prevent unauthorized access to system resources, as a means to manage system access, and ensure the security of patient health information. Using biometric solutions will also enable "much tighter control over physician access to electronic clinical patient records and also will provide tighter audit trails for tracking physician order entry for laboratory tests or prescriptions" (Perrin, 2002, p. 86). Mentioned previously, biometric technology can also help bring the health care industry into compliance with federal regulations such as HIPAA. Creating complexity for authentication in protecting patient health information and complying with HIPAA, biometric technology also presents a multi-layered approach.

Integrating biometric technology into the health care industry helps in many different ways. For example, care givers would be able to implement biometric technology that automatically indexes, searches, and retrieves patient health information. Biometric technology can also be integrated to use as a means of physical access to certain areas of the hospital. One progressive idea for recognition is through gait analysis. Simply put, a physician, or other hospital staff member, is walking down a hospital hallway and passes by a camera. The camera feeds the data to a computer which then determines if the person has access to a specific area, based on a set of preconditions. Depending on the answer from the analysis, the doors at the end of the hall will either stay magnetically locked or become unlocked to allow the physician, or other hospital staff member, to pass through. A multi-layered solution would be to use biometric technology to verify an individual's identity, through one or several biometrics, and then finishing the authentication cycle by prompting the user for a password or PIN. One final benefit biometric technology offers the health care industry is the creation of audit trails. Audit trails allow the health care industry a reliable method for identifying the who, the what, the when, the where, the how, and possibly the why of misappropriated behavior by health care personnel.

Implementing biometric technology in the health care industry can also help prevent liability issues from materializing in regards to security breaches or governmental compliance regulations. Compliance with HIPAA requires the type of multi-layered approach that implementing biometric technology can offer the health care industry. Violating any HIPAA regulation carries serious consequences. Simple, opportunistic, violations could carry up to a fee of $100,000 with a 5 year prison sentence under HIPAA. More complex and malicious violations, those were information is used to defraud, could carry up to a fee of $250,000 with a 10 year prison sentence. Implementing a biometric solution could address the standards required for securing electronic transactions, the privacy of individual health information, and the standards used to protect electronic networks and devices used to transport patient health information.

FUTURE RESEARCH DIRECTIONS

The need for research in biometric data analysis results and its potential application in the health-care industry has been addressed. Bala (2008) noted that "biometric security is [*sic*] emerging as the most foolproof method of automated personal identification in today's highly computer dependent world" (p. 66). Bala also noted that "biometrics…cannot be stolen or misplaced it is unique to every individual" (p. 66). The uniqueness of biometric data and its use in information systems permeates Bala's key points. Joyce (2008) validated the reliability of biometric data and described the process by which biometrics is used to verify "an individual based on unique physiological or behavioral characteristics" (p. 16). Ensuring that biometric data is collected correctly will help identify the algorithms to use that would properly address key areas of security concerning patient health information. Kanneh and Sakr (2008) discussed how inaccurate biometric data can be using the false accept rate and the false reject rate. The correct framework by which to test biometric reliability is also important. Bromme and Kronberg (2002) tested algorithms against biometric data using a framework developed for performance measures and usability concerning iris-biometrics. The series of tests performed resulted in algorithms developed to trend unreadable biometric data such as user behavior and environmental conditions.

Identifying someone by signature or gait may yield useful information that can be used to positively identify health care professionals, create audit trails for use in records and breach discovery, and help create secure "zones" within hospitals that should only be accessed by certain individuals. Ramachandra et al. (2009) posited that their algorithm used cross-validation graphs for positive biometric identification. Annadhorai, Guenterberg, Barnes, Haraga, and Jafari (2008) used real-time wireless sensors to collect gait biometric data. The gait biometric data was then broken into gait cycles used to identify individuals. Goffredo, Bouchrika, Carter, and Nixon (2008) also collected gait biometric data however used a multi-camera surveillance system to do so. The analysis results of the gait biometric data from the studies by both Annadhorai et al. and Goffredo et al. could possibly be used to develop algorithms that identify individuals for secure "zones" in hospitals.

Voice biometric data analysis can also prove useful in securing patient health information. Di Crescenzo, Cochinwala, and Shim (2007) discussed the importance of building identity management architectures using voice biometric data. Likewise, Markowitz (2000) discussed technologies used to verify speakers and also speaker identification using voice biometric data. While Markowitz discussed the broad topic of identifying individuals through voice biometric identification, Di Crescenzo et al. actually modeled cryptographic properties of voice to search for algorithms in identifying an individual. Di Crescenzo et al.'s intent was to provide useful information that would help towards the development of voice-based protocols. When professionals learn how unique, consistent, and pattern driven different types of biometric data is, then using that biometric data as a means of security and compliance in the health care industry seems more plausible today than ever before.

CONCLUSION

Other avenues also remain open for biometric integration. Since biometrics is making great strides in the technological world, the perception of how integrated biometrics will become remains to be seen. Continuous threats to security in many organizations, especially the health care industry,

will help maintain the momentum of more secure information systems. The measured success of biometric technology integration, along with the benefits biometric integration brings, was documented from the various stories presented. While the idea for using biometric data to positively identify an individual is not a new concept, getting that technology integrated into the health care industry remains to be elusive at best.

Keeping in mind the advantages and disadvantages to implementing biometric technology in the health care industry will help the industry understand the importance of fulfilling the obligation to protect patient health information. Health care executives can ensure that all personnel are aware of and committed to "the importance of patient information security and the potential repercussions for violations" (Lafferty, 2007, p. 17). Health care executives also need to ensure that all departments in the organization understand a zero tolerance stance policy for violations of regulations concerning patient confidentiality. Given the sudden rise in medical identity theft, many different law enforcement agencies, including the US government, have responded by enacting legislation governing patient health information.

The problem with acceptance still resides in public perception of biometric technology and personal privacy. If the public perception hinders the ability to implement a biometric solution, then the likelihood the solution will be used as originally intended or is deemed as a success will be diminished. Health care professionals revealed a greater acceptance rate of biometric technology than did any other individual. Health care professionals also differentiated from individuals in regards to how best to implement biometric technology. Implementation of biometric technology should be disclosed on a very basic level if the technology will experience full mainstream implementation. Federal and state requirements for securing patient health information will always play a pivotal role in how standards and legislation will change in direct response to consumers' attitudes. Expanding biometric technologies will bring about new change and cause important issues to develop in the future.

Finally, the integration of biometric technology in securing patient health information will continue to suffer, as long as, there is no support from within the health care industry. Health care professionals should be prepared to address existing consumer concerns regarding the potential use of biometric technology in securing patient health information and preventing far worse problems associated with medical identity theft such as, insurance fraud, medical mishaps, and patient registration difficulties. Biometric technology integration has the potential to help facilitate cost reductions, enhance information security, and improve accessibility. Biometric technology in the health care industry will not reach its full potential until the trust of both the health care professional and consumer have understood its use does not threaten the privacy of personal information.

REFERENCES

Annadhorai, A., Guenterberg, E., Barnes, J., Haraga, K., & Jafari, R. (2008). *Human indentification by gait analysis*. Paper presented at the HealthNet '08.

Bala, D. (2008). Biometrics and information security. *Information security curriculum development: Proceedings of the 5th annual conference on Information security curriculum development*, 64-66.

Boatwright, M., & Lou, X. (2007). *What do we know about biometrics authentication?* Paper presented at the Information Security Curriculum Development Conference '07.

Bromme, A., & Kronberg, M. (2002). *A conceptual framework for testing biometric algorithms within operating systems' authentication*. Paper presented at the SAC '02.

Deybach, G. (2007). Identity theft and employer liability. *Risk Management, 54*(1), 14–17.

Di Crescenzo, G., Cochinwala, M., & Shim, H. (2007). *Modeling cryptographic properties of voice and voice-based entity authentication*. Paper presented at the DIM '07.

Federal Trade Commission. (2003). *Overview of the identity theft program*. Washington, DC: Federal Trade Commission.

Goffredo, M., Bouchrika, I., Carter, J., & Nixon, M. (2008). *Performance analysis for gait in camera networks*. Paper presented at the AREA '08.

Hoffman, S., & Podgurski, A. (2007). Securing the HIPAA secure rule. *Journal of Internet Law, 10*(8), 5–16.

Holtfreter, R., & Holtfreter, K. (2006). Gauging the effectiveness of US identity theft legislation. *Journal of Financial Crime, 13*(1), 56–64. doi:10.1108/13590790610641215

Identity Theft 911. (2010). *Medical identity theft goes high-profile*. Retrieved February 21, 2010, from http://www.identitytheft911.org/articles/article.ext?sp=10863

Joyce, M. (2008). The challenges and future of biometric-based security systems. *Internal Auditing, 23*(2), 14–22.

Kanneh, A., & Sakr, Z. (2008). *Biometric user verification using haptics and fuzzy logic*. Paper presented at the MM '08.

Lafferty, L. (2007). Medical identity theft: The future threat of health care fraud is now. *Journal of Health Care Compliance*, 11-20.

Markowitz, J. (2000). Voice biometrics. *Communications of the ACM, 43*(9), 66–73. doi:10.1145/348941.348995

Perrin, R. (2002). Biometrics technology adds innovation to healthcare organization security systems. *Healthcare Financial Management, 56*(3), 86–88.

Practices, F. (2009). XLVI FL. *Stat*, 817–568.

Ramachandra, A., Pavithra, K., Yashasvini, K., Raja, K., Venugopal, K., & Patnaik, L. (2009). *Offline signature authentication using cross-validated graph matching*. Paper presented at the Compute '09.

Sukhai, N. (2004). *Access control & biometrics*. Paper presented at the InfoSec CD Conference '04.

US Department of Health and Human Services. (2010). *Personal health records and the HIPAA privacy rule*. Retrieved on February 15, 2010, from http://www.hhs.gov

US Department of Justice. (2010). *Identity theft*. Retrieved on February 20, 2010, from http://www.justice.gov/criminal/fraud/websites/idtheft.html

ADDITIONAL READING

Anonymous,. (2002). Beyond doors: Securing records with finger flick. *Security*, *39*(7), 57.

Ballard, L., Kamara, S., Monrose, F., & Reiter, M. K. (2008). *Towards practical biometric key generation with randomized biometric templates*. Paper presented at the CCS '08.

Bedi, H., Yang, L., & Kizza, J. (2009). *Fair electronic exchange using biometrics*. Paper presented at the CSIIRW '09.

Bhargav-Spantzel, A., Squicciarini, A. C., Modi, S., Young, M., Bertino, E., & Elliott, S. J. (2007). Privacy preserving multi-factor authentication with biometrics. *Journal of Computer Security*, *15*, 529–560.

Briggs, P., & Olivier, P. (2008). *Biometric daemons: Authentication via electronic pets*. Paper presented at the CHI '08.

Brunelli, R., & Falavigna, D. (1995). Person identification using multiple cues. *IEEE Transactions on Pattern Analysis and Machine Intelligence*, *17*(10), 955–966. doi:10.1109/34.464560

Chandra, A., & Calderon, T. (2005). Challenges and constraints to the diffusion of biometrics in information systems. *Communications of the ACM*, *48*(12), 101–106. doi:10.1145/1101779.1101784

Chandra, A., Durand, R., & Weaver, S. (2008). The uses and potential of biometrics in health care: Are consumers and providers ready for it? *International Journal of Pharmaceutical and Healthcare Marketing*, *2*(1), 22–34. doi:10.1108/17506120810865406

Drugescu, C., & Etges, R. (2006). Maximizing the return on investment of information security programs: Program governance and metrics. *Information Systems Security*, *15*(6), 30–40. doi:10.1080/10658980601051482

Greenstadt, R., & Beal, J. (2008). *Cognitive security for personal devices*. Paper presented at the AISec '08.

Guinier, D. (1990). Identification by biometrics: An introduction and a survey. *SIGSAC Review*, 1-11.

Hall, J., & Liedtka, S. (2007). The Sarbanes-Oxley Act: Implications for large-scale IT outsourcing. *Communications of the ACM*, *50*(3), 95–100. doi:10.1145/1226736.1226742

Hess, R. (2005). Biometrics: It's not in the cards. *Record*, *17*(11), 30.

Jain, A., Hong, L., & Pankanti, S. (2000). Biometric identification. *Communications of the ACM*, *43*(2), 91–98. doi:10.1145/328236.328110

Jones, L., Anton, A., & Earp, J. (2007). *Towards understanding user perceptions of digital identity technologies*. Paper presented at the ACM Workshop on Privacy in the Electronic Society.

Juliet, L. (2006). Trends in biometrics. Retrieved 02/11/10, from http://www.libertysecurity.org/article1191.html

Kekre, H. B., & Bharadi, V. A. (2009). Adaptive feature set updating algorithm for multimodal biometrics. *International Conference on Advances in Computing, Communication and Control*, 277-282.

Messmer, E. (2004). Healthcare looks to biometrics. *Network World*. Retrieved from http://www.networkworld.com/news/2004/121304biometrics.html

Michigan Legislative Council. (2004). *Act 452 C.F.R.* Identity Theft Protection Act.

Morrissey, J. (2002). Access denied. *Modern Healthcare*, *32*(47), 22–25.

Nanavati, A., & Nanavati, M. (2002). *Biometrics: Identity verification in a networked world*. New York, New York: John Wiley & Sons, Inc.

National Science and Technology Council. (2006). Privacy & biometrics: Building a conceptual foundation. 1-57. Washington DC: National Science and Technology Council

Phillips, P., Martin, A., Wilson, C., & Przybocki, M. (2000). An introduction to evaluating biometric systems. *Computer*, *33*(2), 56–63. doi:10.1109/2.820040

Reid, P. (2004). *Biometrics for network security*. Upper Saddle River, New Jersey: Prentice Hall.

Rustad, M., & Koenig, T. (2007). Negligent entrustment liability for outsourced data. *Journal of Internet Law*, *10*(10), 3–6.

Stajano, F., & Anderson, R. (1999). *The resurrecting duckling: Security issues for ad-hoc wireless networks*. Paper presented at the 7th International Workshop on Security Protocols.

Vijayan, J. (2004). Corporate america slow to adopt biometric technologies. *Computerworld*. Retrieved from http://www.computerworld.com/s/article/95111/Corporate_America_Slow_to_Adopt_Biometric_Technologies

Yang, L., Winters, K., & Kizza, J. (2008). *Biometrics education with hands-on labs*. Paper presented at the ACM Southeast Conference '08.

Section 3
Ethical Implications of Security Monitoring in Health Care

Chapter 12
Ubiquitous Use of RFID in the Health Industry

Mary Brown
Capella University, USA

ABSTRACT

Radio Frequency Identification (RFID) technologies are becoming ubiquitous in a variety of settings and industries. The healthcare industry has adopted the use of RFID as a means of tracking equipment, managing inventory, to locating human resources including controversial applications involving injecting chips into humans as a means of authentication. There are a variety of ethical implications to the use of this technology as well as potential health concerns that will be explored in this chapter.

WHAT IS RFID?

One of the seminal works on Radio Frequency Identification (RFID) technology was first published by Stockman (1948) in conference proceedings for an International Radio Engineers conference. The idea that energy can be reflective and respond to a stimulant is at the root of how RFID works today.

RFID has been around since World War II when it combined radar with radio technology and was used by the British to differentiate friendly aircraft from enemy aircraft. This was accomplished by attaching a transponder to friendly aircraft which could be picked up by the allies. Landt (2005) suggests that following the recognition of how RFID might be made to work, the application of the technology was delayed as much as 30 years by the lack of other supporting technologies including transistors, integrated circuits and networking technologies. It is the integration of RFID to these other technologies that have resulted in the dramatic range of ways that RFID is currently being used or considered for use. The advent of

DOI: 10.4018/978-1-60960-174-4.ch012

these supporting technologies also means that the infrastructure to support RFID is becoming ubiquitous (wireless, satellites, communication technologies etc) creating an environment where the potential use of this technology in different applications continues to grow and expand.

RFID technology is being used in a wide range of activities these days, and there are some basic components that exist in all implementations of this technology. One of these basic components is an RFID tag or sensor that is typically located on a computer chip, although good progress has been made in the development of RFID tags that are printed onto a surface rather than manufacturing an actual chip. Subramanian and et al (2005) review some of the advancements in the creation of printed RFID tags which are thought to be capable of lowering the cost of the tags. It is the cost of tags that are one of the most significant barriers to adoption for large scale applications in areas such as manufacturing and shipping.

These RFID tags, regardless of their format, are programmed with a specific payload in the form of data. When a reader designed to stimulate and discharge the payload is applied to the sensor it transmits this data to the reader. The data that is fed to the reader using back spatter and is then transmitted, generally through wireless networks, to a backend database. According to Clampitt (2006) RFID technology is similar to bar code technology with the exception that, RFID tags are typically smaller and more durable than a typical bar code. The most important differentiator between an RFID tag and a bar code is that the bar code can tell someone in the supply chain that the item on which the code is attached is a certain type of peanut butter. If that same jar of peanut butter was instead attached to an RFID chip, the response would identify that unique instance of the certain type of peanut butter. It is this ability to use RFID to uniquely identify an object to which it has been attached that has created much interest in how this technology can be applied in the healthcare industry. It is also the crux at which

privacy experts see the opportunity for serious ethical implications in how the technology is used. For example, imagine a reader embedded in an anti-theft gateway of a high end department store. The customer is scanned as they pass into the store. The reader activates all of the tags embedded in the shoes, the skirt, the jacket, the purse of the customer and sends that information to an expert system database. The system analyzes the data from the tags, compares it with the inventory system and sends a personalized coupon to the customer on their cell phone. There are those who would embrace this kind of interaction and there are others for whom it would be just plain creepy.

Imagine that these same customer tags were sent to the cell phone of the sales rep with an analysis and recommendation that, based on the credit check done by validating the credit card chip in the purse, as to how much time and attention the sales person should spend on them.

These are examples of just two of the many different ethical and legal issues that can be associated with the use of RFID. The society has currently determined that health data is private based on the HIPAA and HITECH legislation (hhs.gov, 2010). The use of RFID within the health industry must include consideration of how these laws impact the security and privacy of the subject of health data.

RFID chips can be combined, as an example, with sensors used to measure temperature. Clampitt (2006) identifies important functionality that can be added to an RFID chip including the ability to register environmental conditions and other measurements that are capable of documenting the environment through which an RFID chip has travelled over space and time. For example, perishable items being transported can have an RFID chip and sensor attached to the packaging and, through the use of onboard memory that is updated along the way, can literally tell the person at the other end to what temperatures that package was exposed along the way.

RFID is being considered for use within the healthcare industry involving an array of activities and there are potential risks and impediments that are important to consider as part of exploring the use of this technology. Like cell phones, RFID technology involves emitting signals in an environment where sensitive medical equipment can be impacted and that can pose a risk to patient safety. Van der Togt & et al (2008) conducted a study that suggests significant interference that can occur between RFID technologies and some kinds of medical devices including respirators. There has been some challenge to this research including an editorial in the same journal in which the Van der Togt & et al study was published. In this editorial, Berwick (2008) challenges some of the methodologies that were used to create the study. He does, however, agree with the authors of the study that the results demonstrate that the introduction of technology into the complex healthcare environment must be done with an eye towards potential conflicts and incompatibilities that can threaten the health and welfare of patients.

Bennett and Osinski (2009) discuss research being done to enhance the research conducted by Berwick (2008) and to establish safety guidelines for the use of this technology in the acute healthcare setting. This creates concern and demonstrates a need for awareness and further research. This is particularly true given the voracity with which the healthcare industry has embraced this technology and the speed with which it is being integrated into healthcare environments.

CATEGORIES OF TYPICAL RFID USE IN HEALTHCARE

RFID is being used in an array of healthcare activities. It would be impossible to speak to all of the efforts underway using this technology. What this chapter will do is attempt to consider categories of use that are becoming typical to healthcare and to offer some examples that demonstrate how this technology is being used by healthcare providers around the globe.

Among the categories of activities that involve using RFID within healthcare are:

- **Patient and employee management:** Typically involves RFID chips injected into a patient or attached to a patient or their possessions with the goal of tracking their movements within a hospital or nursing home. An alternate use for RFID is tracking employee location and attendance through the use of RFID embedded access control cards.
- **Track medical assets:** RFID is attached to medical and surgical equipment with the objectives of improving patient safety and eliminating theft of expensive assets.
- **Track medical records:** RFID tags are attached to the medical record with the objective of being able to locate the record if misfiled or otherwise misplaced. Use of an RFID chip implanted into a patient that can be interrogated to gain access to the medical record has been piloted but this concept appears not to be gaining any traction in the general populace.
- **Track medication and medical supply charges:** RFID tags are attached to medical supplies, including medications, either at the vendor or as part of intake at the site of the provider. These tags can be combined with the tag that is embedded within the wrist bracelet of the patient creating an expense record within the patient billing system.
- **Improve infection control:** RFID tags implemented to provide oversight of caregiver hand washing activities. Tags are also associated with reusable surgical equipment such as scopes or other invasive equipment to validate sterilization activities between uses.

These categories represent a good sampling of some of the ways that RFID is being used primarily by healthcare providers. There are other projects underway in the homecare industry, the pharmaceutical industry and even a pilot to track artificial limbs that are representative of some of more specialized efforts that are outside of the scope of this paper.

RFID USE TO MANAGE PATIENTS AND EMPLOYEES

In 2004 VeriChip (2009) received FDA approval to begin injecting patients with a glass ampule that contains an RFID chip which is programmed with a unique 16 digit number. The idea is that this 16 digit number would be associated with the medical chart of the patient who would act as a kind of human interface to the computerized electronic record. This technology had previously been used widely by veterinarians who injected these chips into their furry patients in hopes that if they ran away from home they would be found and returned to their owner.

It is not surprising that this proposed use of RFID technology has been controversial and has created a range of discussions as to the risks and benefits of widespread injection of RFID chips as a means of identifying patients within the healthcare system. Albrecht and McIntyre (2005) were among the first to publically challenge the use of this technology as questionable and who charged that it presents an unacceptable risk to personal privacy.

The opposition to the use of the VeriChip as it was originally marketed generated a need for the company to rethink their strategy and to develop a new approach to marketing their product. One population that was targeted early on as a potential market for receiving a chip was the elderly. Sharp (2009) is among those who have worked in geriatric care and who have identified wandering behaviors as one of the most challenging aspects of caring for demented individuals. Long term care facilities had traditionally used physical and chemical restraints to combat wandering, a practice that became increasingly unacceptable to regulating industries and forcing these industries to look for more creative options. Holmerova & et al (2007) and Yamamoto and Aso (2009) describe some of the legal, ethical and moral issues that revolve around the practice of applying physical and chemical restraints to manage wandering behaviors in a demented population. Technology that can help to minimize some of the negative aspects of managing wandering and enhance personal freedom appears to be a useful tool to consider. Additional research may indicate, however, that using inject able RFID technology to track and contain demented patients to a particular location does not just introduce privacy issues, but may pose health risks as well.

The first health risk that came to the surface as possible through the use of injected RFID chips was a bit ironic. The original scenario used to market VeriChip technology was one where an unconscious patient is brought into an emergency room and the technology is then used to identify this patient and prevent potential problems such as allergic reactions and the like. The fact that someone had an embedded RFID chip is likely not something the typical emergency room doctor or nurse is going to consider making the scenario impractical. VeriChip attempted to deal with this by giving away readers to select providers so they might have one available in the event that they did think to scan for the unlikely event that the patient would have such a chip.

Privacy advocates responded that the well established Medic Alert (2009) bracelet system would serve the same purpose. Albrecht and McIntyre (2005) publicized widely that use of the chip to replace the Medic Alert system would not work because the presence of the chip is considered to be one of the conditions for which a patient, who, if found unconscious, cannot be placed in an MRI machine, so would need to wear a Medic

Alert bracelet. Murray (2004) suggests that while true, there are a range of medical implants and devices such as artificial joints and pacemakers that also may not be immediately apparent but would require that hospital staff avoid the use of MRI technology. He also suggests that opponents to RFID are perhaps using a double standard in how they apply logic to this particular technology and that they are not demanding that manufacturers stop making artificial joints because of the potential incompatibility with MRI technology. Another irony, one of the current ways that RFID chips are being applied is to embed them in those very artificial joints so they have the capacity to store historical information on the chip. These chips do not have any particular protections embedded in them meaning that anyone with access to a reader is able to discharge and read any information that is stored on that particular tag. This is an example of the impact that design can play in the potential security and privacy issues surrounding this technology. The ability to discharge the information on an RFID tag is trivial and inexpensive to do. Storing sensitive or personal information on the tag itself generates significantly different levels and types of risk than if the tag is merely used as a pointer to a record within a secure database.

A perhaps more serious charge related to the potential health impacts of injecting RFID into living creatures has recently begun to get attention. Recent studies point to the potential connection between the use of injected RFID chips and the presence of tumors. Lewan (2007) suggests that there were ample lab studies done in the 1990s that suggested a connection between RFID and the presence of cancerous tumors in lab mice and rats. He further suggests that this information must have been available to the FDA when they were reviewing the VeriChip request in 2004 to allow the use of this technology in human beings. He suggests that there may have been political alliances that may have prevented the FDA from rejecting the proposal or requiring further test-

ing into the potential cause and effect between implanted RFID and cancer.

The controversy surrounding the injection of RFID chips into patients has had an impact and it would appear that the vast majority of efforts currently underway involve the use of RFID chips that are attached to the patient in the form of a wrist band or some other device rather than actually embedding the chip inside of the patient. Those proponents of the injectable chip claim that demented patients are likely to remove their clothing which makes embedding the chip or attaching the chip to their clothing not a viable option.

Foreshew (2009) describes a system implemented in an Australian nursing home that has RFID gateways at the exits of the facility that alarm when a patient wearing an RFID chip embedded in a bracelet tries to pass through a doorway. Megan (2009) reports on an English City Council in Nottingham England that introduced RFID chips in the form of buttons that will be distributed to caregivers of demented residents for use in differentiating the clothing of each individual in hopes of solving yet another problem common to those who work in the long term care industry.

Demented patients are one common population that had the attention of the RFID technology industry. Another population that has been targeted by the RFID industry is newborns and newborn safety. Kidnapping of a newborn from a nursery is not a frequent event; however it is a significant concern for hospitals who apply a number of solutions to prevent this from ever happening. RFID technologies embedded into the wrist band of the mother and the infant can prevent the rare but disastrous impact of having infants switched or stolen. The technology differs in terms of available functionality. For example, Swedberg (2008) describes a solution that will not only alert if a tag is removed from an infant but will also alert if a tag is moved near unapproved doorways. Additionally the solution would shut and lock any doors that sense a tag nearby in an attempt to move into an unauthorized area. This is another good example of how complex and sophisticated solutions being developed can be using RFID combined with other technologies into an integrated solution.

There can be little doubt that RFID technology offers practical solutions for some stubborn problems within the healthcare industry involving managing patients who are unable to always fend for themselves. Albrecht and McIntyre (2005) warn that this may be the first step on the slippery slope and that surveillance technologies are introduced into society a bit at a time and then suffer from scope creep over which we, as a society, seem inept at recognizing and preventing until it becomes stifling and personally restrictive. One example is the use of RFID in transponders attached in our cars as a way of paying road tolls without having to stop and pay along the way. The fact that this information might become part of a divorce case or an employee lawsuit or some other criminal action through issuance of a subpoena is not something to which most of us have given much thought yet this is just one of the small ways in which we choose to surrender a piece of our privacy in exchange for convenience.

Although RFID technologies have been around for a long time, the ways in which it is being implemented is growing rapidly. Society will benefit from recognizing the risks as well as the benefits of using RFID to track human beings for a wide array of reasons and will take care to consider the impact on human freedom and dignity when deciding appropriate use of this technology.

Another group of individuals that are being impacted by the use of RFID technology are healthcare employees. Bacheldor (2008) describes how RFID access controls are being used in a Bangladesh hospital to track employee movements throughout the facility and to document their attendance. Srivastava (2005) describes some of the advantages that can be gained by the ability to track human assets. There is an additional benefit when RFID is associated with a caregiver, a patient and a billable asset tag to allow for item charging in a

more automated fashion than would be possible without benefit of RFID information integration. Gruber (2007) describes some of the ways that this technology may potentially be abused and may result in the violation of employee privacy rights. This technology is not unique in presenting a range of ethical issues that are situational and that are impacted more significantly by how the technology is implemented than by the implementation of the technology itself.

There are examples of organizations that have chosen to use inject able RFID chips as a means of access control however these are extreme examples. For the most part employee tracking is accomplished through the use of short range RFID chips embedded within an access card typically worn around the neck. Given the potential health issues being considered related to the use of inject able RFID, wearing this technology close to the skin for long periods of time may present some of the same concerns for employees required as a function of their employment to do so.

RFID USE TO TRACK MEDICAL ASSETS

Another widespread use of RFID technology within the healthcare industry involves the tracking of medical assets. Theft of medical equipment is a problem for many healthcare providers and, in particular, for hospitals. Scott (2006) and Wicks, Visich, & Li (2006) both describe some of the issues that hospitals in particular experience with the loss and theft of expensive medical equipment. They further describe a trend going on in hospitals to integrate RFID technologies with the enterprise wireless networks to track things like wheelchairs and other more high tech equipment. The basic idea behind these implementations is similar in nature. Valuable assets are, as a general practice, assigned inventory tags through the general accounting process. A challenge in most hospitals is that there are multiple entrances and exits and limited staff to secure these doorways. It has been easy work for someone to wander off with popular items such as wheelchairs or computers. Facilities interested in leveraging RFID technology implement a variation on the basic theme of RFID described at the beginning of this chapter. They install readers at the doorways that they want to control. They add to their procedures for intake of medical assets a step for adding an RFID tag to the asset. It is important that these tags be either well hidden or that they be of a type that will cause the system to alert if they are removed. Because RFID can be programmed to be far more sophisticated, as in the earlier example related to infant protection, when a thief tries to remove an asset that has been tagged, the reader in the doorway will send an alert and, if implemented to do so, can bar the doorway preventing the tag, the object to which the tag is attached, and the person driving both of them from leaving the facility.

Another variation on tracking assets using RFID includes tracking instruments and sponges during surgery to ensure that they are all removed from the patient at the end of the operation. There are so many examples of surgical sponges left behind inside of patients after surgery that there is actually a diagnosis for it which is a 'gossypiboma.' Berkowitz, Marshall, and Charles (2007) cites a study that claims the frequency of gossypibomas to be 1000 in every 18,000 operations.. The idea is that all of the sponges used during surgery are tagged with an RFID chip that is the size of a grain of sand. The reader is passed over the patient prior to the patient being surgically closed and any sponges that might remain inside of the patient will alert at the passing of the reader notifying the surgeon to look a little further before continuing. Roger, Jones and Oleynikov (2007) published a study describing the benefits of using RFID tagged sponges to prevent human error involving sewing up patients with sponges still inside of them. They compare the $5000 cost of the RFID reader

against the potentially multi-million dollar lawsuit that could result from an accident or death caused by failure to remove all of the surgical sponges from a patient. Adoption of various types of technology within the healthcare industry, as in most industries, soon become sufficiently integrated that it becomes the best practice or industrial norm. RFID embedded sponges are but one example of the way that RFID technologies begin through small isolated projects and grow to become one of those industry norms.

A less frequent but nonetheless significant problem is also retention of surgical instruments within the body of the patient. Berkowitz, Marshall, and Charles (2007) cite several studies that all estimate the problem to be one instrument left behind for every 1,500 or so operations. They identify particularly high risk situations such as surgery of a morbidly obese patient or in emergent or unexpected changes in routine procedures as situations that increase the risk of losing surgical instruments. The same technology that can be used to track and find surgical sponges can also be applied to surgical instruments. There are particular kinds of RFID tags that will not only prevent instruments from being left behind but that as De Martini (2008) indicates can be programmed to both withstand the temperatures of the sterilization process that is used to clean surgical instruments and to provide reports that validate that the instrument experienced the proper temperatures for the proper amount of time to ensure that it is properly sterile. One of the important advancements being explored by RFID manufacturers is to develop highly robust tags that can tolerate great extremes and still allow for re-use. The cost of RFID tags is a significant barrier to their use and, when combined with other technologies, these costs can become prohibitive. The ability to re-use the tags helps to defray some of the expense.

RFID USE TO TRACK MEDICAL RECORDS

A more recent use of RFID in the healthcare industry is tracking medical records. Bacheldor (2006) describes a large project involving the U.S. Army and an attempt to better track and manage access to the medical files of the soldiers who serve at Fort Hood. Medical files are tagged with passive ID tags and readers are placed at strategic locations within the file room which are able to read these tags and report on them electronically allowing staff at half dozen clinics visibility into the location of charts across all of the clinics. Ferguson (2006) also writes about this implementation and adds that one of the objectives of this implementation includes the elimination of typical human errors such as misfiling and creation of duplicate records. It is expected that as the industry moves from paper charts to electronic health record systems the need to track these paper charts will eventually be phased out of normal procedures by most providers.

Another form of integrating RFID and medical records comes in the form of a smart card which is similar to a credit card however contains an RFID chip and is used to store health updates that are then given to the patient allowing them access to their information. SmartCardAlliance (2006) documents several hospitals conducting pilots that involve the use of smart cards on which health information is updated at each patient visit. It is clear in some of these circumstances how the issue of having a compatible device with which to read the information on the card is being handled and in some cases it is not. It is important however to remember that the RFID chip is only one of the necessary components of this technology and that distribution of a compatible reader is also necessary as part of a successful implementation. An additional concern with moving the care of the medical record to the subject of the data is lack of the same kinds of redundant and backup systems that has been the case with provider controlled health data. Will patients who lose their smart cards have any means by which to restore or recreate that data? If the data is stored in redundancy with the provider then has the impact been to create yet another copy of the data that has to be protected from potential abuse or misuse?

RFID USE TO TRACK MEDICATION AND MEDICAL SUPPLIES

A common challenge for hospitals and clinics is tracking and charging the correct patients for medical supplies that are used in the course of their treatment. Hospitals have used everything from billing sheets to stickers in an attempt to get busy caregivers to devote sufficient time and attention to the use of supplies and to charging them to the proper patients. This is particularly true in extreme situations such as those often found within emergency and operating rooms where the attention is on saving the life of the patient and where the largest use of medical supplies is likely going on in consecutive fashion. The presence of a reader within these emergency treatment spaces can be used to identify and record the presence of the provider who is using the supplies, the patient on whom the supplies are being used and the supplies themselves, all through combining the data that the reader obtains through automatic interrogation of each of the RFID chips and transmitting that information to a backend database. Anonymous (adaptinfo2.com, 2010) describes one example of an RFID system capable of offering this kind of functionality to an organization sufficiently motivated to implement it. Walton (2003) describes a similar system using bar codes in place of RFID and represents a more commonly used approach that is slowly being replaced with the more sophisticated, yet more expensive RFID based systems.

When combined with Computerized Provider Order Entry (CPOE) systems RFID tracking of medication is an effective means of secondary checking. Checking identity of a patient twice has become one of the hallmarks of safe medication administration. Scanning the medication tag and the tag on the bracelet of the patient also provides an audit trail that includes what was given, what time it was given, who it was that gave the drug. Because the medication itself is not the item to which the tag is attached, it is still possible for those who are motivated to collect inaccurate data to be able to do so.

As is true with collection of audit information in general, the information gathered through the association of several RFID tags can prove both harmful and beneficial to the organizations that collect it. For example, if a lawsuit including the audit information gathered by the RFID system reveals that a patient who died received the wrong medication or medication that was late or early, that might just as well work against the organization as much as if it reveals that everything was done properly.

RFID USE TO IMPROVE INFECTION CONTROL

An interesting and complex application of RFID is the monitoring of health staff and the frequency with which they wash their hands. Dynamic Computing Corporation (2009) published a white paper that includes data that supports the importance of proper hand washing by hospital staff in the prevention of infections. Ray (2009) describes an effort by a Miami health center to use RFID in this fashion as a means of enhancing infection control. Staff members that interact with patients are given a badge that contains an RFID chip within it. Those in possession of one of these badges walks up to a soap dispenser that contains a reader that reads the identity contained in the data stored on the badge. It then transmits that information back to a backend database. As the staff member then approaches the bedside of patients, there is also a reader that will determine the length of time

that has passed between the time when the badge was read by the soap dispenser and will make a determination whether or not the caregiver is in compliance with the infection control policy. If it is determined that there has been too much time that has passed, or if the caregiver appears at the bedside of another patient without first approaching a soap dispenser, the technology will issue a verbal reminder to this caregiver to first wash their hands before continuing with their activities. There were no conclusions drawn in these examples what the impact may be on the poor patient who may find comfort in this electronic snitch or may find the whole idea disconcerting.

CONCLUSION

This chapter has addressed a variety of ways in which RFID technology is being integrated into the day to day activities of the healthcare industry. The use of RFID to facilitate the flow of inanimate objects in inventory and billing activities and to protect medical assets from theft or loss are reasonably uncontroversial and can be reasonably seen to add value to the healthcare industry. It is the association of RFID with individuals that creates controversy and introduces a range of ethical issues that cannot be ignored.

Injected RFID solutions have been embraced by small groups of individuals for a range of activities. The circumstances that would require this approach as opposed to a less invasive approach of attaching a tag to an individual are rare and resulted in an overall rejection of this form of RFID implementation. The potential health risks that have been raised including an increase in tumors and a concern as to what would happen to a chip if a patient were inadvertently put into an MRI machine have contributed to the rejection of this approach to RFID monitoring of patients in healthcare.

The practice of using RFID to track staff and patients through the use of RFID embedded bracelets and access control cards is much more common and is the approach that is more likely to become even more commonplace over time. Controlling the movements of demented patients and ensuring the security of infants inside of the hospital are just two of the more obvious ways that the technology is believed to be beneficial. While there may be a perception of privacy violations through the tracking of staff through the use of RFID, the reality is that many rational individuals acknowledge that an employee is an agent of their employer and that the employer has the right to set work rules. There are very few individuals who feel strongly enough about the privacy implications of this technology to jeopardize their employment by refusing to cooperate with an employer who insists on its use. Despite some of the potential risks to health and privacy that are currently under review, there are no laws, either state or federal that would prohibit an employer from requiring that an employee wear an RFID tracking system as a condition of their employment.

RFID was, in the past, perceived as relatively simplistic technology with a limited application. As manufacturers add sophistication to the technology such as creating tags that are both able to withstand sterilization procedures and also to report on events associated with the items to which the tag has been attached, there is opportunity to introduce combined functionality that further leverages this technology to solve stubborn healthcare problems. Dix (2006) describes an incident at a VA hospital where improper sterilization of endoscopic equipment resulted in the transference of Hepatitis between an infected patient and those who were not infected. Use of RFID tags that validate the time and temperatures under which equipment is cleaned may have prevented this unfortunate incident.

RFID technology has the potential to do much good in the healthcare industry. As is true with all technologies it also has the potential to be misused making it important for those implementing this technology to consider what controls can be used to limit or avoid misuse. If someone were to spend time researching RFID technology stakeholders they would find little information or attention relative to the ethical and privacy implications of using this technology. There are those including Albrecht and McIntyre (2005) who make a compelling argument for the wisdom of tackling these tough issues at the outset and formulating rules and strategies for mitigating the concerns rather than putting them in the background in hopes that inattention will somehow make them less of an issue in the long run.

RFID is not unique in that it is just one of a number of technologies that rely on information security controls in order to ensure the privacy of the information. What is unique is that most data, particularly health data that is considered particularly sensitive, is protected through the use of access and authentication controls that involve an owner or steward of the data granting me overt permission through creation of a user account or other security control. The vast majority of RFID chips, due to the need to keep the cost per chip as low as possible and because of a lack of industry norms or standards, can be interrogated and the data on the chip read by anyone with access to a reader which according to Anonymous (Intermec, 2010) are freely available on the Internet.

There are a range of controls that are available to those providers who choose to pay for the extra functionality. These include chips that will only respond to authorized readers or which otherwise limit the ability of a rogue reader to gain access to data. Another useful tool for those implementing these technologies is to limit the information that is physically stored on the chip itself. By using the chip merely as a pointer to a row in the database it is possible to rely on another range of security controls that are typically used to secure data at rest in a database.

Encryption is a technology that is applied in limited fashion. RFID chips have a limited amount of space (known as gates) into which data can be read or written. Manufacturers and those who use the chips have been loath in general to using any of that available space for the purposes of security and privacy.

If the recent past is any indicator, the use of RFID will expand, both within the healthcare industry, and within society in general. The use of this technology to track inanimate objects has been slowly increasing as some of the early technical issues have been resolved through the efforts of early adopters and those who see the potential savings that might be gained once the technology stabilizes. The early adopters of this technology, according to Weier (2008) includes Wal-Mart that proposed in 2008 to begin applying a $2 surcharge to their Sam's Club suppliers for every pallet that was shipped to them without benefit of RFID tracking.

For privacy experts it is not these pallet level shipping applications of RFID that create concern but application of tags to individual packaging and the potential implications of customers taking those tags, associated with items they have bought, out of the stores and into their homes. When the items to which these tags are associated include health related items such as specific medications or other medical supplies that may be private in nature, there is a certain level of risk of exposure of this information. How extreme is that risk or what the potential impact could be is unknown. Privacy experts would like to see any application of RFID that could lead to tracking the activities or movements of an individual be evaluated for the potential security and privacy implications and that manufacturers and users of these tags be required to mitigate any risks that are identified.

Despite a number of characteristics involving the use of RFID that have created opposition or concern as to how it is being used, it is, nonetheless, being used increasingly for a broad range of applications. The growth of this technology is occurring in large part through a wide range of pilot or small projects or, in the case of Wal-Mart and the Department of Defense, in a slice of a particular sector. It is expected that these pilot projects, if they are able to demonstrate the kinds of cost savings that are expected within the supply chains of the early adopters, are likely to breed even more pilot projects. If history is an example as to how this growth is going to occur it would suggest that healthcare providers who want to leverage these benefits are well advised to address the security and privacy implications of their projects prior to experiencing an unhappy incident involving the loss or exposure of sensitive data.

REFERENCES

Albrecht, K., & McIntyre, L. (2005). *SpyChips: How major corporations and government plan to track your every move with RFID* (1st ed.). Nashville, TN: Thomas Nelson, Inc.

Anonymous. (2010). *How RFID tracking helps hospitals and patients.* Retrieved May 24, 2010, from http://www.adaptinfo2.com/software/how-rfid-tracking-helps-hospitals-and-patients

Anonymous. (2010). *–Department of Health and Human Services-health information privacy.* Retrieved May 25, 2010, from http://www.hhs.gov/ocr/privacy/

Anonymous. (2010). *Scalable RFID from the industry experts.* Retrieved May 24, 2010, from http://www.intermec.com/products/rfid/index.aspx?utm&gclid=COGcqevdr6ICFWE45wodqWpl4g

Bacheldor, B. (2006). *Fort hood to RFID-tag medical records.* Retrieved 9/28, 2009, from http://www.rfidjournal.com/article/articleview/2536/1/1/

Bacheldor, B. (2008). *RFID takes root in Bangladesh early adopters include Apollo hospitals Dhaka and the Bangladesh army.* Retrieved 9/28, 2009, from http://www.rfidjournal.com/article/print/3852

Berkowitz, S. BSC, Marshall, H., & Charles, A., MD, FRCSI. (2007). Retained intra-abdominal surgical instruments: Time to use nascent technology? *The American Surgeon, 73*(11), 1083. Retrieved from http://proquest.umi.com.library.capella.edu/pqdweb?did=1419318761&Fmt=7&clientId=62763&RQT=309&VName=PQD

Berwick, D. M. (2008). Taming the technology beast. *Journal of the American Medical Association, 299*(24), 2898–2899. doi:10.1001/jama.299.24.2898

Brenner, B. (2009). 6 ways we gave up our privacy. *CSOonline*, 1-3.

Clampitt, H. (2006). The RFID handbook. Retrieved from http://www.rfidhandbook.blogspot.com/.

De Martini, C. (2008). Brothers in arms. *Health Management Technology, 29*(9), 40. Retrieved June 7, 2010, from http://proquest.umi.com.library.capella.edu/pqdweb?did=1554990491&Fmt=7&clientId=62763&RQT=309&VName=PQD

Dix, K. (2006). *Best practices for scope reprocessing endoscope-related infections and keeping the numbers negligible.* Retrieved September 28, 2009, from http://www.infectioncontroltoday.com/articles/651cover.html

Dynamic Computer Corporation. (2009). *RFID-integrated technologies for infection control: Background and technology comparison on key adoption considerations.* White Paper. Farmington Hills, MI: Dynamic Computer Coporation.

Ferguson, R. B. (2007). *Army taps 3M for RFID tracking of medical records.* Retrieved September 28, 2009, from http://www.eweek.com/c/a/Mobile-and-Wireless/Army-Taps-3M-for-RFID-Tracking-of-Medical-Records/

Foreshew, J. (August 25, 2009). AGED-CARE provider PresCare investigated a range of electronic aids for residents at its newest Queensland site. *AustalianIT.News.com.*

Holmerová, I., Jurasková, B., Kalvach, Z., Rohanová, E., Rokosová, M., & Vanková, H. (2007). Dignity and palliative care in dementia. *The Journal of Nutrition, Health & Aging, 11*(6), 489. Retrieved from http://proquest.umi.com.library.capella.edu/pqdweb?did=1402659161&Fmt=7&clientId=62763&RQT=309&VName=PQD.

Landt, J. (2005). The history of RFID. *IEEE Potentials*, 8-11.

Lewan, T. (September 8, 2007). Cancer fears raised over chip implants. *USA Today.*

MedicAlert. (2009). *About us.* Retrieved September 25, 2009, from http://www.medicalert.org/Main/AboutUs.aspx

Murray, C. (2004). *Chip for humans a blessing to some, a curse to others.* Retrieved from http://www.embedded.com/news/embeddedindustry/54201016?_requestid=152134

PublicTechnology. (2009). *Nottingham city council to use RFID to improving care for citizens.* Retrieved September 25, 2009, from http://www.publictechnology.net/modules.php?op=modload&name=News&file=article&sid=17599&mode=thread&order=0&thold=0

Ray, B. (2009). *Miami health centre starts RFID soap snooping.* Retrieved November 28, 2009, from http://www.theregister.co.uk/2009/08/18/rfid_soap_monitoring/

Rogers, A., Jones, E., & Oleynikov, D. (2007). Radio frequency identification (RFID) applied to surgical sponges. *Surgical Endoscopy, 21*(7), 1235. Retrieved from http://proquest.umi.com.library.capella.edu/pqdweb?did=1297025351&Fmt=7&clientId=62763&RQT=309&VName=PQD. doi:10.1007/s00464-007-9308-7

Scott, M. (2006). So that's where it is. *Hospitals & Health Networks, 80*(4), 28. Retrieved from http://proquest.umi.com.library.capella.edu/pqdweb?did=1033282571&Fmt=7&clientId=62763&RQT=309&VName=PQD.

Sharp, D. PhD, RN. (2009). Evidence-based protocols for managing wandering behaviors. *Nursing Education Perspectives, 30*(4), 258. Retrieved from http://proquest.umi.com.library.capella.edu/pqdweb?did=1850876381&Fmt=7&clientId=62763&RQT=309&VName=PQD

SmartCardAlliance. (2006). *Smart card applications in the U.S. healthcare industry.* Retrieved September 28, 2009, from http://www.smartcardalliance.org/newsletter/february_2006/feature_0206.html

Stockman, H. (1948). Communication by means of reflective power. [IRE]. *Proceedings of the Institute of Radio Engineers, 36,* 1196–1204.

Subramanian, V., Frechet, J. M. J., Chang, P. C., Huang, D. C., Lee, J. B., & Molesa, S. E. (2005). Progress toward development of all-printed RFID tags: Materials, processes, and devices. [Berkeley, CA.]. *Proceedings of the IEEE, 93*(7), 1330–1338. doi:10.1109/JPROC.2005.850305

Swedberg, C. (2008). *Tamper-resistant RFID infant-tracking system improves security.*

Van Oranje, C., Schindler, R., Valeri, L., Vilamovska, A. M., Hatziandreu, E., & Conkin, A. (2009). *Study on the requirements and options for radio frequency identification (RFID) application in healthcare (RFID No. TR-608-EC).* Cambridge, UK: Rand Europe.

VeriChip. (2009). *About us.* Retrieved September 25, 2009, from http://www.verichipcorp.com/about_us.html

Walton, G. (2003). *Medication administration: A wireless safety net.* Retrieved from http://www.ehealthinternational.org/pdfs/Walton.pdf

Weier, M.H. (January 19, 2008). Wal-Mart gets tough on RFID. *InformationWeek.*

Wicks, A. M., Visich, J. K., & Li, S. (2006). Radio frequency identification applications in hospital environments. *Hospital Topics, 84*(3), 3. Retrieved from http://proquest.umi.com.library.capella.edu/pqdweb?did=1086998281&Fmt=7&clientId=62763&RQT=309&VName=PQD. doi:10.3200/HTPS.84.3.3-9

Yamamoto, M., & Aso, Y. (2009). Placing physical restraints on older people with dementia. *Nursing Ethics, 16*(2), 192. Retrieved from http://proquest.umi.com.library.capella.edu/pqdweb?did=1651874511&Fmt=7&clientId=62763&RQT=309&VName=PQD. doi:10.1177/0969733008100079

Chapter 13
Caught in the Web:
The Internet and the Demise of Medical Privacy

Keith A. Bauer
USA

ABSTRACT

The social consequences of the internet are profound. Evidence of this can easily be found in the enormous body of literature discussing its impact on democracy, globalization, social networking, and education. The implications of the internet for medicine have likewise received a great deal of attention from policy makers, clinicians and technology theorists. Medical privacy, in particular, has garnered the lion's share of attention. Nevertheless, research in this area has been lacking because it either fails to unpack the conceptual and ethical complexities of privacy or overestimates the power of technology and policy to protect our medical privacy. The aims of this chapter are twofold. The first is to provide a nuanced explication of the concept of privacy, and, second, to argue that e-medicine and the policies supposedly designed to protect the privacy and confidentiality of personal health information fail to do so and in some instances make their violations easier to commit.

INTRODUCTION

The internet is increasingly being employed to provide medical services to patients (clinical uses)[1] and to manage, store, and transmit patient health information (non-clinical or administrative uses). The relatively new application of the internet within the field of medicine has come to be known as electronic medicine or *e-medicine*.[2] E-medicine is a subset of telemedicine, which

DOI: 10.4018/978-1-60960-174-4.ch013

the Institute of Medicine (IOM) defines in the following manner:

Telemedicine is the use of telecommunications and information technologies to share and to maintain patient health information and to provide clinical care and health education to patients and professionals when distance separates the participants (Field, 1996).

The IOM's definition can be made more specific, by (a) emphasizing a particular technology such as the internet, (b) making a distinction between clinical and non-clinical applications, and (c) conceiving telemedicine either as an integrated system of healthcare delivery or a mere collection of electronic tools.

For our purpose, e-medicine will primarily refer to the electronic medium of the internet and those patients and consumers who access healthcare information from medical websites or have portions of their healthcare managed online by healthcare professionals (Bashshur, Sanders, et al. 1997). Common examples of e-medicine include (a) online-accessible electronic health records (EHR), (b) electronic mail (e-mail), and (c) internet-based networks that link insurance companies, hospitals, individual healthcare professionals, and patients.

Furthermore, e-medicine is not simply medicine's use of information and communication technologies (ICTs); rather, in the context of e-medicine, ICTs such the internet *are* medical technology. According to the Office of Technology Assessment (OTA), medical technology includes "the drugs, devices, and medical and surgical procedures used in medical care and the organization and support systems within which such care is provided" (Lashof, 1981). Because the internet as well as other information and communication technology can be subsumed under "the organization and support systems within which such care is provided," the internet can be

broadly construed as a type of medical technology under the OTA's definition.

E-medicine has a number of already proven benefits, including improvements in health care quality; prevention of medical errors; reduced health care costs; increased administrative efficiencies; decreased paperwork, and expanded access to healthcare (HHS, 2008). However, the continued adoption of computerized patient records and the expanding use of the internet by patients and healthcare professionals as a place to post, find, store, and transit health-related information have only led to even greater concerns about the integrity of medical privacy and confidentiality and who should have access to health-related information. This in turn has raised additional concerns over the potentially deleterious results for healthcare quality, provider-patient relationships, and patients' overall confidence in our healthcare system(s) (Bauer, 2004).

THE CONCEPT OF PRIVACY

But what exactly are we talking about when we discuss *privacy*? Answering this question may appear intuitively straightforward, but the fact of the matter is that defining *privacy* and privacy-related concepts such as *confidentiality* is not as straightforward as it appears, as there is no universally accepted definition, theory, or justification for privacy within the philosophical, legal, and public policy literature. Because of the nebulous nature of privacy, the identification and analysis of important privacy issues associated with internet-based healthcare can be difficult. Despite this limitation, privacy can be analyzed in terms of (1) the nature of privacy, (2) the coherence and distinctiveness of privacy, (3) the contingency or cultural relativity of privacy, and (4) the normative status of privacy (Schoeman 1984). These elements of privacy are important in understanding what is meant by *privacy* and why it is ethically significant in the context of e-medicine.

The Nature of Privacy

Questions about the nature of privacy typically center on (a) examining competing definitions of privacy and (b) determining whether privacy is a moral right. Three definitions of privacy are common (Schoeman 1984). First, privacy can be defined as a *moral right* or *entitlement* that individuals have to determine what personal information may be disclosed or communicated to others.[3] Second, privacy can be defined as the *control* persons have over (a) personal information, (b) intimacies of personal identity, or (c) who has sensory access to them. Third, privacy can be defined as the *state or condition of limited access by others to a person's* (a) information, (b) thoughts, and/or (c) body. As I shall explain, all three definitions of privacy have strengths and weaknesses.

First, defining privacy as a moral right or entitlement assumes that privacy is morally significant, but fails to identify exactly what is morally significant about it. What is needed in this definition, but lacking, is an account of why privacy is important to persons. One could argue that privacy's importance is intuitively self evident and requires no explanation. The epistemologically problem with this position is that not everyone shares the same intuitions about privacy's importance. As such, the subsequent problem is determining how and by what criteria conflicting intuitions about privacy's importance should be adjudicated. As a form of knowledge, intuition has a place, but it also has significant limitations that should not be dismissed.

Second, to make privacy synonymous with *control* over (a) personal information, (b) personal identity, or (c) who has sensory access to us, does specify what is morally significant about privacy and avoids the problem of simply stipulating that privacy is an individual moral right. Yet, the problem with defining privacy this way is that there are clear cases in which persons can have privacy without having control and other cases in which persons can have control without having privacy. In the first instance, a person stranded alone on a desert island has privacy, but does not have control over personal information and who has sensory access to himself. In the second instance, persons can freely disclose to others their most intimate thoughts. Here, persons have control over the intimate thoughts they divulge to others, but they no longer have privacy (Rachels 1984; Schoeman 1984).[4]

Third, to define privacy as the state or condition of limited access that others have to a person's (a) information, (b) thoughts, and/or (c) body, is superior to the other definitions of privacy because it allows us to remain agnostic about privacy's status as a moral right and to evaluate infringements of privacy independent of a person's control. Under this definition, persons have privacy to the extent that others have limited access to them. But a central problem with this approach is in reaching a consensus on what will count as the states and conditions of limited access by others, for example, in one's home or the workplace. Under what conditions is it ethically permissible for the police and employers to violate one's privacy in these contexts?

The Coherence and Distinctiveness of Privacy

Thus far, it has been assumed that privacy is both a coherent and distinctive moral value. The *coherence thesis of privacy* holds that diverse privacy claims and issues have in common the fundamental moral value of privacy (Schoeman 1984). The *distinctiveness thesis of privacy* holds that there are moral values and principles distinct from privacy that can be used to defend privacy claims (Schoeman 1984). For theorists who favor these two theses, privacy, as a coherent and distinct moral value, unites seemingly disparate privacy issues and reflects a unique and diverse social reality that other values, such as *autonomy* and *respect for persons*, fail to do. There are, however, theorists who reject both of the aforementioned theses of privacy. Their general argument is that the coherence thesis should be rejected because different privacy claims or issues actually reflect different and unrelated moral values (e.g., autonomy, the right to property), which very often do not cohere with each other.

In addition, because of this lack of coherence, many of the some theorists argue that the distinctiveness thesis ought to be rejected because privacy can be reduced to other more basic legal and moral values and principles. Following this line of reasoning, instead of talking about a person's right to privacy, it would better to understand privacy and its violations in terms of the more basic values of autonomy and respect for persons and the better established rights of property.[5]

The Historical Relativity of Privacy

Arguments for and against the cultural and historical relativity of privacy typically involve two theses: (1) *the thesis of historical variation*, which includes the consideration of whether any notion of privacy is recognized, and (2) *the thesis of the privacy criterion* (Schoeman 1984).

The *historical variation* thesis centers on determining whether all cultures and societies throughout history have valued privacy. To the chagrin of some privacy theorists, evidence of privacy's cultural and historical contingency is fairly well established. In fact, before Warren and Brandeis penned their famous 1890 law review article on privacy, the legal right to privacy remained undifferentiated from the right to property and was not a central concern for American society (Warren & Brandeis 1984). Regarding this point, Amitai Etzioni writes that "American society only had a vague social concept of privacy, albeit one that was not embedded in a distinct legal doctrine or constitutional right" (Etzioni, 1999). An explicit concern for privacy only emerged as a result of the political, social, and technological changes that sweep across America during the late nineteenth and early twentieth centuries.

If accepted, what are the implications of the cultural and historical contingency of privacy? One consequence is that there is no natural or absolute right to privacy and that definitions of privacy, the values they reflect, and what counts as public and private are plastic and subject to regular modification. However, even if we believe that particular right to privacy are culturally and historically contingent, it does not follow that the right to privacy is itself contingent. Instead, it may mean that some persons, cultures, and societies have just failed to recognize privacy's inherent value.

The *privacy criterion thesis* centers on determining whether there are items, conditions, and aspects of personal and social life that are inherently, rather than conventionally, private. Unlike the *thesis of historical and cultural variation*, this thesis is not concerned with how cultures, past and present, deal with privacy; rather, it is concerned with identifying and establishing standards for judging what *ought* to be private. One major problem with this approach is that any criterion of privacy is subject to revision and modification. For example, we could take as the criterion of privacy those areas of one's life that are of no consequence to the interests of others (e.g., medical information, one's home). However, as soon as one's personal medical information and home is deemed to affect the interests of others in some significant way (e.g., public health, medical research, and child abuse prevention) they cease to be inherently private.

The Normative Nature of Privacy & Its Ethical Justification

The fourth privacy issue pertains to its normative status and ethical justification. In the majority of the telemedicine literature on privacy, a particular definition of privacy is usually stipulated and functions to describe what information and spaces are to be protected and secured. This, of course, is very important to the success of e-medicine. What is missing, however, in a descriptive approach to privacy are normative considerations of what counts as the ethically appropriate and ethically inappropriate items, conditions, and means of securing privacy.

The concept of privacy implicitly denotes the existence of *legitimate* barriers; illegitimate barriers are seen as fostering concealment or secrecy, terms that imply illicit, if not illegal behavior. That is, both the scope of privacy and the nature of the specific acts that are encompassed by definitions of privacy (e.g., sexual behavior, voting) rather than excluded (e.g., office mail, including e-mail, the private lives of public figures) reflect a society's particular values (Etzioni, 1999). If we accept this position, then what one considers private automatically privileges some values, subordinates others, and possibly overlooks other values altogether. Here, privacy is a social category. As such, notions of privacy not only describe various social relations, practices, and norms, but also have normative functions that prescribe, usually implicitly, what social relations, practices, and norms are ethically appropriate and permissible (Benn & Gaus, 1983). Therefore, from a normative standpoint, the issue is not that there are barriers to one's privacy, but rather which barriers are ethically legitimate and which are not.

To date, the majority of the telemedicine literature remains normatively a-theoretical, as it makes no explicit ethical commitments justifying privacy. Nonetheless, e-medicine practitioners and policy makers tacitly engage in ethical decision making and justification when weighing the respective harms and benefits to patient privacy and confidentiality associated with the practice of cybermedicine. In most cases, a mixture of consequentialist and deontological justifications are employed.

From a consequentialist perspective, privacy and confidentiality have *instrumental value*, are a means to an end, because they serve to promote important social goals, including the enhancement of individuality, self-determination, and the freedom to cultivate intimate relationships free from public life (Rachels, 2005). Without a clear demarcation between public and private domains, autonomous individuals, and voluntary relationships would be difficult, if not impossible, to achieve (Edwards 1988). Without a clear demarcation between public and private domains, the autonomous individuals, families, voluntary associations, and homes that constitute liberal democracies would not be possible (Habermas 1989).

In the healthcare realm, a consequentialist justification of privacy and confidentiality has ethical significance because it addresses specific goals such as the promotion of provider-patient relationships and the protection of patients' social status. More generally, privacy and confidentiality have instrumental value because they can help to maximize good patient care and minimize potential patient harm. These two ends are encapsulated in the ethical principles of *beneficence* (i.e., promote the medical good of patients) and *non-malfeasance* or *primum non nocere* ("first of all, do no harm" to patients). Healthcare institutions and individual providers that fail to protect patient privacy and confidentiality violate these fundamental principles.

Unlike a consequentialist approach, a deontological approach (i.e., rule- or duty-based ethics), does not ethically justify privacy and confidentiality by their utility, that is, their instrumental value to maximize good consequences and to minimize bad consequences for patients.[6] Instead, deontological justifications justify privacy and confidentiality in terms of *respect for persons*, which is grounded in the more fundamental principle of *autonomy* (Kant, 1991). From a deontological standpoint, privacy and confidentiality and claims against unauthorized access to patient information are justified in terms of the *intrinsic value* and dignity of autonomous persons, not their instrumental value and the ends they serve. Stated differently, privacy and confidentiality help to protect the moral agency of patients by allowing them to live their lives as they choose (Walters, 1982). In light of these deontological considerations, many countries and international treaties consider privacy to be a fundamental and unalienable right. For example, both the UN Declaration of Human Rights and the International Covenant on Civil and Political Rights recognize the right to privacy. In these treaties, privacy is recognized as a form of autonomy—a way to ensure protection from "arbitrary interference" (United Nations, 1948).

THE CONCEPT OF CONFIDENTIALITY

Confidentiality is similar to privacy to the extent that both concepts generally refer to limiting the access that others have to one's body, thoughts, feelings, documents, and living spaces. Confidentiality is also like privacy in that both concepts generally refer to what is out of the public domain. It is these shared characteristics that explain why privacy and confidentiality are sometimes confused and used interchangeably. These two notions, however, are very different from each other (Walters, 1982).

First, privacy, broadly construed, pertains to the bodies, thoughts, feelings, documents, information, and living spaces of persons, while confidentiality is best understood as a complex of moral, social, and legal practices for protecting privacy.

Second, confidentiality requires at least one person to give up his or her personal privacy to another person in the context of a trust- and promise-based relationship. Disclosure may occur, for example, in professional relationships among healthcare providers and their patients, among lawyers and their clients, or in the informal and non-professional relationships existing among

friends and intimates. Thus, unlike privacy, confidentiality is always relational and must include at least two persons or agents, one of whom discloses private information to the other with the expectation that the disclosed information will remain confidential.

In cybermedicine, disclosures and confidentiality may not always directly involve two persons. This occurs, for example, when patients complete online health forms or give health information to online interactive software designed to diagnose depression and anxiety. According to the Science Panel on Interactive Communication and Health, these sorts of health disclosures will become more common:

In the near future, personal health information will be generated during clinical and non-clinical encounters in disparate settings, such as schools, mobile immunization clinics, public places, and the home. In fact, many health encounters may not even involve a health professional or a person, but rather, an intelligent software agent may be the intermediary (Robinson, Patrick, Eng & Gustavson, 1999).

Therefore, as long as these patients have good reasons to expect their disclosures to remain confidential, confidentiality, in the context of e-medicine, does not require two persons (Winslade, 1995).

Breaching Confidentiality

According to the Hippocratic Oath, healthcare professionals have a moral obligation or duty to protect patient confidences:

What I may see or hear in the course of treatment or even outside of the treatment in regard to the life of men, which on no account one must spread abroad, I will keep to myself holding such things shameful to be spoken about (Edelstein, 1943).

However, unlike Hippocrates and the vast majority of western medicine's history, the duty of patient confidentiality in contemporary healthcare is not thought of as a sacred obligation or absolute rule:

The principle of confidentiality was deemed sacred, and the possibility of breaching this trust was diminished by the limited record-keeping practices of the early 20th century: the typical health record was simply a small ledger card with entries showing the dates of the patient's visits, treatment prescribed, and service fees (Bruce, 1984).

Change in confidentiality's status is due to a number of converging social and technological factors, which include increased medical knowledge, professional specialization, need for greater specificity of information to improve public health and medical research, as well as advances in information and communication technologies. What have been the results of these changes in confidentiality's status?

First, when patients disclose private health information today, the expectation of confidentiality is weaker because it is likely that many more authorized parties will have access to patient information, which makes it more difficult to determine who is responsible for subsequent disclosures. This will is clearly the case for e-medicine, which relies on the electronic transmission of more patient health information and involves more persons and institutions in patient care.

Second, medical confidentiality is today generally viewed as a *prima facie* moral rule that allows for exceptions when other moral values or social goods, such as public health, are at stake. For e-medicine, this means that even though there are potentially greater risks to the privacy and confidentiality interests of individuals, they will need to be balanced against other medical goals and the common good. Disagreements remain over the finer points of when it is morally permissible to breach confidentiality with patients, but

a general consensus has emerged that healthcare professionals should keep in confidence all information about their patients unless (1) the patient has given authorization to his/her healthcare provider or medical institution to disclose his/her medical information to a third party; (2) the healthcare provider is required by law to do so as in cases of communicable diseases, child abuse, and gunshot victims; (3) there is a specific clear and present danger to the life of the patient and/or other persons; and (4) there is a likely threat of serious bodily or psychological harm to the patient and/or other persons (Edwards & Graber, 1988).

In addition, healthcare professionals should *ethically justify* exceptions to medical confidentiality by evaluating the respective harms and benefits of keeping and breaching confidentiality in specific cases. In doing so, healthcare professionals ought to (1) consider all other less drastic means of promoting and protecting competing moral values; (2) reasonably believe that a violation of patient confidentiality or trust will actually promote or protect competing values; (3) reasonably believe that the combined values of breaking confidentiality will trump the combined disvalues of maintaining confidentiality (Edwards & Graber, 1988).

The aforementioned principles and professional guidelines for confidentiality have received judicial acknowledgment and support in *Tarasoff v. Regents of the University of California*, 17 Cal.3d 425,131 Cal.Rptr. 14, 551 P.2d 334 (1976) (Furrow, Greany, et al. 1997). This case deals with a psychotherapist at the University of California whose patient, Podder, had explicitly threatened to harm his former girlfriend during sessions. No one, including the therapist, attempted to warn the woman, Tarasoff, and Podder eventually killed her. Most health professions and healthcare institutions promise to protect patient confidentiality, but *Tarasoff* established legal precedent for the protection of third parties by requiring disclosure of patient information by healthcare professionals and healthcare institutions to identified third parties when they have information about a patient's intent to harm that third party (i.e., someone outside the traditional provider-patient relationship).

As discussed above, confidentiality had been historically treated as inviolate feature of the provider-patient relationship and had been considered to be in the best interest of the patient. Moreover, disclosure of patient information to third parties by healthcare professionals exposes them to legal liability and is avoided for reasons of self-protection. Under *Tarasoff*, however, physicians and other healthcare professionals now have an affirmative legal duty to protect identified third parties by warning them of the likely harmful actions of their patients. Now, if they fail to disclose such information to third parties when there is a credible threat of harm, they could be subject to liability (Furrow, Greany et al. 1997).

Procedural Criteria for Privacy and Confidentiality

As discussed, before exceptions to privacy and confidentiality are made, the specific harms and benefits of doing so should be considered (Kongehl 1999). But in order to ascertain the specific harms and benefits of breaching medical privacy and confidentiality, we must have some understanding of what conditions, states, and items are and ought to be private and confidential. The problem, however, is the likelihood of identifying necessary and sufficient conditions for privacy and confidentiality which are universally agreed to and applicable to diverse settings is highly unlikely.

The good news is that complete agreement on the conditions of privacy and confidentiality are not required for e-medicine. Instead, we can adopt *procedural criteria* to determine what ought to remain private and confidential in the context of cybermedicine by letting individual patients decide, within the limits of the law, what they want kept private and confidential. The strength of this approach is that it not only respects the autonomy of patients (consistent with the law), but is also

practicable, allowing for considerable latitude in determining what should be private and confidential in cybermedicine (Wasserstrom, 1984).

If a procedural approach is adopted, it will still be necessary to avoid a simplistic understanding of privacy and confidentiality that overlooks competing moral values, interests, and social goods. The following statement underscores this concern and provides useful guidance for attaining a consensus on the nature and scope of privacy and confidentiality in e-medicine:

We agree that the flexibility native to the concept of privacy makes it desirable to provide a tighter meaning. This objective is particularly germane for policies regarding which forms of access to which persons will constitute losses that are violations of privacy. We are, however, reluctant to castrate the concept to make it serviceable for policy. Instead, we recommend that those who propose policies carefully specify conditions of restricted access that will and will not count as a loss or violation of privacy. The policy should accurately define the zones that are considered private and not to be invaded, and it should also state interests that may legitimately be balanced against privacy interests. Often the focus will be informational privacy and restricting modes of access to information about persons; but in other cases policies will govern privacy in making decisions, in intimate relationships, and the like (Beauchamp & Childress, 1994).

Therefore, before e-medicine can be evaluated as either an ethically appropriate or an ethically inappropriate mode of healthcare, before useful procedural criteria can be adopted, the scope and meaning of privacy and confidentiality must be guided by and should reflect the concrete conditions and norms that are unique to providing telemedical services. This, as I discuss below, will require a more refined understanding of privacy for e-medicine.

PHYSICAL, INFORMATIONAL, AND DECISIONAL PRIVACY

Privacy is not a singular or uniform concept, but rather a plural notion that includes *informational privacy, physical privacy,* and *decisional privacy*. As will be discussed subsequently, e-medicine will have different consequences for these three types of privacy, often requiring that tradeoffs among them be made.

Physical privacy generally refers to the restricted access that others have to our bodies, relationships, and living spaces. Physical privacy is ethically significant because it allows for intimacy, solitude, personal control, and peace of mind (Allen, 1995). In the context of cybermedicine, physical privacy is significant because it has the potential to reduce the number of unwanted in-person intrusions by healthcare workers. For example, as teleconsultation and telemonitoring increasingly substitute for in-home visits, it may be possible for patients and family caregivers to gain more control over their homes, personal relationships, and daily schedules.

Overall, the greater physical privacy afforded by telemedicine has the potential to protect the intimate and non-public sphere of the home and to enhance the autonomy and well-being of patients and families at a time when much in their lives is out of control. In the future, patients and their families may decide to have more in-person visits than televisits, willingly sacrificing a measure of privacy for security and greater social interaction, but e-medicine might give them options to enhance their physical privacy that don't currently exist in hospital settings.

Informational privacy refers to the *confidentiality* and *security* of identifiable patient health information and clinical data found in patient records and in communications among healthcare professionals and patients (Allen, 1995). As I previously discussed, *confidentiality* is the protection of private information, once it has been disclosed by a patient (e.g., during a medical examination or

taking of a medical history by a healthcare professional), from being shared with others within or outside healthcare settings not directly involved in the patient's care. Confidentiality restricts who can see and use that information.

The *security* of patient health information, which includes considerations of its *accuracy, reliability,* and *quality*, refers to the human, legal, and technical means of preventing the unauthorized or accidental disclosure of confidential health information. Common technological mechanisms include the use of electronic passwords, firewalls, digital signatures and time stamps, and data encryption software that allow health information to be encoding and decoded for transmission and storage (Collmann & Silvestre, 1998).

Decisional Privacy is closely related to the two aforementioned types of privacy, but can be distinguished from them, applying generally to those situations in which persons have secure environments to discuss matters, weigh options, and reach decisions without undue influence by healthcare professionals. For some theorists, however, decisional privacy is not really privacy at all, but rather an aspect of autonomy, freedom, or liberty that has been poorly defined (Allen, 1995). Although the exact status of decisional privacy continues to be debated, as a practical matter decisional privacy has gained general acceptance within the legal system of the United States.

E-medicine creates new threats and new opportunities for the informational, physical, and decisional privacy of patients and family caregivers. Although security violations are relatively uncommon, the potential for harm is great for telemedicine patients, especially when the security of socially stigmatizing health information is breached. Patients may not only lose their privacy, they may be subject to social ostracism, job discrimination, loss of insurance, and social control in the form of blackmail (Shea, 1994).

Total informational, physical, and decisional privacy is not realistic for cybermedicine and healthcare generally. First, other goods like medical research and public health require that limits be placed on the privacy of health information. Second, in order to treat and cure their patients, healthcare professionals must sometimes compromise or enter the informational, physical, and decisional privacy of their patients.

Healthcare professionals must be able to touch their patients and obtain information about the intimate details of their patients' lifestyles and personal habits. Depending on the site or point of care (e.g., hospitals, ambulatory clinics, and patients' homes), patients will have more or less informational, physical, and decisional privacy.

Unfortunately, much of the telemedicine literature on privacy simply fails to distinguish among informational, physical, and decisional privacy. A lack of adequate distinctions should not be construed as a simple semantic problem. If such distinctions are not recognized, many of the privacy issues that should be considered when formulating privacy laws and guidelines for e-medicine will be overlooked. Furthermore, even when distinctions among physical, informational, and decisional privacy are acknowledged in the telemedicine literature, the focus often remains entirely on informational privacy and the confidentiality of identifiable health information.

A good example of this can be seen in the Institute of Medicine's *Telemedicine: A Guide to Assessing Telecommunications in Health Care*. Initially, the IOM distinguishes between and physical and informational privacy, but focuses on informational privacy in its assessment of telecommunications in healthcare. Although recognized by the IOM, physical privacy is not explored in any depth and there is no discussion of the potential impact of telemedicine on the decisional privacy of patients (Field, 1996). Again, the current emphasis on informational privacy over both physical and decisional privacy is problematic when it comes to assessing the benefits and harms of e-medicine and for educating patients about the need for potential tradeoffs among these types of privacy.

PUBLIC CONCERNS

There are a number of specific means by which personal health information (PHI) can be compromised in the practice of e-medicine. First, there is the threat of cookies and spy ware, which allow unauthorized persons to monitor computer use and track online activities, such as the websites patients visit (Buckovich & Rippen, 1999). Second, there is the threat that hackers will gain illicit access to patient records simply because they can do so or for more nefarious ends such identity theft.[7] Third, there is always the possibility that patient information will be accidentally transmitted to unauthorized persons or even the World Wide Web (Collmann & Cooper, 2007). Fourth, and probably the greatest threat to privacy involves the human element, in particular, poorly designed security measures and the inadequate training of staff (Sax & Mandl, 2005). Lastly, there are multiple privacy standards and incompatible security measures among entities that have access to patient information, making it more likely that patients' health-related information will fall into the wrong hands.[8]

A 2000 survey of Internet users found that 75% of respondents were worried that health sites shared information without consent, and that a full 17% would not even seek health information on the web due to privacy concerns. The same poll also found that 61% of Americans felt that too many people have access to their medical records (EPIC, 2008). Little has changed since that poll was conducted. In June 2008, for example, a Harris poll concluded that millions of Americans believe medical records have been compromised (Government Technology, 2008). Is this simply an irrational fear unsubstantiated by evidence? The short answer is no. There are numerous cases in which identifiable patient health information has been compromised.

One case occurred in March of 2008, when a researcher's laptop computer was stolen. The laptop contained the health data of 2,500 subjects, who were participating in a medical trial conducted by the National Institutes of Health (New York Times, 2008). Prior to our ability to store health information on laptops in a digital format, it would have been virtually impossible for someone to steal at one time the health data of 2,500 patients. Moreover, unlike traditional paper record keeping, digitally stored data can be easily replicated and transmitted on the World Wide Web, from where it can be downloaded to a limitless number of personal computers. It should be noted that this case is a not a matter of failed technology; rather, it is clear example of human error and neglect.

In a second case of compromised patient confidentiality, researchers found that implantable cardiac defibrillators and pacemakers equipped with wireless technology (i.e., telemetry-capable medical devices), which permit remote device checks and the transmission of a patient's vital signs over the internet, can be hacked into allowing unauthorized individuals to gain access to an individual's PHI. Equally disturbing is that once security has been breached, a hacker can reprogram these devices without the knowledge and consent of patients (Federal Telemedicine News, 2008).

In a highly publicized third case of compromised medical privacy, Kaiser Permanente (KP) employees accidentally mailed 800 patients' personally identifiable health information (e.g. appointment details, answers to patients' questions, medical advice) to other patients and employees within the KP network. According to KP, the breach occurred at KP's web-enabled healthcare portal and was the result of a systemic problem within the KP organization. The systemic problem included the architecture of the information system, the motivations of individual staff members, differences among the subcultures of individual groups within the organization, as well as technical and social relations across the Kaiser Permanente IT program (IC3, 2003).

With the above cases in mind, it is no wonder that many patients and healthcare profession-als alike have a skeptical and jaundice view of e-medicine and the threat it posses to medical privacy and confidentiality.

MISUSES OF PATIENT HEALTH DATA

Threats to the privacy and confidentiality of personal health data are not new. What is new with the rise of e-medicine is the scope and magnitude of the threats. Digitalization and the exponential growth of the internet in medicine has simply made it easier for authorized and unauthorized persons to collect, store, replicate, and transmit acquired patient data. Once personal health information has been collected, legally or illegally, there are a number of ways in which this information can be misused.

First, patient health-related information could be commercially misused. In recent years, an extensive data market has developed, driven largely by data aggregators, who repackage and sell information without the knowledge or consent of the original information owner. Commercial misuses of data can have several serious consequences for individuals, leading for example to a denial of insurance coverage or credit, or to invasive unsolicited marketing programs (Brenner & Clark, 2005).

Second, criminals can misuse patient health-related information. Identify theft represents a particularly serious problem. In 2003, the FTC estimated that 10 million Americans (nearly 5% of the adult population) were victims of some form of identity theft (FTC, 2007). According to the FBI, the Internet Crime Complaint Center received more than 100,000 complaints regarding identity theft in the five-year period between its opening in 2000 and 2005 (IC3, 2007).

The third and most serious threat comes from our own government. According to a 2004 report issued by the Government Accounting Office (GAO), 52 federal agencies and departments reported 199 data mining efforts, of which 68 were planned and 131 were operational (GAO, 2004). The most common reasons cited by the GAO for data mining included 1) improvements in service or performance, 2) detection of fraud, waste, and abuse, 3) analysis of scientific and research information, 4) management of human resources, 5) detection of criminal activities or patterns, and 6) analysis of intelligence and detecting terrorist activities.

The GAO report also identified the Department of Defense as having the largest number of data mining efforts aimed at analyzing intelligence and detecting terrorist activities followed by the Departments of Homeland Security, Justice, and Education. The Department of Education reported the largest number of efforts aimed at detecting fraud, waste, and abuse. Data mining efforts for detecting criminal activities or patterns, however, were spread relatively evenly among the reporting agencies (GAO, 2004).

In addition, out of all 199 data mining efforts identified, 122 used personal information. For these efforts, the primary purposes were detecting fraud, waste, and abuse; detecting criminal activities or patterns; analyzing intelligence and detecting terrorist activities; and increasing tax compliance. Personal information collected from other federal agencies and the private sector included credit reports, credit card numbers and transactions, student loan application data, bank account numbers, and taxpayer identification numbers. As discussed below, movement toward a nationwide health records system will provide additional opportunities for government to more easily mine, aggregate, and misuse personal health information if it should elect to do so (GAO, 2004).

FAIR INFORMATION PRACTICES

In 1980, the Organization for Economic Cooperation and Development (OECD) released eight guidelines to protect individual privacy while facilitating the free flow of personal data between countries in the conduct of commerce (OECD, 1980). The United States approved the eight OECD guidelines, which are also known as "fair information practices" (FIPs), and incorporated them into subsequent privacy regulations promulgated by the Department of Health and Human Services (HHS) in 2003 (IHF, 2003) under the Health Insurance Accountability and Portability Act of 1996 (HIPAA, 1996). The eight guidelines address 1) collection limitation, 2) data quality, 3) specification of purpose, 4) use limitation, 5) security safeguards, 6) openness regarding data policies and procedures, 7) individual participation, and 8) accountability.

One thing the FIPs do well is to specify the entities covered by them, including defining "protected health information" (PHI). Essentially, PHI is individually identifiable health information that is transmitted by electronic media, maintained in electronic media, or transmitted or maintained in any other form or medium, excluding some classes of records such mental health records. The regulations define "covered entities" as health plans, health clearinghouses, healthcare providers, and business associates who transmit health information in an electronic format (HIPAA, 1996).

In their inception, the intent was to provide a set of FIPs to govern how personal health information would be used. The problem, however, with the HIPAA privacy regulations is that the consent requirements did very little to enhance patient autonomy and protect patient privacy. First, although individuals will be notified that their information will be disclosed, they do not get to decide whether or not they want their personal health information disclosed. There is a huge difference between notification and consent. Second, individuals have the right to request further protections, but their doctors and others do not have to agree to individuals' requests. Third, individuals do not have an absolute right to get copies of their medical records. Clinicians can refuse to share records in some circumstances. Fourth, individuals can request amendments to their medical records, but clinicians are not required to accept a patient's suggested amendments. Furthermore, the privacy rule gives permission for clinicians, hospitals, health plans and other "covered entities" to distribute identifiable patient information without patient consent for so-called "national priority activities" (HIPAA, 1996).

According to the Institute for Health Freedom, the uses and disclosures for which an authorization is not required include (1) uses and disclosures required by law, (2) uses and disclosures for public health activities, (3) disclosures about victims of abuse, neglect or domestic violence, (4) uses and disclosures for health oversight activities, (5) disclosures for judicial and administrative proceedings, (6) disclosures for law enforcement purposes, (7) uses and disclosures about decedents, (8) uses and disclosures for cadaveric organ, eye or tissue donation purposes, (9) uses and disclosures for research purposes, (10) uses and disclosures to avert a serious threat to health or safety, (11) uses and disclosures for specialized government functions, and (12) disclosures for workers' compensation (HIPAA, 1996).

As critics have rightly claimed, instead of protecting patient privacy, HIPAA and associated privacy rules have more or less eliminated patient autonomy and consent from the practice of medicine.

EVOLUTION OF A NATIONAL HEALTH INFORMATION NETWORK

One portion of HIPAA, *Administrative Simplification* (HIPAA 2006), was intended to facilitate greater interoperability among disparate health information systems and for sharing of medical data electronically by moving the nation toward a National Health Information Network (NHIN), requiring the federal government to create (1) Unique Patient IDs (UPI) - a national medical ID card for every citizen; (2) National Provider IDs (NPI) - a unique identification number for

every doctor, nurse, therapist, hospital, health care facility, and other providers; (3) Employer ID Numbers (EIN) - a unique number for every employer; (4) Payer ID - an identification number for every insurer and health plan; (5) national codes for all health care procedures; (6) national transaction sets; and (7) national security standards for health information (HIPAA 1996).

Subsequently, as a way to expedite the creation of the NHIN, President Bush issued Executive Order 13335 on April 27, 2004, establishing the position of a National Coordinator for Health Information Technology (ONC) within the Office of the Secretary of Health and Human Services (HHS, 2007). The Executive Order mandated the ONC to provide leadership for the development and nationwide implementation of an interoperable health information technology infrastructure by 2014 by bringing together all federal activities in health information technology in a coordinated fashion (NGA, 2008; Pritts, 2002). The strategic plan of the ONC is to improve the quality, efficiency and privacy of health-related information, and make it available to patients for non-medical purposes, as directed by the patient (Gunter, 2005).

As a way of reaching these objectives, the ONC recognized interoperability not only requires a seamless, integrated network of information technology and unique IDs; interoperability and subsequent adoption also require the establishment of an unambiguous NHIN lexicon. Consequently, ONC contracted The Alliance for Health Information Technology (AHIT) to develop a common NHIN language by reaching consensus on definitions for the following terms: Electronic medical record (EMR), electronic health record (EHR), patient health record (PHR), health information exchange (HIE), regional health information organization (RHIO), and health information oversight (HIO) (HHS, 2008).

According to the report issued by AHIT, the term "HIE" is frequently used to describe both the processes of health information exchange and the organizations managing the exchanges. As result, HIEs and RHIOs have tended to be used synonymously. To establish greater clarity, the AHIT redefined "HIE" as the process of exchanging information and created a new term, "HIO," to refer to the organizations governing the exchange of information. Under the new definitions, a RHIO is a now a type of HIO (HHS, 2008).

Under the new definitions, the central difference between an EMR and an EHR is the ability to exchange information interoperably. An EMR does not exchange information interoperably, whereas an EHR does (HHS, 2008). The trend, however, is toward electronic records that are capable of using nationally recognized interoperability standards, which is a key feature of EHRs. By the year 2014, it is anticipated that electronic records not capable of exchanging information interoperably will lose their relevance, and the term "EMR" will become obsolete.

Finally, the control of one's health-related information distinguishes the EHR from the PHR. The information in a PHR, whether derived from an EHR or other sources, is for the patient to manage and use. But, when a patient is granted access to his electronic record maintained and controlled by a provider or payer organization, he is accessing an EHR, not his PHR (HHS, 2008).

PROTECTING MEDICAL PRIVACY AND CONFIDENTIALITY

As discussed earlier, HIPAA privacy rules have at least three significant shortcomings:

1. Patient consent and authorization for the use and disclosure of PHI is almost nonexistent;
2. the number of entities that can be included in the class of "covered entities" is legion;
3. and some non-covered entities that receive PHI by covered entities are not required to protect the information once it has been received.

As an illustration of these shortcomings, the Department of Labor and the U.S. Census Bureau, relying on data from 2000 (ERISA, 2000) and 2004 (US Census Bureau, 2004), calculated that close to 15 million people, as employees of covered entities, could be in a position to access and use PHI.

The fact that millions of people might be authorized to access and potentially to disclose PHI should make us worry. We should, however, be even more worried, given that the establishment of a NHIN by 2014 could give even more individuals access to PHI and exacerbate the already limited consent, use, and disclosure requirements operative under HIPAA. If nothing is done, patient privacy and confidentiality, the ethical cornerstone of medicine, is likely to go the way of the dinosaur by 2014 (Froomkin, 2000; Garfinkel, 2000).

Authorized Abuse and Individualism in HIPAA

As discussed earlier, there is a clear genealogy of privacy legislation from the 1973 Code of Fair Information Practices through HIPAA, which means the defects of earlier privacy legislation are likely to have been inherited by HIPAA. Two potential problems that stand out are (1) the problem of authorized abuse, and (2) the problem of individualism.

First, cases of unauthorized access to medical information tend to be isolated acts, often carried out by one person. Most instances of violations of medical privacy and confidentiality result from persons who have authorized and legal access to another's medical information. Etzioni calls this *authorized abuse*. Most violations of privacy of medical records are the result of the legally sanctioned—or at least tolerated—unconcealed, systematic flow of medical information from the orbit the physician-patient-health insurer and health management corporation to other non-health care parties, including employers, marketers, and the press. I refer here not to the occasional slip-up or mischief of a rogue employee, cases that often violate ethical codes or laws, but to authorized abuse—the daily, continuous, and very numerous disclosures and uses that are legal but of highly questionable moral standing (Etzioni 1999).

Unlike traditional medical settings, it is very likely that more electronic health information will be recorded and transmitted in home-based telemedicine in the form of video consults, e-mail, and the steady flow of physiological data. HIPAA legislation, if passed, will have implications for the regulation of electronic health information that is generated during telemedicine encounters. If Etzioni is correct, this means there could be more opportunities for authorized abuse "that are legal but morally questionable in e-medicine.

Second, most privacy legislation and regulation, according to Etzioni, reflect individualism and after-the-fact punitive measures for privacy violations rather than a policy of prevention. If this is the case then these policies have the potential to undermine the common good by thwarting other healthcare goals of quality control, cost control, and medical research. On this point, Etzioni states the following:

The prevailing suggestions for dealing with the tension between privacy and health care goals and a major source of that tension are based on the same legal-ethical doctrine, that of informed consent. This notion is based on legal, philosophical, and moral individualistic assumptions (Etzioni, 1999).

For example, HIPAA includes the *principle of patient control*, which holds that persons have a legal right to access and amend their health records and to be informed of the purposes for which it is used or disclosed to third parties.

From Etzioni's perspective, this HIPAA principle could be seen as an instance of individualism overriding equally important healthcare goals. For example, if voluntary informed consent for each and every disclosure of patient health information

were the norm, the mere mechanics of getting informed consent from patients could require an enormous expenditure of human and financial resources that would, in turn, retard the pursuit and actualization of other medical goals. Also, a legal right for patients to access and amend their records could give them more autonomy, but it could also burden clinicians by requiring them to avoid using technical language in their record keeping that would confuse the average patient. This, in turn, could have a deleterious effect on healthcare efficiency.

As a means of combating authorized abuse and individualism, Etzioni argues for a new communitarian conception of privacy that avoids the extremes of an individualistic conception of privacy by balancing the interests of individuals with the common good.

HIPAA, however, does acknowledge the ethical tension between personal privacy interests and competing social goods, such as public health and medical research. This is expressed in the *principle of public responsibility*, which holds that individual privacy interests ought not to override national priorities of public health, medical research, preventing health care fraud, and law enforcement.

This does not mean that concerns about authorized abuse and individualism are groundless, but they can be managed by means of appropriate technological, social, and organizational measures. First, in addition to obtaining a patient's consent for various categories of disclosures to third parties in advance, EPRs could be configured to send an automatic notice to patients via e-mail, with the transmission of their record to third parties. Second, the development of professional guidelines and codes of ethics for health professions could prove useful in mitigating some legal abuses of privacy (Baker, Caplan, et al., 1999).

The American Medical Association and the American Medical Informatics Association have already developed practice guidelines for governing e-mail communications with patients

(Kane & Sands, 1998). Similarly, the American Telemedicine Association has formulated general guidelines the address the use of medical web sites (ATA 1999). In some instances, these new professional guidelines for telemedicine and other e-health applications are more stringent than the laws and regulations designed to protect patients and consumers.

When healthcare professionals responsibly use their autonomy to self regulate by setting high standards for e-health and other telemedicine practices, the public benefits. Moreover, if healthcare professionals want to remain autonomous and to maintain the trust of the public, it is in their best interest to set the highest standards. If they do not do this, it is likely that they will gradually lose their professional autonomy as more laws and regulations are required to do what they failed to do.

In order to circumvent the flaws of HIPAA's "protections," as well as meet the potential challenges of a NHIN, it is necessary to retool the existing, but poorly implemented, guidelines, which regulate the privacy and confidentiality of PHI. The following seven principles are derived from existing laws, statutes, and fair information practices (PRC, 1997; Markle Foundation, 2003):

1. **Openness and Transparency:** Patients and consumers should be able to know what information has been collected about them, the purpose of its use, who can access and use it, and where it resides. They should also be informed about how they may obtain access to information collected about them. It is also necessary that individuals know how to exercise control. Laws, transparency, and openness do little to enhance patient control if they cannot find their PHI and control who has access to that information. Thus, under a NHIN, it will not be enough for individuals to have a PHR that they control; they will need to have greater access and control over their EHR.

2. **Purpose Specification:** The purposes for which PHI are collected should be specified at the time of collection, and the subsequent use should be limited to those purposes, or others that are specified on each occasion of change of purpose. By doing so, the informed consent of individuals would be necessary. This, of course, is what HIPAA fails to do.

3. **Collection Limitation:** PHI should only be collected for specified purposes and should be obtained by lawful and fair means. The collection and storage of personal health data should be limited to that information necessary to carry out the specified purpose. Where possible, individuals should have knowledge of data collection or provide consent, for collections.

4. **Individual Participation and Control:** Individuals should be able to control access to their personal information. They should know who is storing what information on them, and how that information is being used. They should also be able to review the way their information is being used or stored.

5. **Data Quality and Security Safeguards:** All personal data collected should be relevant to the purposes for which they are to be used and should be accurate, complete, and up-to-date. Reasonable safeguards should protect personal data against such risks as loss or unauthorized access, use, destruction, modification, or disclosure. As early as 2000, the National Research Council (NRC) recommended that the federal government should take steps to include new *technical features* that will better protect the privacy and anonymity of Internet users. Features identified by the NRC include the use of electronic passwords, firewalls, digital signatures, time and date stamps, and encryption software that allows patient health information to be encoded and decoded for transmission and storage. According to the

NRC, "the features include mechanisms to protect the anonymity of Internet users, to keep patient information secure, to validate the identity of users participating in confidential online transactions, and to track users of databases" (Kirnan, 2002).

6. **Accountability and Oversight:** Entities in control of PHI must be held accountable for implementing these principles. An oversight body should be created that is comprised of all stakeholders, including representatives of government, the healthcare industry, vendors and technologists, and consumer, privacy and patient advocates. The oversight body would monitor the effectiveness of the system in accomplishing its goal of benefiting healthcare. It would also review compliance issues and stay current with problems that arise.

7. **Remedies and Sanctions:** Under the NHIN patients should have a right of action for any damages that result from mishandling of their PHI. It is very important that remedies and sanctions exist to address security breaches or privacy violations. The problem is that it is often very difficult to determine who is responsible for a privacy violation. For example, almost 50% of individuals who are victims of identity theft do not even know it (Solove, 2005). Although difficult to enforce, there still ought to be minimum punishments for those individuals who violate the PHI of others.

As mentioned above, these seven privacy principles are derived from existing laws, statutes, and fair information practices. There is, therefore, nothing really new about them. What is new and highly significant is that there is a reduction in the number of covered entities that have access to PHI, and more individual control over how, when, and what PHI will be disclosed and used. The success of these improvements, however, depends upon their effective application and enforcement.

CONCLUSION

E-medicine provides some very real benefits for our healthcare system, including, for example, reduced costs, increased access to services and providers (Bauer, 2003), and reductions in medical errors (Bauer, 2001). These benefits, however, should not blind us to the risks of e-medicine, in particular, privacy violations, unauthorized use and disclosure of PHI, and erosion in the public's trust of our healthcare system. Therefore, it is absolutely essential that future privacy regulations significantly reduce the number of entities that have legal and authorized access to PHI as well as provide individuals greater access and control over their PHI. It is also necessary that adequate security measures be implemented in order to minimize the risk of unauthorized access the PHI.

Also, the creation of a NHIN will make it easier for authorized individuals to access patients' PHI data. The problem is that a network that can be utilized more easily by authorized individuals anytime and anywhere is a network that potentially makes it easier for unauthorized individuals to breach the privacy and confidentially of PHI anytime and anywhere. Legislation and technology can do much to minimize privacy risks, but the human factor is also vitally important. Healthcare professionals need to be trained in the use of EHRs and related digital technologies, understand the ethical significance of and justifications for maintaining the privacy and confidential PHI, as well as the implications of its misuse. If not, then it is unlikely that PHI will remain private for very long.

REFERENCES

Allen, A. L. (1995). *Privacy in healthcare. Encyclopedia of Bioethics* (pp. 2064–2073). New York: Macmillan Library Reference.

Baker, R. B., Caplan, C. L., Emanuel, L. L., & Latham, S. R. (Eds.). (1999). The American medical ethics revolution: How the AMA's code of ethics has transformed physicians' relationships to patients, professionals, and society. *Ethics, 112*(2), 354–356.

Bashshur, R. L., Sanders, J. H., & Shannon, G. W. (Eds.). (1999). *Telemedicine: Theory and practice.*

Bauer, K. A. (2001). Using the Internet to empower patients and to develop partnerships with clinicians. *The American Journal of Bioethics, 1*(2).

Bauer, K. A. (2003). Distributive justice and rural healthcare: A case for e-health. *The International Journal of Applied Philosophy, 17*(2), 243–254.

Bauer, K. A. (2004). Cybermedicine and the moral integrity of the physician-patient relationship. *Journal of Ethics and Information Technology, 6*, 83–91. doi:10.1007/s10676-004-4591-7

Beauchamp, T.L. & Childress, J.F. (1994). *Principles of biomedical ethics.*

Benn, S. I., & Gaus, G. F. (1983). *The public and the private: Concepts and action*. London: Croom Helm.

Bloch, C. (March 24, 2008). Defibrillators and privacy risks. *Federal Telemedicine News*. Retrieved on November 6, 2008, from http://telemedicine-news.blogspot.com/2008/03/defibrillators-and-privacy-risks.html

Brenner, S., & Clarke, L. (2005). *Should commercial misuse of private data be a crime?* Social Science Research Network. Retrieved on November 4, 2008, from http://ssrn.com/abstract=845845

Bruce, J. A. C. (1984). *Privacy and confidentiality of health information*. Chicago: American Hospital.

Buckovich, S. A., & Rippen, H. E. (1999). Driving toward guiding principles: A goal for privacy, confidentiality, and security of health information. *Journal of the American Medical Informatics Association, 6*, 122–133.

Collmann, J., & Cooper, T. (2007). Breaching the security of the Kaiser Permanente Internet Patient Portal: The organizational foundations of information security. *Journal of the American Medical Informatics Association, 14*, 239–243. doi:10.1197/jamia.M2195

Collmann, J., & Silvestre, A. L. (1998). Building a security capable prganization. In *proceedings, PACMedTek, IEEE Computer Society*, Washington, DC.

Department of Health and Human Services. (2007). *Synopsis of the ONC: Coordinated Federal Health Information Plan: 2008-2012*. Retrieved on November 4, 2008, from http://www.hhs.gov/healthit/resources/HITStrategicPlanSummary.pdf

Department of Health and Human Services. (2008a). *Health Information Technology*. Retrieved on November 4, 2008, from http://www.hhs.gov/healthit/

Department of Health and Human Services. (2008b) *The National Alliance for Health Information Technology, report to the ONC on defining key health Information Technology terms*. Retrieved on November 4, 2008 from http://www.hhs.gov/healthit/documents/m20080603/10_2_hit_terms.pdf

Edelstein, L. (1943). The Hippocratic oath: Text, translation and interpretation. *Bulletin of the History of Medicine, 5*(1), 1–64.

Edwards, R. (1988). Confidentiality in the professions. In Edwards, R., & Garber, G. (Eds.), *Bioethics* (pp. 72–81). San Diego: Harcourt Brace Jovanovich.

Electronic Privacy Information Center. (2008). *Privacy survey*. Retrieved on November 4, 2008, from http://www.epic.org/privacy/survey/

Employee Retirement Income Security Act of 1974. (2000). *Rules and regulations for administration and enforcement; claims procedure; final rule. 65 Fed. Reg. 70246-70271.*

Etzioni. (1999). A contemporary conception of privacy. *Telecommunications and Space Journal, 6*, 81-114.

Federal Trade Commission. (2007). *2006 Identity theft survey*. Retrieved on November 4, 2008, from http://www.ftc.gov/os/2007/11/Synovate-FinalReportIDTheft2006.pdf

Field. (1996). *Telemedicine, telehealth, and health Information Technology*. The American Telemedicine Society.

Froomkin, M. (2000). The death of privacy? *Stanford Law Review, 52*, 1461–1469. doi:10.2307/1229519

Furrow, B.R., Greaney, T.L., Johnson, S.H., Jost, S.T. & Schwartz, L.S. (1997). *Treatise on health law.*

Garfinkel, S. (2000). Review of database nation: The death of privacy in the 21st Century. *Journal of Information, Law and Technology*. Retrieved on November 4, 2008, from http://www2.warwick.ac.uk/fac/soc/law/elj/jilt/2000_1/kelman/

Government Accounting Office. (2004). *Data mining: Federal efforts cover a wide range of uses*. Retrieved on November 4, 2008, from http://www.gao.gov/new.items/d04548.pdf

Government Technology. (2008). *Millions believe personal medical records have been compromised, survey says*. Retrieved on November 4, 2008, from http://www.govtech.com/gt/377526

Gunter, T. D., & Nicolas, T. P. (2005). The emergence of national electronic health record architectures in the United States and Australia: Models, costs, and questions. *Journal of Medical Internet Research, 7*(1), E3. doi:10.2196/jmir.7.1.e3

Habermas, J. (1989). *The structural transformation of the public sphere: An inquiry into a category of bourgeois society*. Cambridge, MA: The MIT Press.

HIPAA. (1996). Health Insurance Portability and Accountability Act of 1996. Pub, L. No. 104-191.

HIPAA. (2006). HIPAA Administrative Simplification, Regulation Text, 45 CFR Parts 160, 162, and 164.

Institute for Health Freedom. (2003). *The final federal privacy rule: The definitive guide*. Retrieved on November 4, 2008, from http://www.forhealthfreedom.org/Publications/Privacy/Rule.html#copy

Internet Crime Complaint Center. (2007). *2007 Internet Crime Report*. Retrieved November 4, 2008, from http://www.ic3.gov/media/annualreport/2007_IC3Report.pdf

Kane, B., & Sands, D. Z. (1998). Guidelines for the clinical use of electronic mail with patients. *Journal of the American Medical Informatics Association, 5*(1), 104–111.

Kant, I. (1991). *Groundwork for the metaphysics of morals.*

Kirnan, V. (2000). Medicine could benefit from internet improvement, report says. *The Chronicle of Higher Education.*

Kongehl. (1999). The electronic health record-a new challenge for privacy and confidentiality in medicine? *Biomedical Ethics, 4*(2):52-3.

Lashof, J. C. (1981). *Government approaches to the management of medical technology*. Paper presented at Annual Health Conference of the New York Academy of Medicine.

Markle Foundation. (2003). *Connecting for health: A public-private collaborative*. Retrieved on November 4, 2008, from http://www.connectingforhealth.org/resources/pswg_report.pdf

National Governors Association. State Alliance for e-health. (2008). *Accelerating progress: Using health Information Technology and electronic health information exchange to improve care.* Retrieved on November 4, 2008, from http://www.nga.org/Files/pdf/0809EHEALTHREPORT.PDF

NY Times staff writer. (March 26, 2008) *Safeguarding private medical data.* New York Times. Retrieved November 4, 2008, from http://www.nytimes.com/2008/03/26/opinion/26wed2.html

Organization for Economic Co-Operation and Development. (1980). *Guidelines on the protection of privacy and transborder flows of personal data.*

Pritts, J. (2002). Altered states: State health privacy laws and the impact of the federal health privacy rule. *Yale Journal of Health Policy, Law, and Ethics, 2*(2), 327–364.

Privacy Rights Clearinghouse. (1997). *A review of the fair information principles: The foundation of privacy public policy.* Retrieved on November 4, 2008 from http://www.privacyrights.org/ar/fairinfo.htm

Rachels, J. (2005). Why privacy is important. *Philosophy & Public Affairs, 4*(4), 323–333.

Robinson, T. N., Patrick, K., Eng, T. R., & Gustavson, D. (1999). *An evidence-based approach to interactive health communication: A challenge to medicine in the information age.* Science Panel on Interactive Health and Communication.

Sax, U., & Mandl, K. D. (2005). Wireless technology infrastructures for authentication of patients: PKI that rings. *Journal of the American Medical Informatics Association, 12,* 263–268. doi:10.1197/jamia.M1681

Schoeman, F. D. (1984). *Philosophical dimensions of privacy: An anthology.* Cambridge, UK: Cambridge University Press. doi:10.1017/CBO9780511625138

Shea, S. (1994). Security versus access: trade-offs are only part of the story. *Journal of the American Medical Informatics Association, 1*(4), 314–315.

Solove, D. J., & Hoofnagle, C. J. (2005). *A model regime of privacy protection.* Public Law Research Paper No. 132, George Washington University Law School. Retrieved on November 4, 2008, from http://papers.ssrn.com/sol3/papers.cfm?abstract_id=681902

United Nations. (1948). *Universal declaration of human rights, article 12.* Retrieved November 4, 2008, from http://www.nps.gov/elro/teach-er-vk/documents/udhr.htm

U.S. Census Bureau. (2004). *Statistics of U.S. businesses: 2004—third party administration of insurance and pension funds.*

Walters, L. (1982). Ethical aspects of medical confidentiality. In Walters, L., & Beauchamp, T. (Eds.), *Contemporary issues in bioethics* (2nd ed., pp. 198–203).

Warren, S. D., & Brandeis, L. D. (1984). The right to privacy. *Harvard Law Review, 4*(5).

Wasserstrom, R. (1984). The legal and philosophical foundations of the right to privacy. In Mappes, T. A., & Zembatty, J. S. (Eds.), *Biomedical Ethics* (pp. 109–116). New York: McGraw-Hill.

Winslade, W. J. (1995). *Confidentiality.* (pp. 451-459). Encyclopedia of Bioethics. New York: Macmillan Library Reference.

ENDNOTES

[1] Two of the most common clinical applications are teledermatology and telepsychiatry.

[2] Other neologisms include *cybermedicine, e-health, telemedicine,* and *telehealth.* I will use these terms synonymously and interchangeably in this paper.

3   Rights to privacy are not limited to individuals, but have been assigned to corporations, organizations, and institutions. The notion of rights, especially corporate rights, remains controversial.

4   Divulging personal information to another person is a prerequisite for confidentiality. I will say more about this later.

5   A good example of questions about privacy's distinctiveness can be found in the debates over decisional privacy. This topic is addressed below with a discussion of informational, physical, and decisional privacy.

6   This does not mean consequences have no significance for deontological justifications; it means only that consequences have a secondary role.

7   See note 5.

Chapter 14

Nursing, Ethics, and Healthcare Policy:
Bridging Local, National and International Perspectives

Marilyn Jaffe-Ruiz
Pace University, USA

Sarah Matulis
Pace University, USA

Patricia Sayre
Pace University, USA

ABSTRACT

This chapter examines and analyzes ethical problems associated with the global nursing shortage, the international recruitment of nurses, and the strategies healthcare systems and governments use to minimize the impact of the nursing shortage within their borders. An argument is made that a more appropriate solution to the U.S. nursing shortage is not to pull from already burdened systems, but rather to recruit and provide financial aid to potential nursing students, especially underrepresented and economically disadvantaged students, from within the United States. Implications for migration, education, and healthcare policy are explored. Resulting challenges for nursing leadership and demands on nursing education are addressed, as well as approaches for addressing the issues of providing safe patient care, a satisfying work environment, and professional development.

DOI: 10.4018/978-1-60960-174-4.ch014

INTRODUCTION

Today there is a wide-ranging shortage of nurses (Buchan & Calman, 2004) and (Kline 2004). That adequate nursing care is a requisite for improving healthcare outcomes worldwide is widely recognized and cannot be overemphasized (Buerhaus, et al., 2005a) and (Chenowethm, Jeon, Goff, & Burke, 2006). The nursing shortage severely impedes the development of world health because nurses are the basis for any healthcare system's ability to provide health services. First, the primary role of nurses is to meet their patients' healthcare needs, while acknowledging, respecting and supporting their patients' values (Chenowethm, Jeon, Goff, & Burke, 2006). Additionally, nurses are vital to improving patient outcomes and enabling patients to utilize medical treatment from their providers. Consequently, this shortage looms as one of the biggest obstacles to achieving improved health and well-being for the world's population.

The nursing shortage severely impedes the implementation and development of a feasible means to improve healthcare and address health disparities worldwide. It is important to note the imbalance in the nurse-to-population ratio, which highlights the scope of the shortage. Though nurses are the 'front line' in most healthcare systems, and their contributions are essential to meeting a minimal standard of healthcare and development goals, there is increasing evidence of nurse supply/demand inequality in many countries, which prevents meeting even the minimum standard of care.

Focusing on specific regions helps to highlight the global discrepancies of the nursing shortage. Europe, for example, has the highest ratio of nurses-to-population and it is 10 times greater than the lowest ratios of Africa and Asia. The average ratio in North America is, likewise, 10 times that of South America. The nurse-to-population ratio in the Caribbean varies from island to island, but is higher on average than Central or South America (Buchan & Calman, 2004.)

Even within a single region, there are discrepancies that need to be evaluated. Within Europe, for instance, Scandinavia has an average nurse-to-population ratio that is twice that of southern Europe. Greece, Portugal and Spain report much lower ratios than Scandinavian countries. Many countries in Africa, Asia, and Latin America are finding it especially challenging to retain a minimal level of nurses in their workforce to keep hospitals and clinics operational. Even within a single nation the nurse-to-population ratios can vary from less than ten nurses per 100,000 people to more than 1,000 nurses for 100,000 people – a difference of one hundredfold. The low availability of nurses in many countries is further exacerbated by a geographically uneven distribution, with even fewer nurses available in rural and remote areas than in cities. Adding to the discrepancy, skills and staff mixes vary among organizations, regions, and countries, and there is no "optimal" mix of nurses that countries may expect to achieve soon.

In the United States, the nurse-to-population ratio is approximately 825 nurses for 100,000 people according to the findings from the 2004 National Sample Survey of Registered Nurses, the latest of such surveys to be released to-date (Health Resources and Services Administration, 2006). The Health Resources and Services Administration study *Projected Supply, Demand, and Shortages of Registered Nurses: 2000-2020* calculated an anticipated 20 percent shortage of nurses by 2015, and a 29 percent shortage by 2020. The current shortage in the United States is expected to reach 12 percent in 2010 (Health Resources and Services Administration, July 2002).

In response to this shortage, and because of the financial rewards offered to those who help hospitals in developed nations to fill the gap, the number of international nurse recruiters has grown significantly and healthcare systems of developed nations now look to nurses from outside their borders; predominantly recruiting candidates from developing countries. Critical nursing shortages in industrialized countries are generating a demand that is fueling international recruitment campaigns to obtain nurses educated abroad and integrate them into the United States healthcare system (Brush, Sochalski, & Berger, 2004) and (Buchan & Sochalski, 2004) and (Xu & Kwak, 2007.) The current shortage is not likely to abate as the elderly population is burgeoning, the nursing workforce is aging, and there is an increasing deficit of new nurses to meet the demand due. In 2004, only 8 percent of the U.S. nursing population was under the age of 30, while 41.1 percent were over the age of 50 (Health Resources and Services Administration, 2006.) Though previous deficits have occurred in the past, this is the worst and longest lasting nursing shortage in 50 years for the U. S. (Buerhaus et al., 2005a).

The shortage of registered nurses in the United States will grow even greater as the supply of nurses in the developed world fails to keep pace with increasing demand. Polsky, Ross, Brush, and Sochalski found that, compared with 1990, new foreign-trained RNs in 2000 were twice as likely to originate from low-income countries and 30 percent more likely to originate from countries with a low supply of nurses. They note that even a small upsurge in the number of nurses from countries with a limited number of nurses may represent a large proportion of those countries' total nurse population. "For example, the 11.1 percent of foreign-trained RNs who entered the United States from Africa between 1990 and 2000 alone represents more than 1 percent of the entire stock of African nurses." (Polsky, Ross, Brush, & Sochalski, May 2007).

Issues of the Nursing Shortage

Buchan and Calman point out three critical challenges that are related to global nursing shortages (Buchan & Calman, 2004). The first is the negative impact of HIV/AIDS in sub-Saharan Africa, both upon the healthcare system by making an increased demand for nurses, and upon the nurse population dying from this disease. Second is the

migration of nurses, especially in recent years as the international recruiting of nurses has become more intensive. Domestic migration also is a factor, since nurses are moving from rural to urban areas, from public sector to private sector, and nursing employment to non-nursing employment, searching for better pay or better opportunities. Third, an overall lack of effective health sector reform and reorganization is hampering the supply of nurses. Indeed, state regulations that allow nurses to be mandated long-hours, tasked with physically demanding workloads, while given an increasing number of patients per nurse while administering potentially fatal medications, makes many experienced nurses opt to leave the bedside for other safer, less stressful opportunities.

These issues are not the only hindrances to expanding the nursing workforce. Danger in the workplace from disease exposure and violence against health workers persists in many countries, with nurses often taking the brunt of these problems because they are the forefront of direct patient care and contact (Kingma, 2001), (Likupe, 2006) and (Muular, Mfutso-Bengo, Makoza, & Chatipwa, 2003). Nurse dissatisfaction accounts for much of the exodus of nurses out of the health workforce. Health economist Stephen Birch noted that the global nursing shortage can be attributed to planners not recognizing the increased stress from the increasing workload of nurses, and the consequential burnout this causes (Armstrong, 2003). A survey study conducted in the U.S. by Buerhaus, Donelan, Ulrich, Kirby, Norman, and Dittus, determined that low job satisfaction for RNs could be predicted with key variables of high stress leading to burnout, an overall negative view of the healthcare system in which they are working in, being burdened by non-nursing tasks, and an increase in the nurse-to-patient ratio. [15]

Furthermore, this research determined that less than half of all the nurses surveyed would recommend nursing as a profession to those who wanted respect in the workplace. Similarly, as Lathan, Hogan and Ringl noted, although the workplace environment is a key aspect of nurse retention, recruitment, and patient safety, "there is ongoing evidence that inadequate communication, intra-professional oppression, and lack of collaboration and conflict resolution continue to disempower nurses and hinder improvement of workforce conditions. (Buerhaus et al., (2005).

Another significant barrier to expanding the population of US nurses is the dearth of nurse educators. As with the general nursing population, there is a growing shortage of nurse educators. Also mirroring the general nursing population, 39.4 percent of nursing educators are over age 55.[5] A 2009 study by the American Association of Colleges of Nursing found 803 staff vacancies reported by 310 schools of nursing. In addition to these reported vacancies 117 schools cited the need to create 279 additional faculty positions to accommodate student demand (Fang & Tracy, 2009).

Ethical Implications for Nursing

Ethical considerations in nursing recruitment and retention are nothing new, but this debate has escalated over the past few years as international nurse recruitment and the demand for nurses have markedly increased. This ethical dilemma has, consequently, been discussed more frequently in the nursing literature in recent years. When considering this, Xu and Zhang contend that the paramount issue required of us to understand in "the ethical standards of international nurse recruitment is to know whose interests they are designed to represent and protect (Xu & Zhang, 2005).

Two primary ethical paradigms often discussed are: (1) the individual right of nurses from developing countries to seek out opportunities and lives they believe to be best for themselves and their families, and (2) the burden the "brain drain" of nurses imposes on already overly burdened healthcare systems in the developing world, countries from where most of nurses being recruited were

born and trained. A common mistake made is deeming these viewpoints as contradictory.

The authors do not challenge the right of the individual to migrate from his or her country or region to another where he or she believes greater opportunities lie. Even before the nursing shortage, migration was part of the human condition (Lane, 2005). Immigration, in fact, is often heralded as allowing regions to experience greater diversity and an influx of ideas. International nursing recruitment, however, goes one step beyond this to entice and obtain human resources from countries and regions where the supply is scarce and the consequences severe, to the few regions that have less of a shortage. Proponents of recruiting foreign nurses argue that recruiting from developing nations helps to alleviate poverty for individuals, especially women who would otherwise be forced to cope with a lifetime of poverty and poor work environments. Moreover, nurses who come to the U.S. to work send money back home, thereby increasing the economic standards for their families and communities, which in turn benefits their countries of origin.

This premise does not fully recognize the severity the loss of each individual nurse imposes upon already burdened health systems. In fact, by recruiting nurses from regions with a disproportionately large nursing shortage, recruiting organizations are worsening the conditions they claim to be rescuing nurses from, thereby making it more problematic and grueling for nurses who choose to stay, and less likely that students will choose to enter the field of nursing. This, in turn, further encourages nurses to leave these desperate situations, forming a downward spiral.

The contentions of proponents of foreign nurse recruitment must be looked at with some skepticism, as recruiting organizations are not charitable, humanitarian organizations fighting for the empowerment of foreign nurses working in impoverished conditions. They are not seeking a means to eradicate poverty nor are they taking steps to help developing nations build-up their nursing workforces.

As noted previously, the right of each individual to seek out his or her best opportunities in life must be acknowledged and respected, and it should be noted that there are "push" factors in nurses leaving their home countries to emigrate. Indeed, the "push" of poor working conditions and low pay for nurses in their home countries already encourages many skilled nurses to seek better options elsewhere. This does not negate the ethical problem that the "pull" of U.S. hospitals and international recruiters cause by further depleting developing nations of vital resources while putting an unfair burden on these countries to educate nurses whose resources will be used elsewhere. For these reasons, De Raeve, the Committee Secretary General of the Standing Committee of Nurses of the European Union (EU), rejected overseas recruitment as a solution for the nursing shortage in developed countries. He noted, "It is, to say at the least, unethical, and in many cases any existing surplus of nurses may be the result of an under-resourced and underdeveloped health service" (De Raeve, 2003) The potentially damaging consequences of overseas recruitment needs to be taken into account in any worldwide strategy that may be developed to tackle the global problem of nursing shortages.

Nursing leaders, then, must consider ways of influencing the global perspective. Key steps taken can help curb the recruitment of international nurses as a short-term solution to a long-term problem. First, nursing leaders must use their collective voice to develop a plan which is ethically and morally responsible. This can only be achieved by discouraging and refraining from engaging in unfair or unethical recruitment practices while advocating for policies to attract more people from domestic resources into nursing. Toward this end, recruitment and finance aid for nursing education for minority and economically disadvantaged students who are underrepresented in the field of nursing would be a valuable first step.

The 2004 National Sample Survey of Registered Nurses found that only approximately 12.2 percent of all RNs self-reported as an ethnic or racial minority, making minority nurses significantly underrepresented in comparison to the distribution of minorities in the general population of the United States. Increasing the diversity of the nurse population would also aid in increasing patient access to culturally competent care. Additionally, National Sample Survey Data suggests that minority nurses are more likely to work full-time in nursing than non-minority counterparts. The report showed that 75.2 - 81.2 percent of employed minority RNs worked full-time, compared to 68.5 percent of employed non-Hispanic White RNs.[5] Additionally, special attention must be given to increasing the number of nurse educators in the United States. Raising the number of new nurses educated in the U.S. cannot occur without first providing ample teachers to do so.

Meanwhile nurse leaders must step up efforts to change and improve health care delivery systems so that nurses are not worn out and, therefore, drop out of the system or discourage others from entering it. Adherence to "Magnet" principles, which keep hospitals accountable for improving the workplace for nurses, is likely to help nurse recruitment and retention. Indeed, "Magnet" principles were first defined in a 1983 research study that identified the characteristics of organizations that were best able to recruit and retain nurses during the nursing shortages of the 1970s and 1980s. Fourteen principles were characterized, including image of nursing, professional development opportunities, quality nursing leadership, and organizational structure (American Nurse Credentialing Center, 2009). Likewise, an increase in resources to support the development of comprehensive human resource strategies and to assess current work patterns and benefits is vital. There must be a development of global health funds to strengthen human resource delivery infrastructures, including education. Finally, forming strategic alliances between governments, donors, agencies, educators, regulators, unions and associations to maximize buy-in of various stakeholders and to expand availability of resources is necessary.

Developed countries can help those that are developing to build capacity in the area of human resource planning and management, build national self-sufficiency to manage domestic issues of supply and demand, and improve access to high-quality technical assistance. Developing countries need to be urged and supported in taking action at the national level. They must consider the range of nursing personnel required to meet national health needs; embrace new models of care, with an emphasis on primary care and new technologies; address issues of skill mix and the delegation/devolution of some tasks to other workers; and improve workloads and working conditions.

CONCLUSION

In a report issued by the Sullivan Commission, former Surgeon General Leon Sullivan issued thirty-seven recommendations to address the root causes of the nation's underrepresentation of minority health professionals, including nurses, doctors and dentists.[23] The Commission found that failure to reverse this trend could place the health of at least one-third of the nation's citizens at risk as health care providers become further disconnected from the minority populations they serve (Sullivan Commission, 2004).

In this article the authors have reviewed various issues of nursing recruitment and retention and the implications of the nursing shortage both upon developing nations and developed nations. Over reliance on foreign educated nurses by the health care industry serves only to postpone efforts to address the needs of nursing students and the United States nursing workforce and further deplete already overly burdened healthcare systems. The U.S. government must engage in health care workforce planning to build a sustainable nursing

and health care workforce and must provide additional funding for domestic schools of nursing to foster sufficient preparation of nurses for the U.S., from within the U.S.

REFERENCES

American Nurse Credentialing Center. (2009). *Forces of magnetism*. Retrieved on October 14, 2009, from http://www.nursecredentialing.org/Magnet/ProgramOverview/ForcesofMagnetism.aspx

Armstrong, F. (2003). Migration of nurses: Finding a sustainable solution. *Australian Nursing Journal*, 11.

Brush, B., Sochalski, J., & Berger, A. (2004). Imported care: Recruiting foreign nurses to U.S. healthcare facilities. *Health Affairs, 23*(3), 78–87. doi:10.1377/hlthaff.23.3.78

Buchan, J., & Calman, L. (2004). *The global shortage of registered nurses: An overview of issues and actions*. International Council of Nurses.

Buchan, J., & Sochalski, J. (2004). The migration of nurses: Trends and policies. *Bulletin of the World Health Organization, 82*(8), 587–594.

Buerhaus, P., Donelan, K., Ulrich, B., Kirby, L., Norman, L., & Dittus, R. (2005a). Registered Nurses' perceptions of nursing. *Nursing Economics, 23*(3), 110–118.

Buerhaus, P., Donelan, K., Ulrich, B., Norman, L., Williams, M., & Dittus, R. (2005). Hospital RNs' and CNOs' perceptions of the impact of the nursing shortage on the quality of care. *Nursing Economics, 23*(5), 214–221.

Chenowethm, L., Jeon, Y., Goff, M., & Burke, C. (2006). Cultural competency and nursing care: An Australian perspective. *International Nursing Review, 53*, 34–40. doi:10.1111/j.1466-7657.2006.00441.x

De Raeve, P. (2003). Nursing powers in the EU: The role and outcomes of the Standing Committee of Nurses of the EU. *Journal of Advanced Nursing, 43*, 4.

Fang, D., & Tracy, C. (2009). *Special survey on vacant faculty positions for academic year 2009-2010.* Washington, DC: American Association of Colleges of Nursing.

Health Resources and Services Administration. (2002). *Projected supply, demand, and shortages of Registered Nurses*: 2000-2020. Washington, DC.

Health Resources and Services Administration. (2006). *The Registered Nurse population: Findings from the 2004 National Sample Survey of Registered Nurses.* Retrieved on October 14, 2009, from http://bhpr.hrsa.gov/healthworkforce/rnsurvey04/3.htm

Kingma, M. (2001). Nursing migration: Global treasure hunt or disaster-in-the-making? *Nursing Inquiry, 8*(4), 205–212. doi:10.1046/j.1440-1800.2001.00116.x

Kline, D. (2003). Push and pull factors in international nurse migration. *Journal of Nursing Scholarship, Second Quarter.*

Lane, M. (2005). Philosophical perspectives on states and immigration. Retrieved on September 19, 2008, from http://www histecon.kings.cam.ac.uk/docs/lane_migration.pdf

Latham, C., Hogan, M., & Ringl, K. (2008). Nurses supporting nurses: Creating a mentoring program for staff nurses to improve the workforce environment. *Nursing Administration Quarterly, 32*(1), 27–39.

Likupe, G. (2006). Experiences of African nurses in the UK National Health Service: A literature review. *Journal of Clinical Nursing,* 15.

Muular, A., Mfutso-Bengo, J., Makoza, J., & Chatipwa, E. (2003). The ethics of developed nations recruiting nurses from developing countries: The case of Malawi. *Nursing Ethics, 10*(4). International Council of Nurses. (2006). *Patient and Public Safety Matter: The Biennial ICN Report, 2004-2006.*

Polsky, D., Ross, S., Brush, B., & Sochalski, J. (2007, May). Trends in characteristics and country of origin among foreign-trained nurses in the United States, 1990 and 2000. *American Journal of Public Health, 97,* 895–899. doi:10.2105/AJPH.2005.072330

Sullivan Commission. (2004). *Missing persons: Minorities in the health professions.* Retrieved on July 22, 2006, from http://www.amsa.org/advocacy/Sullivan_ Commission.pdf

Xu, Y., & Kwak, C. (2007). *Comparative trend analysis of characteristics of internationally educated nurses and U.S.-educated nurses in the United States.* International Council of Nurses.

Xu, Y., & Zhang, J. (2005). One size doesn't fit all: Ethics of international nurse recruitment from the conceptual framework of stakeholder interests. *Nursing Ethics, 12*(6), 571–581. doi:10.1191/0969733005ne827oa

Chapter 15
Why Doesn't Information Systems Vision Exist in the Healthcare Sector?

Matthew W. Guah
Claflin University, USA

ABSTRACT

The nature of healthcare provision has changed dramatically and irreversibly over the past two decades. The focus has shifted from inward-looking supervision of medical care with substantial protection and defensive attitude to globally oriented, patient-centric facilitation of medical care and preventive services. Information technologies are increasingly playing a key role in reforming healthcare globally. How much of this reform addresses the primary goal of healthcare institutions? This chapter questions current expectations that information technology could bring benefits to healthcare sector—for which governments around the world are mandating and increasing investment in IT initiatives. There has been a remarkable expansion of information technology capabilities resulting in many ambitious IT projects in various healthcare institutions. The most sophisticated ones seem to concentrate on relatively simple coordination, resource allocation and documentation aspects of healthcare delivery process. There is little emphasis on the management of treatment process or optimization of resource use because definitive models do not exist for patient treatment processes.

The major question being presented for open discussion here is whether these IT projects coincide with the primary goals of healthcare organizations. Is there an overall vision for IT in healthcare? If so, what is it? How does such vision contribute to the primary objectives of healthcare? Finding answers to these questions increases our understanding of current IT initiatives and considers the implications of the organizing vision for further development and diffusion of healthcare IS.

DOI: 10.4018/978-1-60960-174-4.ch015

INTRODUCTION

A typical hospital—in USA, UK and most Western countries—is available at all hours of the day providing medical attention to a wide variety of patients. Every treatment must be tailored and provided within reasonable time. Combined with substantial increases in the number of people visiting hospitals today, hospital environments have been observed with patients being forgotten in hallways, some have been turned away, medical records have been misplaced and waiting times have been unacceptably excessive. Massive investment in healthcare IT promises to improve the health and political impact of several instigated efforts to ensure patient waiting and treatment times are minimized. Policy makers and healthcare leaders are increasingly looking to IT to play an important role in addressing these issues (Guah & Currie, 2007). How much of the current healthcare reform initiatives typically incorporate industrial engineering principles? Although there have been some degree of success, huge gaps still exist in our understanding of healthcare delivery process. With current overviews of patient flows the facilitation of decision support activities with IT remains elusive. Yet high expectations for the "solution" that IT might bring to healthcare, government mandates and funding for IT initiatives and dramatic expansion of IT capabilities are stimulating ambitious IT projects in various healthcare institutions (Guah, 20011). Could such expectations be reconciled with limited "hard evidence" of true economic value of healthcare IS and substantial barriers to successful adoption and diffusion?

With heightened interest and investment in healthcare reform, a number of huge IT projects have sprung up in the last two decades aimed at improving healthcare delivery quality, reducing cost and better access to patient data. Spending on healthcare accounts for a substantial and growing portion of the gross domestic product (GDP) in many countries. (e.g., 14.1% of American GDP;

average of 8% for 30 countries in the Organization for Economic Cooperation and Development). While the level of financial investment for these systems is very impressive (Baig & Gururajan, 2011; Guah & Currie, 2007) they focus on relatively simple coordination, resource allocation and documentation aspects of hospital operations (Wickramasinghe, 2010; Mark, 2007). *IT initiative* is used here to characterize these projects (Guah, 2007). The focus in this paper is to understand the true vision of these IT initiatives and how they could be organized around different healthcare goals.

An organizing vision incorporates not only IT projects, but also assumptions about organizing healthcare practices and institutions to take advantage of IT capabilities. Does the organizing vision for IT initiative incorporates ideas about coordinated clinical care, reduced medical errors, and improved compliance to clinical standards and guidelines? Despite uncertainties about IT costs, benefits and implications, organizing visions for IT in healthcare can stimulate interest and investment in IT. While the healthcare industry has started to gain experience with unrestrained IT projects, some stakeholders are beginning to raise concerns about the costs and institutional barriers that hinder successful implementations (Baig & Gururrajan, 2011; Currie & Guah, 2007). In contrast to general IT industry innovation processes, government and charity foundations collaboratively play complex and vital roles in the shaping of organizing visions for IT use in the healthcare sector. This has resulted to questions around the unilateral expectation that IT initiatives in healthcare will improve the quality of healthcare delivery. Conflicting goals and priorities among various healthcare actors are also becoming more evident. Beliefs about how IT initiatives in healthcare could improve healthcare delivery quality, reduce cost and improve access to patient data in the face of substantial economic, social and institutional barriers are also being debated as part of IT vision in healthcare (Abrahan et al, 2010).

LOOKING FOR EVIDENCE

IS in healthcare consists of complex organizational technologies; with applications, usages, limitations and implications that have neither clear-cut benefits nor assured projects champions amongst the many actors (Wilson & Tulu, 2010). Clear and convincing ideas about how IS can improve healthcare delivery costs, quality and access are critical to promote adoption and guide successful implementation. Such ideas can be negotiated among various stakeholders, including medical practitioners, executives of healthcare institutions, health department and other government regulatory agencies, as well as IT vendors and consultants working in the healthcare sector. Better understanding of the social construction and interpretive processes through which healthcare IS are developed and communicated is key to anticipating outcomes of IT impact in this critical sector. Such understanding will direct the IT vision and healthcare, *legitimising* various reform initiatives and *mobilizing* the healthcare IT marketplace in ways that facilitate development and diffusion of the IT. A mature marketplace consists of responsible consortiums that develop standards and facilitate the development of complementary products to reassure potential adopters.

IS in our healthcare institutions today attempt to provide a range of support from patient workflow management to electronic patient record facilities. A number of Healthcare IS currently assists with patient tracking, workload management and record handling. Additional functionalities are also provided to these systems through supplementary, particularly wireless, hardware that facilitates patient, patient record, test result and resource tracking. They may be interfaced with handheld tablets that can display patient records or accept nurse and doctor documentation, orders for prescriptions and follow-up instructions. Healthcare IS, for the most part, provide for data entry for triage, nursing assessment, doctor assessment and prescription management. Patient management is usually facilitated by provision of workflow modules that list patients awaiting treatment, their presenting problem and their severity. In theory an integrated healthcare IS can incorporate every step in the patient care process, thus, automating human handoffs in healthcare delivery process. Each step can automatically be logged and tracked. Timing of steps can be determined and acceptable variation in timing and sequencing specified. Human interactions with networked electronic devices such as personal computers, CT scanners, lab systems, telephones, IV pumps, and wireless patient tracking tags can be linked to the system for automation of process control. Physicians entering orders, nurses bar-coding medications, clerks registering patients, and surgeons scheduling surgery can be linked and coordinated automatically as they perform their own specialties. Workflow engines sequence, monitor, track, alert, and reroute any step in each of the patient care processes. While such a vision for IS in healthcare is laudable and are possibly achievable in the future, current healthcare systems fall well short of this image (Guah & Davidson, 2008). Many systems in use today do promote reduction of waiting time, transfer and rework times by improving coordination of staff and resources, but they certainly do not optimise patient flow and resource use, nor do they address decision support for clinical aspects of patient treatment (Wickramasinghe, 2010). Guah (2011) suggest a problem of modelling the accuracy of patient care monitoring in our healthcare institutions to be the result of such inabilities. Models of the patient treatment processes do not exist, so IS cannot predict what the next step in any process is likely to be, greatly handicapping their ability to actively support decision-making in the healthcare sector.

Within the healthcare discourse, IS vision takes shape as a solution to medical problems or issues that are widely recognized within the healthcare sector. The specific *business problem* for which this organizing vision provides a solution is refined, extended, and sometimes redirected as stakeholders in the sector gain experience with the system, and such experiences filter into the discourse. While it may be difficult for an organizing vision to represent a consensus view among all stakeholders in healthcare—where competitive views and perspectives are common—various stakeholders are bound to take positions relative to an evolving vision. Many stakeholders shall actively attempt to shape the organizing vision through the discourse, often to their own advantage (Guah & Davidson, 2008). By so doing, the IS vision acts both as an output of a healthcare discourse and as a shaping influence on that stakeholders

Past attempts to model of healthcare IS simply led to grouping patients according to demographic variables and in a form of high level patient flows using simulation, industrial engineering and medical case mix concepts (Guah, 2011; Porter & Teisberg, 2006). Such views of patients are proving to be difficult because of the complexity of symptoms, range of severities and variety of medical specialisations involved in treatment. Each patient is different in seemingly unpredictable ways so treatment has to be individually customized, thus, the existing difficulties to move healthcare IS beyond the generic ordering, recording and monitoring support for individual patients we see today.

That leaves us with few unanswered questions:

- Is that because these systems design have been based on administrative functions (such as triage, bed or room allocation, nurse and doctor assessments, laboratory, drug and imaging, ordering and coordination, and discharge-related documentations)?
- Is Information System capable of taking a process-centric view of healthcare, where hospital operations are viewed as a series of value-adding functions, with various functions describing the flow of patients through healthcare institutions from arrival to departure?

Answers to the above questions are necessary for proper IS alignment to healthcare functions portraying the inherent sequence of activities. Existing healthcare IS cannot accurately support patient treatment process in the absences of patient group recognition according to process similarity—something Vissers (2005:71) called 'iso-process grouping'. Every patient treatment should be viewed as unique. Any attempt to manage the complexity of the hospital departments by applying additional coordination mechanisms to cater for the variety of patients, treatment locations, staff and resources may lead to a situation where overhead costs for the additional control systems surpass the benefit of efficient coordination of every variant. Some authors have documented particular difficulties with Iso-process grouping of patients due the broad range of demographics and presentations (Vissers, 2005), and this is undoubtedly limiting healthcare IS advances in this regard. Could there be a new technique consisting of self-organised process mining that may allow iso-process grouping of patients?

ORGANIZING VISION FOR IT INITIATIVES

Why are most reform initiatives in healthcare today deemed unsuccessful? Could it be that IS visions in healthcare are non-distinctive and overburdened with implausible expectations for applicability? Have certain IT projects lost support to other visions which may have proven to be more compelling?

Ramiller and Swanson (2003) suggest four characteristics of an organizing vision relating to the ability to influence IS adoption and diffusion:

- The IS vision must be *interpretable* and *informative* about the value of the system.

- The IS vision must be *plausible*, which means free of exaggerated or misplaced claims about expected outcomes for the adopters.

- The IS vision must convey a sense of *importance* to the IT initiatives, not only that the initiative has significant business value but also that it is (or is likely to be) accepted within the marketplace.

- The IS vision must be *distinctive* and valuable, but not substantially discontinuity from existing technologies and practices. If too different, the innovation may be perceived as unreachable.

Using the above, how can we represent IS vision in healthcare? Many references to electronic health records have recently begun to take shape as a vision distinct from related healthcare IT innovations. We also notice IS projects to be attracting significant attention and funding in healthcare, although a clear definition of electronic health records has not emerged amongst healthcare professionals (Abrahan et al, 2010). Little evidence exists demonstrating business problems, technology solutions, and institutional implications have been negotiated within the healthcare discourse to ensure the most analytically useful IS vision emerges. Understanding some form of substance, evolution and influence of an IS vision is important for healthcare managers and policy makers spearheading IT projects. An in-depth, empirical analysis of the IS visions in healthcare is also of interest to management theory, since few studies have examined an IS vision empirically. Such empirical assessment of the IS vision in healthcare would lead to an understanding of how various stakeholders (practitioners, hospitals, insurers, consultants, etc.) may interpret and respond to the current drive for IT projects in healthcare.

We need better understanding of specific IS vision in healthcare to facilitate the assessment of similarities and differences within the general analytic framework for organizing visions. Some aspects of IS processes are common across industries and service sectors. However, variations in the technical and institutional environments of industries can influence the realization of IT vision and its institutional applications in a significant way for healthcare. A good empirical examination of the IS vision will also explore the social and technical boundaries of this theoretic view. This will also conceptualise a framework for healthcare and help to delineate general social construction processes from those specific to the healthcare sector.

Visions coalesce around widely acknowledged problems and issues in the healthcare discourse termed the "business problematic." In most Western countries, reducing the rate of growth of healthcare spending, improving the quality of healthcare delivery, and improving access to quality healthcare are the high-level goals stated (in varying degrees, terms and specificity) for all healthcare IS projects. Most discussions of the benefits of electronic health records are founded on a few common assumptions. For example, that collecting and sharing data electronically can reduce medical errors and duplication of services, which result from lack of information, misinformation, or misinterpretation of information (e.g., illegible handwriting) at the point of care delivery. One related assumption is that by intervening via IT in the health care encounter with practice—guidelines, alerts and reminders—physicians will make more informed and cost-effective decisions. With the advent of many healthcare websites on the Internet and consumer interest in online information, justifications for IT projects sometimes incorporate ideas about sharing data with patients (patient health records) and patients' active involvement in health management.

Using IT to address these widely acknowledged issues in the U.S. healthcare system involves the use of a core set of information technologies as well as organizing and re-organizing healthcare practices and institutions to take advantage of IT capabilities. Assumptions about technologies and practices are interrelated in the IS vision in complex ways. For example, making patient-level clinical data available among loosely coupled healthcare providers via a secure network is core to the vision for IT, because data accessibility and sharing are assumed to be proximate causes of quality problems such as drug interaction. However, identifying a patient's data reliably across multiple providers is challenging not only due to technology problems (e.g., lack of a common patient identifier in disparate systems, lack of system interoperability) but also due to a legal and legislative problem.

Patient records would include integrated access to all patient data, opportunities to provide reminders, alerts and advice to clinicians at the point of care (i.e., built-in care protocols), methods for direct entry of data by clinicians, a vehicle for greater access to clinical knowledge bases, and communication support to all clinicians treating a patient. The technological capabilities that support these functions include a database of patient data, computerized processing systems in clinical departments (e.g., laboratory, pharmacy, radiology), an interface (usually browser-based, more recently wireless and mobile) for clinical order entry and viewing, and an interface engine, utilizing standards for clinical data representation (such as HL7) to integrate data from various sources and devices. This view of patient record assumes a network to link clinical system components together and to administrative systems and to allow access to medical libraries exists.

This IS vision is similar to the emerging vision of electronic health records in that both assume computerized data will be acquired, stored, and accessed at the patient level and that data will be integrated across organizational boundaries. Both also assume that such a system is most valuable if it mediates the clinician-patient interaction at the point of care. That is, the system becomes a third party in care delivery encounter, providing some data and requiring other data be entered during the encounter. Problems with implemented that

are anticipated, or have been encountered, with patient record are a result of these changes in clinical practice. Physicians have resisted direct order entry, citing reduced productivity and time to enter as barriers. Easy-to-use and meaningful representation of non-standardized clinical data also remains a barrier to adoption, though widespread availability of web-based interfaces and mobile devices has lessened interface issues.

WHY HAVE INFORMATION SYSTEMS VISION FOR HEALTHCARE?

Could it be that IS vision is emerging from healthcare institutions' organization-centric visions for hospitals, physician practices or a form of network-centric visions of sharing health information among a variety of healthcare providers? Two recent prominent examples of implementing comprehensive patient information are Patient Support Systems (Santa Barbara, California) and Connecting for Health (England, UK). Both systems cost around $10m each, created a pilot, fully operational peer-to-peer data exchange for participating healthcare providers. Early hopes to promote full-blown systems in both cases were scrapped, due to lack of consensus on vendors and functionality and high initial investment costs to healthcare institutions. The system intervenes at the point of care delivery with relevant patient information, but not with care guideline reminders. Physicians at various levels of IS adoption, can use the data exchange system.

IS vision represents the stakeholder community's negotiated interpretations of these IT projects. The vision changes as stakeholders gain experience with the innovation, particularly as problems and limitations become known. Several major issues have been identified in the healthcare discourse related to IT projects related to the successful adoption and diffusion of patient records. Some issues are common to many emerging technologies, such as lack of standardization that inhibits interoperability and data exchange. Other issues are more specific to the healthcare industry. For example, legislative requirements to maintain patient privacy and confidentially have raised concerns about security and access to networked patient records repositories.

Could finding vision for IS bring an end to so much attention in the healthcare discourse regarding low level of IT adoption in healthcare institutions generally and in general practices in particular? Some of the underlying causes of low adoption are possibly unique to the NHS (UK National Health Service). Another key issue is local primary care trusts are losing out financially as the NHS invests billions of pounds on healthcare. These healthcare institutions not only bear the direct expense of investing in healthcare IT, but also suffer from reduced productivity in patient care as a result of the learning cure for new IT systems as well as any increases in time to enter and maintain electronic patient data.

The current targets of Healthcare IS fail to proactively support patient flow and resource allocation partly because they approach the primary goal of hospital activities—operations—from s semi-clinical rather than process perspective. Thus, patients tend to be grouped according to arrival sequence, urgency, demographic variables and diagnosis. While such groupings may provide insight into patient severity, they do not facilitate decision support activities due to the lack of any type of predictive functions. For example, by knowing a patient's urgency or age does not help determine that patient's treatment or diagnosis, but may only give an indication of resource requirements. Healthcare practitioners also need treatment clusters that combine predictive properties with traditional clinical groupings to provide a high level of decision support. Possibly the greatest impediment to process-based decision support, however, it is generally believed, in medical circles, that definition of treatment process, prediction of resource requirements and delivery specifications are not possible.

With this view of healthcare delivery process, treatments are clusters based on scrupulously maintained hospital records providing a picture of actual treatment being performed in within each department. Classifying patients according to the treatment they receive reduces the uncertainty associated with emergency operations. Where demand (patient arrival) was indeterminate with respect to type of presentation (ailment) a host of methods are now available to predict what treatment the next patient is likely to need and what procedure any patient is likely to need next. The current view is that treatment of patient needs to be tailored to every patient. Would that require placing patients into treatment classes that can be measured and managed using the idea of a focused information factory? A decision support system loaded with information about the pathways patients are expected to follow should be able to provide several views of hospital departmental operations.

As different groups of healthcare IS users gain experience, and such experiences are reported in the public discourse, ideas about the possibilities and limitations of IT use in healthcare will evolve and possibly be transformed. The concept of an IS vision provides a useful theoretic framework to examine the social construction processes through which systems are developed, adopted and applied in the healthcare sector. Investments in healthcare IT are increasing globally, especially amongst Western governments. An understanding of these social processes will help healthcare practitioners to interpret the potential and the reality of IS and informs policy setting and action. Such research will be valuable to healthcare leaders and managers, as it identifies and synthesizes issues in the discourse related to patient records and their implications for healthcare policy. The research will also contribute to general management theory by applying, testing, and conceptualising the IS vision framework through its empirical application in the healthcare sector.

A 'GOOD FOR HEALTHCARE' LABEL

This paper proposes a need for new method to extract process information and the resulting treatment clusters of self-organised process mining described as well as others. It may be concluded that treatment clusters present an invigorating opportunity for enhancements to healthcare IS. It is also evident that the healthcare industry is necessarily cautious about implementing changes, as may be expected from the imperative to care for patients come paramount (Guah, 2011). There are two essential elements challenging researchers in the healthcare arena:

- First, the confirmation of treatment clusters at hospitals anywhere in the world needs to be research. While initial explorations across multiple hospital campuses are being carried out, the viability of the process approach, in-depth studies have yet to be conducted, and the researcher are actively seeking collaborators in any country who wish to pursue similar explorations.
- Second, area in which this research needs to be extended is in the development and testing of a prototype system. A unique simulation model should be built to support prototype development. This simulation model should be integrated with a decision support system built around the ideas contained in this paper. This will permit the exploration of decision support scenarios in a safe, simulated environment prior to testing in the hospital setting.

A second possibility is that, as healthcare practitioners' experiences with IT projects are interpreted and shared, the Healthcare IS vision may be seen as implausible or too much of a discontinuity from current practices and structures to be feasibly achieved. At a high level, IT use, computerization of medical information, and data sharing are seen as inherently good and their beneficial effects on health care costs and quality are accepted almost as a matter of faith. However, significant causal factors related to healthcare costs and quality has little to do with information collection and sharing. For example, the aging of the "baby boom" generation, with the anticipated consumption of health care services, will not be averted through information use. Development of costly medical technologies and demands for their use also contribute to escalating costs. Several of the sources we reviewed attempted to characterize the tangible financial benefits of HIS, but these analysis were based on broad assumptions with highly variable estimates (such as the IOM's estimates of the rate of medical errors), thus these financial analysis are at best questionable. Quantifying economic and productivity effects of IT investments, particularly at aggregate levels of analysis, is difficult to do in any industry. In the healthcare industry, financial benefits that do accrue may go to stakeholders who will not necessarily pass on savings (e.g., 3rd party payers), or they may dissipate among a broad range of stakeholders, so that aggregate effects are negligible. To effectively legitimate and mobilize the adoption process, the Healthcare IS organizing vision must develop and be articulated in a way that provides a clearer cause-effect path from investment to savings. Programs should also be put into place to evaluate costs and savings, so that the credibility of the vision can grow.

The HIS vision may presents substantial structural and practice discontinuities as well as technological challenges to the healthcare sector. Some of these discontinuities exist at the institutional level of the NHS (Currie & Guah, 2007). But to be effective at promoting IS adoption in healthcare sector this vision must mobilize various stakeholders to organize in ways that promote experience sharing and support to smaller institutions. Medical professional bodies (like British Medical Associations and Royal Society of Nursing) and consulting organizations would definitely play key roles in this aspect of the patient record vision.

Low adoption rates in both UK and USA are in sharp contrast with certain nations' (i.e. Malaysia, Canada, Singapore, Australia, etc.) experiences with adoption of IT in healthcare. As government healthcare IT investments grows in Western countries, it is possible that many are watching until they see sustained and substantial commitment of resources by the national government or a bandwagon effect begins to develop.

CONCLUSION

This chapter promotes research that focuses on various organizing visions for IT initiatives in the healthcare sector, specifically patient-centric systems. Such visions could build on related organizing visions like electronic medical records, community health information networks, care records service, electronic appointment booking, electronic transmission of prescriptions, and electronic transfer of digital images (e.g. X-rays and scans) and other IT initiatives being supported by national IT infrastructure and network projects. There is a further need to assess the substance and significance of these organizing visions and examine the discourse related to healthcare business, professional and academic reputations. Such analysis should highlight stakeholders' expectations for IT initiatives, both benefits and potential issues. The work should consider how the healthcare IT organizing vision would influence the diffusion and assimilation of IT capacities in specific contexts as well as suggestions for specific theoretic frameworks apply within the institutional environment of healthcare.

There exists a need to present a new approach for the modelling of patient flow in our healthcare institutions and to show how this may be incorporated into decision support systems that enhance existing healthcare IS. Such a model would not only describe how knowledge of patient treatment and subsequent patient flow may be incorporated into IS that extend management of, and deci-sion support for, patient treatment. It would also enhance existing information and evidence for knowledge management and decision support advances in healthcare.

By providing insights into how existing healthcare IS might be extended to provide active decision support, the author has placed healthcare institutions in context of an uncertain and complex environment and went on to review the level of support currently provided by information systems (including networked, wireless and mobile technologies). Opportunities for healthcare IS are not being exploited partly because process-based models do not exists for the core activity of healthcare institutions—patient treatment.

Having IS vision for healthcare can contribute to the following goals:

- Create clarity of purpose of IS in this critical sector
- Unit disparate groups of IS workers currently striving to contribute to a common goal
- Help align priorities and making it easy for healthcare managers to make good decisions
- Attract much needed resources (be it financial, highly skilled HR or technology)
- Inspire and energise both clinical and administrative staff working in healthcare

The IS discipline can benefit as well, both by testing its theories and methods in healthcare settings and through cross-pollination with health informatics expertise." (Wilson & Lankton, 2004). While existence of common and specific treatment processes are exciting from the IS perspective, clinicians may not share the enthusiasm, burdened as they are with the responsibility for human lives. The treatment decision support described in this paper may bring closer healthcare IS the idea of a paperless clinical environment, but such systems can only be developed with the support and sanction of healthcare professionals.

Thus lay major canons of a possible IS vision and framework for the healthcare sector as well as a suggested set of research questions, based on a framework that investigates evolving ideas about patient records. In response to several recent challenge for meaningful IS research (Abrahan, 2010; Guah & Davidson, 2008; Myers et al, 2010; Paul, 2007) the author has described an overall research framework that analyses the discourse related to patient records as a first stage of finding substance of the IS vision in healthcare. The author hopes to follow this chapter by a full research paper that analyses current research with relevance to reforming healthcare delivery processes and management practices.

REFERENCES

Abrahan, C., Akiyama, M., Brown, C., Currie, W., Davidson, E., LeRouge, C., & Strong, D. (2010). *Healthcare IT Adoption under Different Government Models: Debating the HITECH Impacts.* Panel presentation at the International Conference on Information Systems (ICIS2007), December 12-15, 2010, St. Louis, USA.

Baig, A. H., & Gurururajan, R. (2011). *Wireless Technology and Clinical Influences in Healthcare Setting: An Indian Case Study.* Chapter in Guah 2011, Healthcare Delivery Reform and New Technologies: Organizational Initiatives, pp.55-74.

Currie, W. L., & Guah, M. W. (2007). A national programme for IT in the organizational field of healthcare: An example of conflicting institutional logics. *Journal of Information Technology, 22*(3), 235–247. doi:10.1057/palgrave.jit.2000102

Guah, M. W. (2007). *Critical systems diffusion approach in healthcare.* Paper presented at the International Conference of Information Systems, Montreal.

Guah, M. W. (2008). Changing healthcare institutions with large Information Technology projects. *Journal of Information Technology Research, 1*(1), 14–26.

Guah, M. W. (2011). *Healthcare Delivery Reform and New Technologies: Organizational Initiatives*, Preface, pp-xvii.

Guah, M. W., & Currie, W. L. (2007). *Managing vendor contracts in public sector IT: A case study on the UK National Health Service.* Paper presented at the European Conference on Information Systems (ECIS2007), June 7-9, 2007, St. Gallen, Switzerland.

Guah, M. W., & Davidson, E. (2008). *Practicing IS Research in Medical Practice: Opportunities and Dilemmas for Rigors and Relevance in Health IT Research.* Panel presentation at the European Conference for Information Systems (ECIS2008), June 9-11, 2008, Galway, Ireland.

Mark, A. L. (2007). Modernising healthcare–is the NPfIT for purpose? *Journal of Information Technology, 22*, 248–256. doi:10.1057/palgrave.jit.2000100

Myers, M., Baskerville, R., Gill, G., & Ramiller, N. (2010). *Setting Our Research Agendas: Institutional Ecology, Informing Sciences or Management Fashion Theory.* Panel presentation at the International Conference on Information Systems (ICIS2007), December 12-15, 2010, St. Louis, USA.

Paul, R. J. (2007). Changes to Information Systems: Time to change. *European Journal of Information Systems, 16*(3), 193–195. doi:10.1057/palgrave.ejis.3000681

Porter, M. E., & Teisberg, E. O. (2006). *Redefining healthcare: Creating value-based competition on results.* Boston: Harvard Business School Press.

Ramiller, N. C., & Swanson, E. B. (2003). Organizing visions for information technology and the I.S. executive response. *Journal of Management Information Systems, 20*(1), 13–50.

Vissers, J., & Beech, R. (2005). *Health operations management: Patient flow logistics in healthcare care*. UK: Routledge.

Wickramasinghe, N. (2010). The Role for Knowledge Management in Modern Healthcare Delivery. *International Journal of Healthcare Delivery Reform Initiatives, 1*(2), 1–9.

Wilson, E. V., & Lankton, N. K. (2004). Interdisciplinary research and publication opportunities in Information Systems and healthcare. *Communications of the Association for Information Systems, 14*, 332–343.

Wilson, E. V., & Tulu, B. (2010). The rise of a health-IT academic focus. *Communications of the ACM, 53*(5), 147–150. doi:10.1145/1735223.1735259

Compilation of References

104.th Congress of the United States Of America. (1996). Public Law 104-191. In Health Insurance Portability and Accountability Act of 1996. Retrieved July 28, 2009, from http://www.cms.hhs.gov/ HIPAAGenInfo/Downloads/ HIPAALaw.pdf

Abrahan, C., Akiyama, M., Brown, C., Currie, W., Davidson, E., LeRouge, C., & Strong, D. (2010). *Healthcare IT Adoption under Different Government Models: Debating the HITECH Impacts.* Panel presentation at the International Conference on Information Systems (ICIS2007), December 12-15, 2010, St. Louis, USA.

Adams, J. (2007). Risk management: It's not rocket science... It's much more. *Risk Management, 54*(5), 36–40.

Agrawal, R. B., Faloutsos, R., Kiernan, C., Rantzau, J. R., & Srikant, R. (2004). Auditing compliance with a Hippocratic Database. Proceedings of the 30th International Conference on Very Large Databases, 30, 516-527.

Ahlfeldt, R., Erikson, N., & Soderstrom, E. (2009). Standards for information security and processes in healthcare. *Journal of Systems and Information Technology, 11*(3), 295–308. doi:10.1108/13287260910983650

Albrecht, K., & McIntyre, L. (2005). *SpyChips: How major corporations and government plan to track your every move with RFID* (1st ed.). Nashville, TN: Thomas Nelson, Inc.

Alhaqbani, B., Jøsang, A., & Fidge, C. (2009). A medical data reliability assessment model. [from ABI/INFORM Global.]. *Journal of Theoretical and Applied Electronic Commerce Research, 4*(2), 64–78. Retrieved October 11, 2009. doi:10.4067/S0718-18762009000200006

Alhaqbani, B., & Fidge, C. J. (2009). *A time-variant medical data trustworthiness assessment model.* Paper presented at the 11th IEEE International Conference on e-Health Networking, Applications and Services (IEEE HealthCom 2009), 16-18 Dec 2009, Sydney.

Allan, R. (2005). Biometrics wields a double-edged sword. [from Academic Search Premier Database.]. *Electronic Design, 53*(14), 77–81. Retrieved September 10, 2009.

Allen, K. (1999). *Adults with severe disabilities: Federal and state approaches for personal care and other services: HEHS-99-101.* GAO Reports.

Allen, A. L. (1995). *Privacy in healthcare. Encyclopedia of Bioethics* (pp. 2064–2073). New York: Macmillan Library Reference.

AMA Practice Management Center. (2008). *2008 national health insurer report card.* AMA.

Ameri, A. (2004). The five pillars of information security. [from ABI/INFORM Global.]. *Risk Management, 51*(7), 48. Retrieved October 5, 2009.

American Management Association. 2004. *AMA 2004 workplace testing survey: Medical testing.* Retrieved on July 29, 2009 from http://www.amanet.org/ research/pdfs/ medical testing 04.pdf

American Nurse Credentialing Center. (2009). *Forces of magnetism.* Retrieved on October 14, 2009, from http://www.nursecredentialing.org/Magnet/ProgramOverview/ForcesofMagnetism.aspx

Anand, P., & Datta, A. (2004). Protect your IP when outsourcing to India and managing intellectual property. Retrieved September 5, 2009, from Business Source Complete Database.

Angst, C., & Agarwal, R. (2009). Adoption of electronic health records in the presence of privacy concerns: The elaboration likelihood model and individual persuasion. [from Business Source Complete Database.]. *Management Information Systems Quarterly*, *33*(2), 339–370. Retrieved August 12, 2009.

Annadhorai, A., Guenterberg, E., Barnes, J., Haraga, K., & Jafari, R. (2008). *Human indentification by gait analysis*. Paper presented at the HealthNet '08.

Armstrong, F. (2003). Migration of nurses: Finding a sustainable solution. *Australian Nursing Journal*, 11.

Arnold, S., Wagner, J., Hyatt, S., & Klein, G. (2007). Electronic health records: A global perspective. *Healthcare Information and Management Systems Society* (HIMSS). Retrieved December 12, 2009, from http://www.providersedge.com/ehdocs/ehr_articles/Electronic_Health_Records-A_Global_Perspective-Exec_Summary.pdf

Aston, G. (2010). Comparative effectiveness. [from ProQuest Medical Library.]. *Trustee*, *63*(1), 13–14, 19–21. Retrieved May 9, 2010.

Avorn, J. (2009). Debate about funding comparative effectiveness research. *The New England Journal of Medicine*, *360*(19), 1927–1929. doi:10.1056/NEJMp0902427

Bacheldor, B. (2006). *Fort hood to RFID-tag medical records*. Retrieved 9/28, 2009, from http://www.rfidjournal.com/article/articleview/2536/1/1/

Bacheldor, B. (2008). *RFID takes root in Bangladesh early adopters include Apollo hospitals Dhaka and the Bangladesh army*. Retrieved 9/28, 2009, from http://www.rfidjournal.com/article/print/3852

Bacon, P., Jr. (March 18, 2010.). GOP lawmakers, candidates promise to 'repeal it', more than 100 sign pledge to back effort to overturn healthcare bill. *The Washington Post*, A04.

Baig, A. H., & Gurururajan, R. (2011). *Wireless Technology and Clinical Influences in Healthcare Setting: An Indian Case Study*. Chapter in Guah 2011, Healthcare Delivery Reform and New Technologies: Organizational Initiatives, pp.55-74.

Baker, R. B., Caplan, C. L., Emanuel, L. L., & Latham, S. R. (Eds.). (1999). The American medical ethics revolution: How the AMA's code of ethics has transformed physicians' relationships to patients, professionals, and society. *Ethics*, *112*(2), 354–356.

Bala, D. (2008). Biometrics and information security. *Information security curriculum development: Proceedings of the 5th annual conference on Information security curriculum development*, 64-66.

Baldwin-Stried, K. (2006). E-discovery and HIM: How amendments to the federal rules of civil procedure will affect HIM professionals. *Journal of American Health Information Management Association*, *77*(9), 58–60.

Bandyopadhyay, K., & Iyer, R. (2000). Managing technology risks in the healthcare sector: Disaster recovery and business continuity planning. *Disaster Prevention and Management Journal*, *9*(4), 257–270. doi:10.1108/09653560010351899

Barton, T., Shenkir, W., & Walker, P. (2009). The evolution of a balancing act. *Financial Executive*, *25*(10), S10-S12, S14. Retrieved January 13, 2010, from ABI/INFORM Global.

Bashshur, R. L., Sanders, J. H., & Shannon, G. W. (Eds.). (1999). *Telemedicine: Theory and practice*.

Bauer, K. A. (2001). Using the Internet to empower patients and to develop partnerships with clinicians. *The American Journal of Bioethics*, *1*(2).

Bauer, K. A. (2003). Distributive justice and rural healthcare: A case for e-health. *The International Journal of Applied Philosophy*, *17*(2), 243–254.

Bauer, K. A. (2004). Cybermedicine and the moral integrity of the physician-patient relationship. *Journal of Ethics and Information Technology*, *6*, 83–91. doi:10.1007/s10676-004-4591-7

Beasley, M., Frigo, M., & Litman, J. (2007). Strategic risk management: Creating and protecting value. *Strategic Finance*, *88*(11), 24-31, 53.

Beauchamp, T.L. & Childress, J.F. (1994). *Principles of biomedical ethics*.

Benn, S. I., & Gaus, G. F. (1983). *The public and the private: Concepts and action*. London: Croom Helm.

Berkowitz, S. BSC, Marshall, H., & Charles, A., MD, FRCSI. (2007). Retained intra-abdominal surgical instruments: Time to use nascent technology? *The American Surgeon, 73*(11), 1083. Retrieved from http://proquest.umi.com.library.capella.edu/pqdweb?did=1419318761&Fmt=7&clientId=62763&RQT=309&VName=PQD

Bhargav-Spantzel, A., Squicciarini, A., Modi, S., Young, M., Bertino, E., & Elliot, S. (2007). Privacy preserving multi-factor authentication with biometric. *Journal of the Computer Security, 15*(5), 529–560.

Bioethics Committee in Long-Term Care Institutions for the Developmentally Disabled. (2004)... *HEC Forum, 4*(3), 163–173. doi:10.1007/BF00057869

Blitz, C., & Mechanic, D. (2006). Facilitators and barriers to employment among individuals with psychiatric disabilities: A job coach perspective. *Work (Reading, Mass.), 26*(4), 407–419.

Blobel, B. (2004). Authorisation and access control for electronic Health Record Systems. *International Journal of Medical Informatics, 73*(3), 251–257. doi:10.1016/j.ijmedinf.2003.11.018

Bloch, C. (March 24, 2008). Defibrillators and privacy risks. *Federal Telemedicine News*. Retrieved on November 6, 2008, from http://telemedicinenews.blogspot.com/2008/03/defibrillators-and-privacy-risks.html

Blum, D. (2004). Weigh risks of offshore outsourcing. [from Business Source Complete Database.]. *New World (New Orleans, La.), 21*(10), 35–35. Retrieved September 6, 2009.

Blumenthal, D. (2009). Stimulating the adoption of health Information Technology. [from ProQuest Medical Library.]. *The New England Journal of Medicine, 360*(15), 1477–1479. Retrieved May 16, 2010. doi:10.1056/NEJMp0901592

Blumenthal, D. (2010). Launching HITECH. [from ProQuest Medical Library.]. *The New England Journal of Medicine, 362*(5), 382–385. Retrieved May 25, 2010. doi:10.1056/NEJMp0912825

Boatwright, M., & Lou, X. (2007). *What do we know about biometrics authentication?* Paper presented at the Information Security Curriculum Development Conference '07.

Bolevich, Z., & Mules, C. (2009). *A coherent future: Aligning health service and ICT trends.* NZ Ministry of Health. Retrieved from http://www.slideshare.net/HINZ/aligning-health-service-and-ict-trends

Booler, T. (June 16th, 2009). Self-service check. *Sunderland Echo, 1.*

Brailer, D. (2010). Guiding the health Information Technology agenda. [from ProQuest Medical Library.]. *Health Affairs, 29*(4), 586–594. Retrieved May 9, 2010. doi:10.1377/hlthaff.2010.0274

Brenner, J. (2007). ISO 27001: Risk management and compliance. *Risk Management, 54*(1), 24–29.

Brenner, B. (2009). 6 ways we gave up our privacy. *CSOonline*, 1-3.

Brenner, S., & Clarke, L. (2005). *Should commercial misuse of private data be a crime?* Social Science Research Network. Retrieved on November 4, 2008, from http://ssrn.com/abstract=845845

Bristol, N. (2005). The muddle of US electronic medical records. [from Academic Search Premier Database.]. *Lancet, 365*(9471), 1610–1611. Retrieved September 6, 2009. doi:10.1016/S0140-6736(05)66492-6

Britz, J. (2008, May). Making the global information society good: A social justice perspective on the ethical dimensions of the global information society. *Journal of the American Society for Information Science and Technology, 59*(7), 1171–1183. Retrieved September 6, 2009. doi:10.1002/asi.20848

Bromme, A., & Kronberg, M. (2002). *A conceptual framework for testing biometric algorithms within operating systems' authentication.* Paper presented at the SAC '02.

Brooker, R. (2004). Consumers and IT: Setting policy priorities. [from Business Source Complete Database.]. *Consumer Policy Review, 14*(4), 116–125. Retrieved September 6, 2009.

Brouillard, C. P. (2008). *Emergency liability issues specific to healthcare technology.* Retrieved June 17, 2010, from http://www.slidefinder.net/B/Brouillard/13847638

Brown, T. M., Cueto, M., & Fee, E. (2006). The World Health Organization and the transition from "International" to "Global" public health. [from ABI/INFORM Global.]. *American Journal of Public Health, 96*(1), 62–72. Retrieved May 16, 2010. doi:10.2105/AJPH.2004.050831

Brownstein, J., Freifeld, C., & Madoff, L. (2009). Digital disease detection-harnessing the Web for public health surveillance. [from ProQuest Medical Library.]. *The New England Journal of Medicine, 360*(21), 2153–2155, 2157. Retrieved May 17, 2010. doi:10.1056/NEJMp0900702

Bruce, J. A. C. (1984). *Privacy and confidentiality of health information*. Chicago: American Hospital.

Brush, B., Sochalski, J., & Berger, A. (2004). Imported care: Recruiting foreign nurses to U.S. healthcare facilities. *Health Affairs, 23*(3), 78–87. doi:10.1377/hlthaff.23.3.78

Buchan, J., & Calman, L. (2004). *The global shortage of registered nurses: An overview of issues and actions*. International Council of Nurses.

Buchan, J., & Sochalski, J. (2004). The migration of nurses: Trends and policies. *Bulletin of the World Health Organization, 82*(8), 587–594.

Buckovich, S. A., & Rippen, H. E. (1999). Driving toward guiding principles: A goal for privacy, confidentiality, and security of health information. *Journal of the American Medical Informatics Association, 6*, 122–133.

Buehler, J. W., Berkelman, R. L., Hartley, D. M., & Peters, C. J. (2003). Syndromic surveillance and bioterrorism-related epidemics. *Emerging Infectious Diseases, 9*(10), 1197-1204. Retrieved May 15, 2010, from http://ezproxy.library.capella.edu/login?url=http://search.ebscohost.com.library.capella.edu/login.aspx?direct=true&db=aph&AN=11063767&site=ehost-live&scope=site

Buerhaus, P., Donelan, K., Ulrich, B., Kirby, L., Norman, L., & Dittus, R. (2005a). Registered Nurses' perceptions of nursing. *Nursing Economics, 23*(3), 110–118.

Buerhaus, P., Donelan, K., Ulrich, B., Norman, L., Williams, M., & Dittus, R. (2005). Hospital RNs' and CNOs' perceptions of the impact of the nursing shortage on the quality of care. *Nursing Economics, 23*(5), 214–221.

Burris, S. (2002). Disease stigma in U.S. public health law. [from Academic Search Premier Database.]. *The Journal of Law, Medicine & Ethics, 30*(2), 179–190. Retrieved September 6, 2009. doi:10.1111/j.1748-720X.2002.tb00385.x

California, H. C. F. (2009). *An unprecedented opportunity: Using federal stimulus funds to advance health IT in California*. California Healthcare Foundation. Retrieved October 12, 2009, from http://www.chcf.org/

Callahan, J. (2007). *What health care providers need to know about e-discovery. Central New York M.D.* News.

Carter, R., Cobb, J., Earhart, L., & Noblett, A. (2008). *IT compliance management guide: Version 1.0*. Microsoft Corporation. Retrieved October 31, 2009, from http://technet.microsoft.com/en-us/solutionaccelerators/default.aspx

Cats-Baril, W., & Jelassi, T. (1994). The French Videotex system Minitel: A successful implementation of a national Information Technology infrastructure. [from Business Source Complete Database.]. *Management Information Systems Quarterly, 18*(1), 1–20. Retrieved September 6, 2009. doi:10.2307/249607

Causi, S. P. (2009). *Healthcare by 2015*. Canada GHBN. Retrieved from http://www.slideshare.net/GHBN/healthcare-by-2015-mar-2009

CDC. (2009). Safety of influenza A (H1N1) 2009 monovalent vaccines - United States, October 1 - November 24, 2009. *Morbidity and Mortality Weekly Report, 58*, 1-6. Retrieved December 13, 2009 from http://www.cdc.gov/mmwr/preview/mmwrhtml/mm58e1204a1.htm?s_cid=mm58e1204a1_e#tab1

Chan, V., Ray, P., & Parameswaran, N. (2008). Mobile e-Health monitoring: An agent-based approach. *IET Communications, 2*(2), 223–230. Retrieved September 6, 2009. doi:10.1049/iet-com:20060646

Cheek, P., Nikpour, L., & Nowlin, H. (2005). Aging well with smart technology. [from CINAHL with Full Text Database.]. *Nursing Administration Quarterly, 29*(4), 329–338. Retrieved September 6, 2009.

Chenowethm, L., Jeon, Y., Goff, M., & Burke, C. (2006). Cultural competency and nursing care: An Australian perspective. *International Nursing Review, 53*, 34–40. doi:10.1111/j.1466-7657.2006.00441.x

China Daily. (2001). *Patient's privacy rights become an issue in China.* Retrieved September 6, 2009, from http://www.china.org.cn/english/2001/Jul/16178.htm

Christie, J. S. J. (2009). *Electronic discovery for healthcare providers.* Birmingham, AL: Bradley Arant Rose & White LLP.

Ciampa, M. (2005). *Security+ guide to network security fundamentals* (2nd ed.). Boston: Course Technology.

Cintron, A., & Hamel, M. (2006). The effect of a Web-based, patient-directed intervention on knowledge, discussion, and completion of a healthcare proxy. *Journal of Palliative Medicine, 9*(6), 1320–1328. doi:10.1089/jpm.2006.9.1320

Clampitt, H. (2006). The RFID handbook. Retrieved from http://www.rfidhandbook.blogspot.com/.

CMIO. (2009). *HHS requests comments on beefed up HIPAA enforcement abilities.* CMIO Online. Retrieved November 3, 2009, from http://www.cmio.net/index.php?option=com_articles&view=article&id=19372&division=cmio

Collmann, J., & Cooper, T. (2007). Breaching the security of the Kaiser Permanente Internet Patient Portal: The organizational foundations of information security. *Journal of the American Medical Informatics Association, 14,* 239–243. doi:10.1197/jamia.M2195

Collmann, J., & Silvestre, A. L. (1998). Building a security capable prganization. In *proceedings, PACMedTek, IEEE Computer Society,* Washington, DC.

Conn, J. (2007). Invasion of privacy? [from Business Source Complete Database.]. *Modern Healthcare, 37*(29), 20. Retrieved September 12, 2009.

Conn, J. (2006). A real steal. [from ABI/INFORM Global database.]. *Modern Healthcare, 36*(40), 26–28. Retrieved May 31, 2009.

Consumer. (2009, October). *Harm standard violates congressional legislative intent in protecting privacy.* Consumer Watchdog Organization. Retrieved November 3, 2009, from http://www.consumerwatchdog.org/patients/articles/?storyId=30367

Cornell University Law School. (2010). *Federal rules of civil procedure.* Retrieved June 17, 2010, from http://www.law.cornell.edu/rules/frcp/

Corporation, I. B. M. (2006). IBM Hippocratic Database auditing user guide, Version 1.0. Retrieved August 7, 2009, from IBM Corporation Web site: http://www.almaden.ibm.com/cs/projects/iis/hdb/Publications/papers/HDBAuditingUserGuide.pdf

Crowell. (2008). *State laws governing security breach notification.* Crowell & Moring International Law Firm. Retrieved October 21, 2009, from http://www.crowell.com/

Curran, K., & Canning, P. (2007). Wireless handheld devices become trusted network devices. *Information Systems Security, 16*(3), 134–146. Retrieved September 6, 2009. doi:10.1080/10658980701401686

Currie, W. L., & Guah, M. W. (2007). A national programme for IT in the organizational field of healthcare: An example of conflicting institutional logics. *Journal of Information Technology, 22*(3), 235–247. doi:10.1057/palgrave.jit.2000102

D'Allegro, J. (2000). Study: Health websites divulge personal information. *National Underwriter / Life & Health Financial Services, 104*(8), 3. Retrieved September 2, 2009, from Business Source Complete Database.

Data Protection Act. (1998) *Data protection act.* Retrieved August 17, 2009, from http://www.opsi.gov.uk/ACTS/acts1998/ukpga_19980029_en_1

Datasec & NHS Fife. (2009). *eHealth demonstrator project for IT governance.* Edinburgh: Scottish Executive.

Davis, K., Schoenbaum, M., & Audet, A. (2005). A 2020 vision of patient-centered primary care. *JGIM: Journal of General Internal Medicine, 20*(10), 953–957. doi:10.1111/j.1525-1497.2005.0178.x

De Martini, C. (2008). Brothers in arms. *Health Management Technology, 29*(9), 40. Retrieved June 7, 2010, from http://proquest.umi.com.library.capella.edu/pqdweb?did=1554990491&Fmt=7&clientId=62763&RQT=309&VName=PQD

De Raeve, P. (2003). Nursing powers in the EU: The role and outcomes of the Standing Committee of Nurses of the EU. *Journal of Advanced Nursing, 43,* 4.

Department for Culture. Media and Sports. (2008). *Digital Britain: The future of communications.* Retrieved June 16, 2010, from http://webarchive.nationalarchives.gov.uk/+/http://www.culture.gov.uk/reference_library/media_releases/5548.aspx/

Department of Health and Human Services. (2007). *Synopsis of the ONC: Coordinated Federal Health Information Plan: 2008-2012.* Retrieved on November 4, 2008, from http://www.hhs.gov/healthit/resources/HITStrategicPlanSummary.pdf

Detmer, D. E., Lumpkin, J. R., & Williamson, J. J. (2009). Defining the medical subspecialty of clinical informatics. *Journal of the American Medial Informatics, 16*(2), 167–168. doi:10.1197/jamia.M3094

Deursen, T., Koster, P., & Petkovic, M. (2008). *Hedaquin: A reputation-based health data quality indicator.* Paper presented at the 3rd International Workshop on Security and Trust Management (STM 2007), 27 Feb 2008, Dresden, Germany.

Deybach, G. (2007). Identity theft and employer liability. *Risk Management, 54*(1), 14–17.

Di Crescenzo, G., Cochinwala, M., & Shim, H. (2007). *Modeling cryptographic properties of voice and voice-based entity authentication.* Paper presented at the DIM '07.

Dignam, A. J., & Lowry, J. P. (2006). *Company law* (Dignam, A. J., Ed.). 3rd ed.). Oxford: Oxford University Press.

Dimik, C. (2007). E-discovery: Preparing for the coming rise in electronic discovery requests. *Journal of American Health Information Management Association, 78*(5), 24–29.

Dimitropoulos, L., & Rizk, S. (2009). A state-based approach to privacy and security for interoperable health information exchange. [from ABI/INFORM Global.]. *Health Affairs, 28*(2), 428–434. Retrieved October 10, 2009. doi:10.1377/hlthaff.28.2.428

Dirking, B., & Kodali, R. R. (2008). *Strategies for preparing for e-discovery.* Information Management Journal.

Dix, K. (2006). *Best practices for scope reprocessing endoscope-related infections and keeping the numbers negligible.* Retrieved September 28, 2009, from http://www.infectioncontroltoday.com/articles/651cover.html

Dixon, P. (2005). Electronic health records and the national health information network: Patient choice, privacy, and security in digitized environments. In *testimonial before the NCVHS Subcommittee on Privacy and Confidentiality,* San Francisco.

Dynamic Computer Corporation. (2009). *RFID-integrated technologies for infection control: Background and technology comparison on key adoption considerations.* White Paper. Farmington Hills, MI: Dynamic Computer Coporation.

Edelstein, L. (1943). The Hippocratic oath: Text, translation and interpretation. *Bulletin of the History of Medicine, 5*(1), 1–64.

Edwards, R. (1988). Confidentiality in the professions. In Edwards, R., & Garber, G. (Eds.), *Bioethics* (pp. 72–81). San Diego: Harcourt Brace Jovanovich.

Electronic Privacy Information Center. (2008). *Privacy survey.* Retrieved on November 4, 2008, from http://www.epic.org/privacy/survey/

Eliot, C. W. (1910). Oath of Hippocrates. In P.F. Collier and Son (Ed.), Harvard Classics (vol 38). Boston: Harvard Press.

Elliott, M. (2005). Securing the healthcare border. [from ABI/INFORM Global.]. *Health Management Technology, 26*(9), 32, 34–35. Retrieved November 2, 2009.

Employee Retirement Income Security Act of 1974. (2000). *Rules and regulations for administration and enforcement; claims procedure; final rule. 65 Fed. Reg. 70246-70271.*

Erlen, J. (2004). HIPAA-clinical and ethical considerations for nurses. *Orthopedic Nursing, 23*(6), 410–414. doi:10.1097/00006416-200411000-00014

Etzioni. (1999). A contemporary conception of privacy. *Telecommunications and Space Journal, 6,* 81-114.

European Union. (1995, November 23). Directive 95/46/EC of the European Parliament and of the Council of 24 October 1995 on the Protection of Individuals with Regard to the Processing of Personal Data and on the Free Movement of Such Data. Official Journal of the European Communities of, L(281), 31–50.

Falcone, R., & Castelfranchi, C. (2001). Social trust: A cognitive approach. In Castelfranchi, C., & Tan, Y.-H. (Eds.), *Trust and deception in virtual settings* (pp. 55–99). Kluwer.

Fang, D., & Tracy, C. (2009). *Special survey on vacant faculty positions for academic year 2009-2010*. Washington, DC: American Association of Colleges of Nursing.

Federal Trade Commission. (2007). *2006 Identity theft survey report*. Retrieved September 2, 2009, from http://www.ftc.gov/os/2007/11/SynovateFinalReportIDTheft2006.pdf

Federal Trade Commission. (2003). *Overview of the identity theft program*. Washington, DC: Federal Trade Commission.

Federal Trade Commission. (2007). *2006 Identity theft survey*. Retrieved on November 4, 2008, from http://www.ftc.gov/os/2007/11/SynovateFinalReportIDTheft2006.pdf

Ferguson, R. B. (2007). *Army taps 3M for RFID tracking of medical records*. Retrieved September 28, 2009, from http://www.eweek.com/c/a/Mobile-and-Wireless/Army-Taps-3M-for-RFID-Tracking-of-Medical-Records/

Fickenscher, K. (2005). The new frontier of data mining. [from ABI/INFORM Global.]. *Health Management Technology, 26*(10), 26, 28, 30. Retrieved August 12, 2009.

Field. (1996). *Telemedicine, telehealth, and health Information Technology*. The American Telemedicine Society.

Filipek, R. (2007). Information security becomes a business priority. *The Internal Auditor, 64*(1), 18.

Foreshew, J. (August 25, 2009). AGED-CARE provider PresCare investigated a range of electronic aids for residents at its newest Queensland site. *AustalianIT.News.com.*

Foultz, W. (2004). *The impact of the HIPAA regulation on information technology security in the healthcare industry.* D.P.A. dissertation, University of La Verne, California.

Francis, T. (2009). These men could kill sarbox. *Business Week*. 40-43

Freedman, I. (2007). What does "interoperability" really mean? [from ProQuest Medical Library.]. *Health Management Technology, 28*(10), 50–51. Retrieved May 9, 2010.

Freeman, E. (2004). *Veterans Administration Palo Alto healthcare system*. Retrieved August 15, 2009, from www.csahq.org/pdf/bulletin/issue_6/va_freeman043.pdf

Froomkin, M. (2000). The death of privacy? *Stanford Law Review, 52*, 1461–1469. doi:10.2307/1229519

Fuhrmans, V. (May 31, 2005). Health insurers' new target. *Wall Street Journal*, B1, B4.

Furrow, B.R., Greaney, T.L., Johnson, S.H., Jost, S.T. & Schwartz, L.S. (1997). *Treatise on health law*.

Galt, K., & Johnson, S. (2007). *How many physicians have adopted electronic health records in Nebraska?* EHRNebraska. Retrieved October 17, 2009, from http://ehrnebraska.org/interact/

Gambetta, D. (1990). *Trust: Making and breaking cooperative relations* (pp. 213–238). Basil Blackwell.

GAO Reports. (2007). *Health Information Technology: Early efforts initiated but comprehensive privacy approach needed for national strategy: GAO-07-238*. Retrieved September 6, 2009, from Business Source Complete Database.

Garfinkel, S. (2000). Review of database nation: The death of privacy in the 21st Century. *Journal of Information, Law and Technology*. Retrieved on November 4, 2008, from http://www2.warwick.ac.uk/fac/soc/law/elj/jilt/2000_1/kelman/

Gay, L., Mills, G., & Airasian, P. (2006). *Educational research: Competencies for analysis and applications* (8th ed.). Upper Saddle Creek, NJ: Prentice Hall.

Goffredo, M., Bouchrika, I., Carter, J., & Nixon, M. (2008). *Performance analysis for gait in camera networks.* Paper presented at the AREA '08.

Goldberg, E. (2008). Sustainable utility business continuity planning: A primer, an overview and a proven, culture-based approach. *The Electricity Journal, 21*(10), 67–74. doi:10.1016/j.tej.2008.10.016

Goodman, C. S. (2004). *HTA 101: Introduction to health technology assessment*.

Gordon, L., Loeb, M., Lucyshyn, W., & Richardson, R. (2006). CSI/FBI computer crime and security survey. Retrieved November 11, 2009, from http://i.cmpnet.com/gocsi/db_area/pdfs/fbi/FBI2006.pdf

Gostin, L. O., & Nass, S. (2009). ...*Journal of the American Medical Association, 301*(13), 1373–1375. doi:10.1001/jama.2009.424

Government Accounting Office. (2004). *Data mining: Federal efforts cover a wide range of uses.* Retrieved on November 4, 2008, from http://www.gao.gov/new.items/d04548.pdf

Government Technology. (2008). *Millions believe personal medical records have been compromised, survey says.* Retrieved on November 4, 2008, from http://www.govtech.com/gt/377526

Guah, M. W. (2008). Changing healthcare institutions with large Information Technology projects. *Journal of Information Technology Research, 1*(1), 14–26.

Guah, M. W. (2007). *Critical systems diffusion approach in healthcare.* Paper presented at the International Conference of Information Systems, Montreal.

Guah, M. W., & Currie, W. L. (2007). *Managing vendor contracts in public sector IT: A case study on the UK National Health Service.* Paper presented at the European Conference on Information Systems (ECIS2007), June 7-9, 2007, St. Gallen, Switzerland.

Guah, M. W., & Davidson, E. (2008). *Practicing IS Research in Medical Practice: Opportunities and Dilemmas for Rigors and Relevance in Health IT Research.* Panel presentation at the European Conference for Information Systems (ECIS2008), June 9-11, 2008, Galway, Ireland.

Guah, M. W. (2011). *Healthcare Delivery Reform and New Technologies: Organizational Initiatives,* Preface, pp-xvii.

Gunter, T. D., & Terry, N. P. (2005). The emergence of national electronic health record architectures in the United States and Australia: Models, costs, and questions. *Journal of Medical Internet Research, 7*(1), e3. doi:10.2196/jmir.7.1.e3

Habermas, J. (1989). *The structural transformation of the public sphere: An inquiry into a category of bourgeois society.* Cambridge, MA: The MIT Press.

Hammond, W., Bailey, C., Boucher, P., Spohr, M., & Whitaker, P. (2010). Connecting information to improve health. [from ABI/INFORM Global.]. *Health Affairs, 29*(2), 284–288. Retrieved May 31, 2010. doi:10.1377/hlthaff.2009.0903

Hardy, G. (2006). Using IT governance and COBIT to deliver value with IT and respond to legal, regulatory and compliance challenges. *Information Security Technical Report, 11*(1), 55–61. doi:10.1016/j.istr.2005.12.004

Harris Interactive. (2004). Survey on medical privacy. Retrieved from http://www.harrisinteractive.com/news/newsletters/healthnews/HI_HealthCareNews2004Vol4Iss13.pdf

Hayes, J., & Hannold, E. (2007). The road to empowerment: Historical perspective on the medicalization of disability. *Journal of Health and Human Services Administration, 30*(3), 352–377.

He, D., & Yang, J. (2009). Authorization control in collaborative healthcare systems. [from ABI/INFORM Global.]. *Journal of Theoretical and Applied Electronic Commerce Research, 4*(2), 88–109. Retrieved October 11, 2009.

Health Information Privacy Code. (1994). *HIPC.* Retrieved August 30, 2009, from http://www.privacy.org.nz/health-information-privacy-code-1994/

Health Insurance Portability and Accountability Act. (1996). *Health information privacy.* Retrieved September 1, 2009, from http://www.hhs.gov/ocr/privacy/hipaa/understanding/index.html

Health Resources and Services Administration. (2002). *Projected supply, demand, and shortages of Registered Nurses*: 2000-2020. Washington, DC.

Health Resources and Services Administration. (2006). *The Registered Nurse population: Findings from the 2004 National Sample Survey of Registered Nurses.* Retrieved on October 14, 2009, from http://bhpr.hrsa.gov/health-workforce/rnsurvey04/3.htm

Healthcare Information Management and Systems Society. (2009). *20th annual 2009 HIMSS leadership survey (annual survey No. 20).* HIMSS.

Helping Hands for the Disabled. (2008). *July 2008 board meeting proceedings.*

Hendriks, A. (2007). UN convention on the rights of persons with disabilities. *European Journal of Health Law, 14*(3), 273–298. Retrieved September 8, 2009. doi:10.1163/092902707X240620

Herrod, C. (2006). The role of information security and its relationship to information technology risk management. In M.E. Whitman & H.J. Mattord (Eds.), *Readings and cases in the management of information security* (45-61). Boston: Course Technology.

Heubusch, K. (2006). Interoperability: What it means, why it matters. *Journal of American Health Information Management Association, 77*(1), 26-30. Retrieved January 11, 2010, from http://library.ahima.org/xpedio/groups/public/documents/ahima/bok1_028957.hcsp?dDocName=bok1_028957

Hillestad, R., Bigelow, J., Bower, A., & Girosi, F. (2005). Can electronic medical record systems transform health care? Potential health benefits, savings, and costs. *Health Affairs, 24*(5), 1103. Retrieved May 11, 2010, from http://proquest.umi.com.library.capella.edu/pqdweb?did=899710741&Fmt=7&clientId=62763&RQT=309&VName=PQD

Hiner, J. (2008). SIM survey: Top 10 IT management concerns of 2008. *Techrepublic.* Retrieved from http://blogs.techrepublic.com.com/hiner/?p=882

HIPAA. (1996). Health Insurance Portability and Accountability Act of 1996. Pub, L. No. 104-191.

HIPAA. (2006). HIPAA Administrative Simplification, Regulation Text, 45 CFR Parts 160, 162, and 164.

Hirschfeld, M., & Wikler, D. (2003). An ethics perspective on family caregiving worldwide. *Generations (San Francisco, Calif.), 27*(4), 56–60.

HISPC. (2007, June). *Security and privacy barriers to health information interoperability: Final report for the state of Nebraska.* Health Information Security and Privacy Committee, State of Nebraska. Retrieved October 17, 2009, from http://chrp.creighton.edu/

Hoboken, N. J. (2008). *National survey finds information technology and business alignment a struggle for American companies.* Retrieved Sep 9, 2009, from http://www.stevens.edu/press/pr/pr1206

Hoerbst, A., & Ammenwerth, E. (2009). A structural model for quality requirements regarding electronic health records-state of the art and first concepts. In *Proceedings of the 2009 ICSE Workshop on Software Engineering in Health Care*, (pp. 34-41). Washington, DC.

Hoffman, S. & Podgurski, A. (2007). Securing the HIPPA security rule. *Journal of Internet Law 10*(8), 1, 6-15.

Holmerová, I., Jurasková, B., Kalvach, Z., Rohanová, E., Rokosová, M., & Vanková, H. (2007). Dignity and palliative care in dementia. *The Journal of Nutrition, Health & Aging, 11*(6), 489. Retrieved from http://proquest.umi.com.library.capella.edu/pqdweb?did=1402659161&Fmt=7&clientId=62763&RQT=309&VName=PQD.

Holtfreter, R., & Holtfreter, K. (2006). Gauging the effectiveness of US identity theft legislation. *Journal of Financial Crime, 13*(1), 56–64. doi:10.1108/13590790610641215

Human Rights Commission. (2009). Human rights in New Zealand today. Retrieved September 10, 2009, from http://www.hrc.co.nz/report/chapters/chapter05/disabled02.html

Iakovidis, I. (1998). Towards personal health record: Current situation, obstacles and trends in implementation of electronic healthcare record in Europe. *International Journal of Medical Informatics, 52*(1-3), 105–115. doi:10.1016/S1386-5056(98)00129-4

Identity Theft 911. (2010). *Medical identity theft goes high-profile.* Retrieved February 21, 2010, from http://www.identitytheft911.org/articles/article.ext?sp=10863

Institute for Health Freedom. (2003). *The final federal privacy rule: The definitive guide.* Retrieved on November 4, 2008, from http://www.forhealthfreedom.org/Publications/Privacy/Rule.html#copy

Internet Crime Complaint Center. (2007). *2007 Internet Crime Report.* Retrieved November 4, 2008, from http://www.ic3.gov/media/annualreport/2007_IC3Report.pdf

Isaacs, S., Jellinek, P., & Ray, W. (2009). The independent physician-Going, going... [from ProQuest Medical Library.]. *The New England Journal of Medicine, 360*(7), 655–657. Retrieved May 25, 2010. doi:10.1056/NEJMp0808076

Ismail, R., & Jøsang, A. (2002). *The Beta reputation.* Paper presented at the 15th Electronic Commerce Conference, 17-19 June 2002, Bled, Slovenia.

Itakura, Y., & Tsujii, S. (2005). Proposal on a multifactor biometric authentication method based on cryptosystem keys containing biometric signatures. *International Journal of Information Security, 4*(4), 288–296. doi:10.1007/s10207-004-0065-5

ITGI. (2008). *Aligning COBIT 4.1, ITIL V3 and ISO/IES 27002 for business benefits*. Retrieved August 16, 2009, from http://www.itgi.org

Jecker, N. (2002). Taking care of one's own: Justice and family caregiving. *Theoretical Medicine and Bioethics, 23*(2), 117–133. doi:10.1023/A:1020323828931

Jin, J., Ahn, G., Hu, H., Covington, M. J., & Zhang, X. (2009). Patient-centric authorization framework for sharing electronic health records. In *Proceedings of the 14th ACM Symposium on Access Control Models and Technologies*, (125-134). Stresa, Italy. NY: ACM.

Jirotka, M., Luff, P., & Buscher, M. (2009). *EPSRC: Research cluster on innovative media for a digital economy*. Retrieved June 16, 2010, from http://www.oerc.ox.ac.uk/research/digital-economy

Johnson, V. (2008). Data security and tort liability. *Journal of Internet Law, 11*(7), 22–31. Retrieved from http://search.ebscohost.com.library.capella.edu.

Johnson, T. D. (2010). Health officials use new means to trace sources of food illness. *Nation's Health, 40*(4), 1-12. Retrieved May 16, 2010, from http://ezproxy.library.capella.edu/login?url=http://search.ebscohost.com.library.capella.edu/login.aspx?direct=true&db=aph&AN=50140933&site=ehost-live&scope=site

Jones, R. (2009). The role of health kiosks in 2009. *International Journal of Environmental Research and Public Health, 6*(6), 1818–1855. doi:10.3390/ijerph6061818

Jøsang, A. (2001). A logic for uncertain probabilities. *International Journal of Uncertainty. Fuzziness and Knowledge-Based Systems, 9*(3), 279–212. doi:10.1142/S0218488501000831

Jøsang, A. (1997). *Artificial reasoning with subjective logic*. Paper presented at the 2nd Australian Workshop on Commonsense Reasoning, Dec 1997, Perth, Australia.

Jøsang, A., & Pope, S. (2005). *Semantic constraints for trust transitivity*. Paper presented at the the Asia-Pacific Conference of Conceptual Modeling (APCCM), Feb 2005, Newcastle, Australia.

Jøsang, A., AlZomai, M., & Suriadi, S. (2007). *Usability and privacy in identity management architectures*. Paper presented at the the Australasian Information Security Workshop: Privacy Enhancing Technologies (AISW 2007), 31 Jan 2007, Ballarat, Australia.

Jøsang, A., Bhuiyan, T., & Cox, C. (2008). *Combining trust and reputation management for Web-based services*. Paper presented at the 5th International Conference on Trust, Privacy and Security in Digital Business (TrustBus2008), 4-5 Sept 2008, Turin, Italy.

Jøsang, A., Luo, X., & Chen, X. (2008). *Continuous ratings in discrete Bayesian reputation systems*. Paper presented at the the Joint iTrust and PST Conferences on Privacy, Trust Management and Security (IFIPTM 2008),18-20 June 2008, Trondheim, Norway.

Joyce, M. (2008). The challenges and future of biometric-based security systems. *Internal Auditing, 23*(2), 14–22.

Kabler, J. (2010). *Wellpoint kiosks: Instant access to health*. Retrieved June 16, 2010, from http://www.wellpointgroup.com/

Kahn, J., Aulakh, V., & Bosworth, A. (2009). What it takes: Characteristics of the ideal personal health record. *Health Affairs, 28*(2), 369–376. doi:10.1377/hlthaff.28.2.369

Kamvar, S., Schlosser, M., & Garcia-Molina, H. (2003). *The Eigentrust algorithm for reputation management in P2P networks*. Paper presented at the 12th International Conference on World Wide Web (WWW '03), 20-24 May 2003, Budapest, Hungary.

Kane, B., & Sands, D. Z. (1998). Guidelines for the clinical use of electronic mail with patients. *Journal of the American Medical Informatics Association, 5*(1), 104–111.

Kanneh, A., & Sakr, Z. (2008). *Biometric user verification using haptics and fuzzy logic*. Paper presented at the MM '08.

Kant, I. (1991). *Groundwork for the metaphysics of morals*.

Kanter, A. (2007). The promise and challenge of the United Nations convention on the rights of persons with disabilities. [from Business Source Complete Database.]. *Syracuse Journal of International Law & Commerce, 34*(2), 287–321. Retrieved September 7, 2009.

Kaplan-Leiserson, E. (2001). The tremendous issues of technology. *T+D, 55*(11), 27. Retrieved September 6, 2009, from Academic Search Premier Database.

Kaufmann, D., Kraay, A., & Zoido-Lobatón, P. (2000). Governance matters: From measurement to action. *Finance & Development, 37*(2).

Kaushal, R., Bates, D., Jenter, C., Mills, S., Volk, L., & Burdick, E. (2009). Imminent adopters of electronic health records in ambulatory care. [Retrieved from Academic Search Premier database.]. *Informatics in Primary Care, 17*(1), 7–15.

Kay, R. (2005). Biometric authentication. *Computerworld, 39*(14), 26.

Keller, S., Powell, A., Horstmann, B., Predmore, C., & Crawford, M. (2005). Information security threats and practices in small businesses. *Information Systems Management, 22*(2), 7–19. Retrieved from http://search.ebscohost.com.library.capella.edu. doi:10.1201/1078/45099.22.2.20050301/87273.2

Khandelwal, A. (2006). E-health governance model and strategy in India. *Journal of Health Management, 8*(1), 145–155. doi:10.1177/097206340500800111

Kingma, M. (2001). Nursing migration: Global treasure hunt or disaster-in-the-making? *Nursing Inquiry, 8*(4), 205–212. doi:10.1046/j.1440-1800.2001.00116.x

Kirnan, V. (2000). Medicine could benefit from internet improvement, report says. *The Chronicle of Higher Education.*

Kline, D. (2003). Push and pull factors in international nurse migration. *Journal of Nursing Scholarship, Second Quarter.*

Knapp, K., & Boulton, W. (2006). Cyber-warfare threatens corporations: Expansion into commercial environment. [from Business Source Complete Database.]. *Information Systems Management, 23*(2), 76–87. Retrieved September 6, 2009. doi:10.1201/1078.10580530/45925.23.2.20060301/92675.8

Kongehl. (1999). The electronic health record-a new challenge for privacy and confidentiality in medicine? *Biomedical Ethics, 4*(2):52-3.

Kontzer, T. (2009). Why IT and business can't get in sync. *CIO Insight.* Retrieved from http://www.cioinsight.com/index2.php?option=content&task=view&id=882683&pop=1&hide_ads=1&page=0&hide_js=1

Korst, L. M., Signer, J. M. K., Aydin, C., & Fink, A. (2008). Identifying organizational capacities and incentives for clinical data-sharing: The case of a regional perinatal information system. *Journal of the American Medical Informatics Association, 15*(2), 195–197. doi:10.1197/jamia.M2475

Kuehn, B. (2009). IT vulnerabilities highlighted by errors, malfunctions at veterans' medical centers. [from CINAHL.]. *JAMA: Journal of the American Medical Association, 301*(9), 919–920. Retrieved September 10, 2009. doi:10.1001/jama.2009.239

Lafferty, L. (2007). Medical identity theft: The future threat of healthcare fraud is now. [from Business Source Complete Database.]. *Journal of Health Care Compliance, 9*(1), 11–20. Retrieved May 31, 2009.

Landt, J. (2005). The history of RFID. *IEEE Potentials,* 8-11.

Lane, M. (2005). Philosophical perspectives on states and immigration. Retrieved on September 19, 2008, from http://www histecon.kings.cam.ac.uk/docs/lane_migration.pdf

Lashof, J. C. (1981). *Government approaches to the management of medical technology.* Paper presented at Annual Health Conference of the New York Academy of Medicine.

Lassetter, J. (2010). HIEs to transform. [from ProQuest Medical Library.]. *Health Management Technology, 31*(1), 18. Retrieved May 9, 2010.

Latham, C., Hogan, M., & Ringl, K. (2008). Nurses supporting nurses: Creating a mentoring program for staff nurses to improve the workforce environment. *Nursing Administration Quarterly, 32*(1), 27–39.

Lefevre, K., Agrawal, R., Ercegovac, V., Ramakrishnan, R., Xu, Y., & Dewitt, D. (2004). Limiting disclosure in Hippocratic Databases. Proceedings of the 30th International Conference on Very Large Databases, 30, 108-119.

Leung, J. (2006). The emergence of social assistance in China. *International Journal of Social Welfare, 15*(3), 188–198. doi:10.1111/j.1468-2397.2006.00434.x

Levey, N. N. (February 4, 2010). Soaring cost of healthcare sets a record: Spending was 17.3% of the economy last year. The share paid by the U.S. will soon exceed 50%, a study says. *Los Angeles Times,* pp. 1.

Lewan, T. (September 8, 2007). Cancer fears raised over chip implants. *USA Today.*

Likupe, G. (2006). Experiences of African nurses in the UK National Health Service: A literature review. *Journal of Clinical Nursing, 15.*

Lobree, B. (2003). IT security: A tactical war. [from Academic Search Premier Database.]. *Information Systems Security, 12*(3), 9. Retrieved September 6, 2009. doi:10.1201/1086/43327.12.3.20030701/43622.3

Logue, K., & Selmrod, J. (2008). Genes as tags: The tax implications of widely available Genetic information. [from Business Source Complete Database.]. *National Tax Journal, 61*(4), 843–863. Retrieved September 6, 2009.

Lorenzi, N., Kouroubali, A., Detmer, D., & Bloomrosen, M. (2009). How to successfully select and implement electronic health records (EHR) in small ambulatory practice settings. *BMC Medical Informatics and Decision Making, 9,* 1–13. doi:10.1186/1472-6947-9-15

Lueng (2006) characterizes the Chinese support system as disjoint and decentralized.

Luftman, J. (2000). Assessing business-IT alignment maturity. *Communications of AIS, 4*(14).

Macios, A. (2009). Who's watching what? Data mining raises privacy issues. *Radiology Today, 10*(1), 20.

Maharaja, A. (2009). *Use of the electronic health record in private medical practices.* Ed.D. dissertation, Duquesne University.

Marden, S. (2005). Technology dependence and health-related quality of life: A model. *Journal of Advanced Nursing, 50*(2), 187–195. doi:10.1111/j.1365-2648.2005.03378.x

Margolis, P., & Halfon, N. (2009). Innovation networks. A strategy to transform primary health care. *Journal of the American Medical Association, 302*(13), 1461–1462. doi:10.1001/jama.2009.1428

Mark, A. L. (2007). Modernising healthcare–is the NPfIT for purpose? *Journal of Information Technology, 22,* 248–256. doi:10.1057/palgrave.jit.2000100

Markle Foundation. (2003). *Connecting for health: A public-private collaborative.* Retrieved on November 4, 2008, from http://www.connectingforhealth.org/resources/pswg_report.pdf

Markowitz, J. (2000). Voice biometrics. *Communications of the ACM, 43*(9), 66–73. doi:10.1145/348941.348995

Mavhunga, C. (2009). The glass fortress: Zimbabwe's cyber-guerilla warfare. [from Academic Search Premier Database.]. *Journal of International Affairs, 62*(2), 159–173. Retrieved September 6, 2009.

McBride, R. (2009). Health information exchanges the health IT inside. *CIMO.net Online Magazine.* Retrieved November 29, 2009, from http://epubs.democratprinting.com/publication/?i=26411

McCain, J. (2009). Applying the privacy act of 1974 to data brokers contracting with the government. [from ABI/INFORM Global.]. *Public Contract Law Journal, 38*(4), 935–953. Retrieved October 11, 2009.

McCaughey, B. (2009). *Ruin your health with the Obama stimulus plan.* Bloomberg. Retrieved October 18, 2009 from http://www.bloomberg.com/apps/news?pid=2060 1039&sid=aLzfDxfbwhzs# McGraw, D., Dempsey, J., Harris, L., & Goldman, J. (2009). Privacy as an enabler, not an impediment: Building trust into health information exchange. *Health Affairs, 28*(2), 416-27. Retrieved October 10, 2009, from ABI/INFORM Global.

McCormick, D., Woolhandler, S., Bose-Kolanu, A., Germann, A., Bor, D. H., & Himmelstein, D. U. (2009). U.S. physicians' views on financing options to expand health insurance coverage: A national survey. *JGIM: Journal of General Internal Medicine, 24*(4), 526–531. doi:10.1007/s11606-009-0916-x

McDonald, C. (2009). Protecting patients in health information exchange: A defense of the HIPAA Privacy Rule. [from ABI/INFORM Global Database.]. *Health Affairs, 28*(2), 447–449. Retrieved June 1, 2009. doi:10.1377/hlthaff.28.2.447

McGraw, D., Dempsey, J. X., Harris, L., & Goldman, J. (2009). Privacy as an enabler, not an impediment: Building trust into health information exchange. [from ABI/INFORM Global database.]. *Health Affairs, 28*(2), 416–427. Retrieved May 31, 2009. doi:10.1377/hlthaff.28.2.416

McKinney, M. (2010, April). 'Huge potential' for EHRs and comparative effectiveness. [from ProQuest Medical Library.]. *Hospitals & Health Networks, 84*(4), 41–42. Retrieved May 9, 2010.

McLaughlin, J. Gustafson, C., Sutton, M., Stone, E., & Davis, N. (1984). *Developmentally disabled infants can be hard to trace.* Retrieved August 20 2009 from http://www.ncbi.nlm.nih.gov/pubmed/6199152

MedicAlert. (2009). *About us.* Retrieved September 25, 2009, from http://www.medicalert.org/Main/AboutUs.aspx

Merlis, M. (2009). *Simplifying administration of health insurance.* Retrieved May 11, 2010, from http://www.rwjf.org/files/research/merlisadmin.pdf

Merrill, M. (2009, November). Iowa first to receive matching funds for EHR incentive program. *Healthcare Finance News.* Retrieved November 29, 2009, from http://www.healthcarefinancenews.com/news/iowa-first-receive-matching-funds-ehr-incentive-program

Microsoft Corporation. (2008). *Securing a better future for electronic medical records.* Retrieved July 24, 2009, from http://www.microsoft.com/business/peopleready/business/relationshps/insight/digitalrecords.aspx

Miller, A. R., & Tucker, C. E. (2009). *Electronic discovery and electronic medical records: Does the threat of litigation affect firm decisions to adopt technology?* Retrieved June 17, 2010, from http://www.ftc.gov/be/seminardocs/090430amiller.pdf

MIPSA. (1999). *Setting information age parameters for medical privacy.* Retrieved September 1, 2009 from http://leahy.senate.gov/press/199903/990310b.html

Monegain, B. (2006, March). Healthcare data exchange moves from theory to proof. *Healthcare IT News.* Retrieved November 3, 2009, from http://www.healthcareitnews.com/news/healthcare-data-exchange-moves-theory-proof

Morin, D., Tourigny, A., Pelletier, D., Robichaud, L., Mathieu, L., & Vézina, A. (2005). Seniors' views on the use of electronic health records. *Informatics in Primary Care, 13*(2), 125–133.

Morrissey, J. (1999). Integration sacrificed for Y2K preparation. [Retrieved from CINAHL with Full Text database.]. *Modern Healthcare, 29*(18), 31.

Mui, L., Mohtashemi, M., Ang, C., Szolovits, P., & Halberstadt, A. (2001). *Rating in distributed systems: A Bayesian approach.* Paper presented at the Workshop on Information Technologies and Systems (WITS), 15-16 Dec 2001, New Orleans.

Muir, R. (2007). *eHealth governance, security and privacy. the UK perspective.* UK: slideshare.net. Retrieved from http://www.slideshare.net/HINZ/ehealthgovernance-security-and-privacya-uk-perspective

Mullaney, J. (2006). The digital doctor logs off. *Business Week, 3983,* p12-15.

Murray, C. (2004). *Chip for humans a blessing to some, a curse to others.* Retrieved from http://www.embedded.com/news/embeddedindustry/54201016?_requestid=152134

Muular, A., Mfutso-Bengo, J., Makoza, J., & Chatipwa, E. (2003). The ethics of developed nations recruiting nurses from developing countries: The case of Malawi. *Nursing Ethics, 10*(4). International Council of Nurses. (2006). *Patient and Public Safety Matter: The Biennial ICN Report, 2004-2006.*

Myers, M., Baskerville, R., Gill, G., & Ramiller, N. (2010). *Setting Our Research Agendas: Institutional Ecology, Informing Sciences or Management Fashion Theory.* Panel presentation at the International Conference on Information Systems (ICIS2007), December 12-15, 2010, St. Louis, USA.

National Alliance for Health Information Technology. (2008). *Defining key health information technology terms.* Retrieved October 3, 2009 http://healthit.hhs.gov/portal/server.pt/gateway/PTARGS_0_10741_848133_0_0_18/10_2_hit_terms.pdf.

National Governors Association. State Alliance for e-health. (2008). *Accelerating progress: Using health Information Technology and electronic health information exchange to improve care.* Retrieved on November 4, 2008, from http://www.nga.org/Files/pdf/0809EHEALTHREPORT.PDF

Netschert, B. (2008). *Information security readiness and compliance in the healthcare industry.* Ph.D. dissertation, Stevens Institute of Technology, New Jersey.

Network World. (2007, January 8). *Year ahead to bring risks, opportunities.* Retrieved September 6, 2009, from Business Source Complete Database.

Nevada, N. R. S. (2009). *Chapter 603A: Security of personal information.* Retrieved October 21, 2009, from http://www.leg.state.nv.us/NRS/NRS-603A.html#NRS603ASec010

News Staff. (2010). *'Meaningful use' rule needs significant modifications, says AAFP.* Retrieved from http://www.aafp.org/online/en/home/publications/news/news-now/practice-management/20100304mean-use-ltr.html

NIH. (2009). *Protecting privacy in health research.* Research portfolio online reporting tool, U.S. Department of Health and Human Services. Retrieved November 3, 2009, from http://projectreporter.nih.gov/project_info_description.cfm

Nikolai, B. (2008). *Medical records: The interoperability conundrum.* University of British Columbia - School of Library, Archival & Information Studies. Retrieved January 11, 2010, from http://www.bound2leap.com/media/med_records.pdf

NIST. (July, 2009). *Risk management framework: Helping organizations implement effective information security programs.* ITL Security Bulletin. Retrieved October, 10, 2009, from http://csrc.nist.gov/publications/PubsITLSB.html

NY Times staff writer. (March 26, 2008) *Safeguarding private medical data.* New York Times. Retrieved November 4, 2008, from http://www.nytimes.com/2008/03/26/opinion/26wed2.html

Office of the National Coordinator for Health IT. (2008). *The ONC-coordinated federal health information technology strategic plan: 2008-2012.* Retrieved on June 8, 2009, from http://healthit.hhs.gov/portal/server.pt/gateway/PTARGS_0_10731_848084_0_0_18/HITStrategicPlanSummary508.pdf

O'Hara, P. (2009). *Joined-up health and social care: Challenging times.*

Olmsted, S., Grabenstein, J., Jain, A., & Lurie, N. (2006). Patient experience with, and use of, an electronic monitoring system to assess vaccination responses. *Health Expectations, 9*(2), 110–117. doi:10.1111/j.1369-7625.2006.00378.x

Olowu, D. (2006). A critique of the rhetoric, ambivalence, and promise in the protocol to the African Charter on Human and People's Rights on the Rights of Women in Africa. [from Academic Search Premier Database.]. *Human Rights Review, 8*(1), 78–101. Retrieved September 6, 2009. doi:10.1007/s12142-006-1017-4

Organization for Economic Co-Operation and Development. (1980). *Guidelines on the protection of privacy and transborder flows of personal data.*

Patient Handoffs. (2008). *H&HN: Hospitals & Health Networks.* Retrieved September 14, 2009, from Academic Search Premier Database.

Paul, R. J. (2007). Changes to Information Systems: Time to change. *European Journal of Information Systems, 16*(3), 193–195. doi:10.1057/palgrave.ejis.3000681

Paul, R. (2007). *Top US government research labs infiltrated by hackers.* Retrieved October 12, 2009, from http://arstechnica.com

Perrin, R. (2002). Biometrics technology adds innovation to healthcare organization security systems. *Healthcare Financial Management, 56*(3), 86–88.

Pew Internet and American Life Project. (2003). *Who's not online: Several demographic factors are strong predictors of Internet use.* Retrieved September 7, 2009, from http://www.pewinternet.org/Reports/2003/The-EverShifting-Internet-Population-A-new-look-at-Internet-access-and-the-digital-divide/02-Who-is-not-online/03-Several-demographic-factors-are-strong-predictors-of-Internet-use.aspx

Poirier, J. (2009). *Lawmaker urges regulations for file-sharing.* Thomson Reuters Wire Service. Retrieved August 1, 2009, from http://www.reuters.com

Polsky, D., Ross, S., Brush, B., & Sochalski, J. (2007, May). Trends in characteristics and country of origin among foreign-trained nurses in the United States, 1990 and 2000. *American Journal of Public Health, 97,* 895–899. doi:10.2105/AJPH.2005.072330

Porter, M. E., & Teisberg, E. O. (2006). *Redefining healthcare: Creating value-based competition on results.* Boston: Harvard Business School Press.

Powner, D. (2006). *Health Information Technology: HHS is continuing efforts to define its national strategy: GAO-06-1071T.* GAO Reports. Retrieved September 6, 2009, from Business Source Complete Database.

Practices, F. (2009). XLVI FL. *Stat, 817–568.*

Prescott, B. (2009, May). *Patients reveal a willingness to trade hands-on medical care for computer consultations.* Beth Israel Deaconess Medical Center Web Site. Retrieved November 3, 2009, from http://www.bidmc.org/News/InResearch/2009/May/PatientsandComputers.aspx

PriceWaterhouseCooper. (2008). *IT governance global status report 2008.* USA: IT Governance Institute. Retrieved from http://tais3.cc.upv.es/V/BEA6QVG8VHQP-KT7UMV26BICX9F7VFJXNB5GINHXXF77Y2N-LQUP-00908?func=quick-1

Prince, K. (2008). *A comprehensive study of healthcare data security breaches in the United States from 2000-2007.* Perimeter eSecurity. Retrieved October 21, 2009, from http://www.privacyrights.org/ar/ChronDataBreaches.htm.

Pritts, J. (2002). Altered states: State health privacy laws and the impact of the federal health privacy rule. *Yale Journal of Health Policy, Law, and Ethics, 2*(2), 327–364.

Privacy Rights Clearinghouse. (1997). *A review of the fair information principles: The foundation of privacy public policy.* Retrieved on November 4, 2008 from http://www.privacyrights.org/ar/fairinfo.htm

Professional Practices. (n.d.). Disaster Recovery Institute (n.d.). *Professional practices.* Retrieved September 8, 2009 from https://www.drii.org/professionalprac/prof_prac_details.php

PublicTechnology. (2009). *Nottingham city council to use RFID to improving care for citizens.* Retrieved September 25, 2009, from http://www.publictechnology.net/modules.php?op=modload&name=News&file=article&sid=17599&mode=thread&order=0&thold=0

Quibria, M., Tschang, T., & Reyes-Macasaquit, M. (2002). New information and communication technologies and poverty: Some evidence from developing Asia. *Journal of the Asia Pacific Economy, 7*(3), 285–309. doi:10.1080/1354786022000007852

Rachels, J. (2005). Why privacy is important. *Philosophy & Public Affairs, 4*(4), 323–333.

Ramachandra, A., Pavithra, K., Yashasvini, K., Raja, K., Venugopal, K., & Patnaik, L. (2009). *Offline signature authentication using cross-validated graph matching.* Paper presented at the Compute '09.

Ramiller, N. C., & Swanson, E. B. (2003). Organizing visions for information technology and the I.S. executive response. *Journal of Management Information Systems, 20*(1), 13–50.

Ray, B. (2009). *Miami health centre starts RFID soap snooping.* Retrieved November 28, 2009, from http://www.theregister.co.uk/2009/08/18/rfid_soap_monitoring/

Read, T. (2007). *Architecting availability and disaster recovery solutions: Sun blueprints online.* Retrieved September 8, 2009, from http://www.sun.com/blueprints/0406/819-5783.pdf

Rebelo, M. J. (2007). *E-discovery in health care litigation.* Physician's News Digest.

Reeves, R. (2010). *Heath and well being: The role of the state.* Retrieved June 16, 2010, from http://www.dh.gov.uk/en/Publichealth/index.htm

Resnick, P., & Zeckhauser, R. (2002). Trust among strangers in Internet transactions: Empirical analysis of eBay's reputation system. In Baye, M. R. (Ed.), *The Economics of the Internet and E-commerce* (pp. 127–157). Elsevier. doi:10.1016/S0278-0984(02)11030-3

Reynolds, R. (2008). *A study to determine first year medical students' intention to use electronic health records.* Ed.D. dissertation, Memphis State University.

Richardson, D. (2009). *Correlationally assessing the relationship of information technology investments in electronic medical records to business value.* Ph.D. dissertation, Capella University.

Richey, W. (March 23, 2010). Attorneys General in 14 states sue to block healthcare reform law. *The Christian Science Monitor.*

Ridgely, M. S., & Jerrell, J. M. (1996). Analysis of three interventions for substance abuse treatment of severely mentally ill people. *Community Mental Health Journal, 32*(6), 561. Retrieved May 8, 2010, from http://proquest.umi.com.library.capella.edu/pqdweb?did=10347436&Fmt=7&clientId=62763&RQT=309&VName=PQD

Riemer-Reiss, M. (2000). Vocational rehabilitation counseling at a distance: Challenges, strategies and ethics to consider. [from Academic Search Premier Database.]. *Journal of Rehabilitation, 66*(1), 11–17. Retrieved September 6, 2009.

Rishel, W., Riehl, V., & Blanton, C. (2007) *Summary of the NHIN prototype architecture contracts.* Gartner, Inc. Retrieved on June 1, 2009 from http://healthit.hhs.gov/portal/server.pt/gateway/PTARGS_0_10731_848093_0_0_18/summary_report_on_nhin_Prototype_architectures.pdf

Roberts, J. G. J. (2006). *Federal rules of civil procedure.* Retrieved June 17, 2010, from www.supremecourt.gov/orders/courtorders/frcv10.pdf

Robertson, L., Smith, M., Castle, D., & Tannenbaum, D. (2006). Using the Internet to enhance the treatment of depression. *Australasian Psychiatry, 14*(4), 413–417.

Robeznieks, A., & Conn, J. (2006). GAO blasts HHS on IT, privacy. [from Academic Search Premier Database.]. *Modern Healthcare, 36*(36), 8–9. Retrieved September 6, 2009.

Robinson, T. N., Patrick, K., Eng, T. R., & Gustavson, D. (1999). *An evidence-based approach to interactive health communication: A challenge to medicine in the information age.* Science Panel on Interactive Health and Communication.

Rodwin, M. A. (2009). The case for public ownership of data. *Journal of the American Medical Association, 302*(1), 86–88. doi:10.1001/jama.2009.965

Rogers, A., Jones, E., & Oleynikov, D. (2007). Radio frequency identification (RFID) applied to surgical sponges. *Surgical Endoscopy, 21*(7), 1235. Retrieved from http://proquest.umi.com.library.capella.edu/pqdweb?did=1297025351&Fmt=7&clientId=62763&RQT=309&VName=PQD. doi:10.1007/s00464-007-9308-7

Ross, Katzke, Johnson, Swanson, & Stoneburner (2008). Managing risk from information systems: An organizational perspective. *National Institute of Standards and Technology. NIST Special Publication 800-39.* U.S. Department of Commerce.

Rothstein, M., & Talbott, M. (2007). Compelled authorizations for disclosure of health records: Magnitude and implications. *The American Journal of Bioethics, 7*(3), 38–45. doi:10.1080/15265160601171887

Safran, C., Bloomrosen, M., Hammond, E., Labkoff, S., Markel-Fox, S., & Tang, P. C. (2007). Toward a national framework for the secondary use of health data: An American Medical Informatics Association White Paper. *Journal of the American Medical Informatics Association, 14*(1), 1–9. doi:10.1197/jamia.M2273

Sample, D. (2003). *TriWest answers questions on stolen computer info, increased security.* American Forces Press Service. Retrieved November, 8. 2009, from http://www.defenselink.mil/news/newsarticle.aspx?id=29491

Santiago, A. (2010). *The medicus firm physician survey: Health reform may lead to significant reduction in physician workforce.* Retrieved May 9, 2010, from http://www.themedicusfirm.com/pages/medicus-media-survey-reveals-impact-health-reform

Sax, U., & Mandl, K. D. (2005). Wireless technology infrastructures for authentication of patients: PKI that rings. *Journal of the American Medical Informatics Association, 12,* 263–268. doi:10.1197/jamia.M1681

Schackow, T., Palmer, T., & Epperly, T. (2008). EHR meltdown: How to protect your patient data. [from ABI/INFORM Global.]. *Family Practice Management, 15*(6), A3–A8. Retrieved October 10, 2009.

Schein, E. (1992). *Organizational culture and leadership*. San Francisco: Jossey-Bass, Inc.

Schein, E. (n.d.). *Kurt Lewin's change theory in the field and in the classroom: Notes toward a model of managed learning*. Retrieved September 8, 2009, from http://www.a2zpsychology.com/articles/kurt_lewin's_change_theory.htm

Schneider, J., Kortuem, G., Jager, J., Fickas, S., & Segall, Z. (2000). Disseminating trust information in wearable communities. *Personal and Ubiquitous Computing, 4*(4), 245–248. doi:10.1007/BF02391568

Schoeman, F. D. (1984). *Philosophical dimensions of privacy: An anthology*. Cambridge, UK: Cambridge University Press. doi:10.1017/CBO9780511625138

Schwartz, A., Pappas, C., & Sandlow, L. J. (2010). Data repositories for medical education research: Issues and recommendations. *Academic Medicine, 85*(5), 837–843. doi:10.1097/ACM.0b013e3181d74562

Schwartz, P., & Janger, E. (2007). Notification of data security breaches. *Michigan Law Review, 105*(5), 913–984. Retrieved from http://search.ebscohost.com.library.capella.edu.

Scott, M. (2006). So that's where it is. *Hospitals & Health Networks, 80*(4), 28. Retrieved from http://proquest.umi.com.library.capella.edu/pqdweb?did=1033282571&Fmt=7&clientId=62763&RQT=309&VName=PQD.

Scottish Government. E. P. (2009). *eHealth demonstrator project of IT governance at NHS in Scotland*. Scotland, UK: NHS Scotland annual conference 2009. Retrieved from http://www.nhsslearning2009.scot.nhs.uk/poster-gallery.aspx

SearchSecurity. (n.d.) *PKI*. Retrieved on June 12, 2009, from http://searchsecurity.techtarget.com/sDefinition/0,sid14_gci214299,00.html

Sharp, D. PhD, RN. (2009). Evidence-based protocols for managing wandering behaviors. *Nursing Education Perspectives, 30*(4), 258. Retrieved from http://proquest.umi.com.library.capella.edu/pqdweb?did=1850876381&Fmt=7&clientId=62763&RQT=309&VName=PQD

Shea, S. (1994). Security versus access: trade-offs are only part of the story. *Journal of the American Medical Informatics Association, 1*(4), 314–315.

Shortliffe, E. H. (2005). Strategic action in health Information Technology: Why the obvious has taken so long. [from ABI/INFORM Global.]. *Health Affairs, 24*(5), 1222–1233. Retrieved May 31, 2010. doi:10.1377/hlthaff.24.5.1222

Silvius, A. J. G. (2007). *Business & IT alignment in theory and practice*. Paper presented at the 40th Hawaii International Conference on Systems Science (HICSS-40 2007).

Simonsson, M., & Johnson, P. (2006). Defining IT governance-a consolidation of literature. *18th Conference on Advanced Information Systems Engineering CAiSE '06*, Luxembourg.

Slattery, F. (2008). Medicine and the Internet. *The OECD Observer. Organisation for Economic Co-Operation and Development, 268*, 31–32.

SmartCardAlliance. (2006). *Smart card applications in the U.S. healthcare industry*. Retrieved September 28, 2009, from http://www.smartcardalliance.org/newsletter/february_2006/feature_0206.html

Solove, D. J., & Hoofnagle, C. J. (2005). *A model regime of privacy protection*. Public Law Research Paper No. 132, George Washington University Law School. Retrieved on November 4, 2008, from http://papers.ssrn.com/sol3/papers.cfm?abstract_id=681902

Sondheimer, N., Katsh, E., Clarke, L., Osterweil, L., & Rainey, D. (2009). Dispute prevention and dispute resolution in networked health information technology. In S. A. Chun, R. Sandoval, and P. Regan (Eds.) *Proceedings of the 10th Annual international Conference on Digital Government Research: Social Networks: Making Connections between Citizens, Data and Government*. (pp. 240-243).

Stamatiadis, D. (2005). Digital archiving in the pharmaceutical industry. *Information Management Journal, 39*(4), 54-56, 59. Retrieved October 15, 2009, from ABI/INFORM Global.

Stevenson, G. (2007). *HIPAA security: Intercultural perspectives of health information technology professionals and clinicians*. Ph.D. dissertation, University of Illinois at Chicago, Health Sciences Center.

Stockman, H. (1948). Communication by means of reflective power. [IRE]. *Proceedings of the Institute of Radio Engineers, 36*, 1196–1204.

Strecha, D., Persad, G., Marckmann, G., & Danis, M. (2009). Are physicians willing to ration health care? Conflicting findings in a systematic review of survey research. *Health Policy Journal, 95*(2), 113–124. doi:10.1016/j.healthpol.2008.10.013

Subramanian, V., Frechet, J. M. J., Chang, P. C., Huang, D. C., Lee, J. B., & Molesa, S. E. (2005). Progress toward development of all-printed RFID tags: Materials, processes, and devices. [Berkeley, CA.]. *Proceedings of the IEEE, 93*(7), 1330–1338. doi:10.1109/JPROC.2005.850305

Sukhai, N. (2004). *Access control & biometrics.* Paper presented at the InfoSec CD Conference '04.

Sullivan Commission. (2004). *Missing persons: Minorities in the health professions.* Retrieved on July 22, 2006, from http://www.amsa.org/advocacy/Sullivan_Commission.pdf

Swanson, R., & Holton, E. (2005). *Research in organizations: Foundations and methods of inquiry.* San Francisco: Berrett-Koehler.

Swanson, M., Bartol, N., Sabato, J., Hash, J., & Graffo, L. (2003). *Security metrics guide for information technology systems.* NIST Special Publication 800-55. Retrieved October 12, 2009, from http://webharvest.gov/peth04/20041027033844/csrc.nist.gov/publications/nistpubs/800-55/sp800-55.pdf

Swartz, N. (2008). Partnerships advance e-health records. *Information Management Journal, 42*(3), 10–14.

Swartz, N. (2005). Electronic health records could save $81 billion. [from ABI/INFORM Global.]. *Information Management Journal, 39*(6), 6. Retrieved October 15, 2009.

Swedberg, C. (2008). *Tamper-resistant RFID infant-tracking system improves security.*

Symantec Corporation. (2007). *Managing electronic-messaging and E-discovery for healthcare providers.* Retrieved June 17, 2010, from http://eval.symantec.com/mktginfo/enterprise/white_papers/ent-whitepaper_managing_messaging_healthcare_11-2007.en-us.pdf

Tang, P. (2002). AMIA advocates national health information system in fight against national health threats. *Journal of the American Medical Informatics Association, 9*(2), 123-124. Retrieved January 10, 2010, from http://jamia.bmj.com/content/9/2/123.full

Teacy, W., Patel, J., Jennings, N., & Luck, M. (2006). TRAVOS: Trust and Reputation in the Context of Inaccurate Information Sources. *Autonomous Agents and Multi-Agent Systems, 12*(2), 183–198. doi:10.1007/s10458-006-5952-x

Teich, J., Wagner, M., Mackenzie, C., & Schafer, K. (2002). The informatics response in disaster, terrorism, and war. *Journal of the American Medical Informatics Association, 9*(2), 97-104. Retrieved January 10, 2010, from http://jamia.bmj.com/content/9/2/202.full

Tenczar, J., Lemme, M., & Stanfield, S. (2009). *Microsoft surface, experience it, showcase.* Retrieved June 9, 2010, 2010, from http://www.microsoft.com/surface/en/us/Pages/Experience/Showcase.aspx

The Disability Social History Project. (2009). Disability history timeline. Retreived August 15, 2009, from http://www.disabilityhistory.org/timeline_new.html

The Economist. (2005). The no-computer virus - IT in the health-care industry. *The Economist, 375*(8424), 65-67.

TheBigOptOut.org. (2009). *About the campaign.* Retrieved September 10, 2009, from http://www.thebigoptout.com/?page_id=3

Thielst, C. (2007). The future of healthcare technology. [from ABI/INFORM Global.]. *Journal of Healthcare Management, 52*(1), 7–9. Retrieved October 10, 2009.

Thru-group. Managing sensitive records in health care: Industry solution profile.

Tillmann, G. (2007). Will biometric authentication solve corporate security challenges? *Optimized, 6*(2), 24.

Tomes, J. P. (2009). You are not a HIPPA Covered entity–you may be a red flag covered entity as well. *Journal of Health Care Compliance, 11*(1), 5–13.

Trochim, W. (2006). *Qualitative validity.* Research Methods Knowledge Base. Retrieved October 20, 2009, from http://www.socialresearchmethods.net/kb/qualval.htm

Truffer, C., Keehan, S., Smith, S., Cylus, J., Sisko, A., & Poisal, J. (2010). Health spending projections through 2019: The recession's impact continues. [from ABI/IN-FORM Global.]. *Health Affairs, 29*(3), 522–529. Retrieved May 13, 2010. doi:10.1377/hlthaff.2009.1074

Tschida, M. (2000). Prior-IT-ies (health information and management systems society survey on information technology). *Modern Physician*. Retrieved from http://www.accessmylibrary.com/article-1G1-62408652/prior-ies-health-information.html

U.S. Census Bureau. (2004).*Statistics of U.S. businesses: 2004—third party administration of insurance and pension funds.*

U.S. Department Of Commerce. (2009). Safe Harbor privacy principles.

U.S. Department of Health and Human Services. (2010). *NHIN exchange.* Retrieved 2010, May 17, from http://healthit.hhs.gov/portal/server.pt?open=512&objID=1407&parentname=CommunityPage&parentid=8&mode=2&in_hi_userid=11113&cached=true

U.S. Department of Health and Human Services. (2010). *Health information security and privacy collaboration.* Retrieved 2010, May 17, from http://healthit.hhs.gov/portal/server.pt?open=512&mode=2&cached=true&objID=1240

U.S. Department of Health & Human Services. (2005). *HHS awards contracts to develop nationwide health information network.* Retrieved on June 8, 2009, from http://www.hhs.gov/news/press/2005pres/20051110.html

United Nations Office of Legal Affairs. Convention on the Rights of Persons with Disabilities, (2006). *U.N. Doc A/RES/61/.* Retrieved September 1, 2009, from http://www.un.org/esa/socdiv/enable/opsigola.htm

United Nations. (1948). *Universal declaration of human rights, article 12.* Retrieved November 4, 2008, from http://www.nps.gov/elro/teach-er-vk/documents/udhr.htm

United States Department of Education Family Educational Rights and Privacy Act (FERPA). (1974). *Family Policy Compliance Office (FPCO) home.* Retrieved September 7, 2009, from http://www.ed.gov/policy/gen/guid/fpco/ferpa/index.html

United States Department of Education - Individuals with Disabilities Education Act. (2004). *Building the legacy: IDEA 2004.* Retrieved September 7, 2009, from http://idea.ed.gov/

United States Department of Health and Human Services - Center for Disease Control and Prevention. (2009). *Single gene disorders and disability.* Retrieved September 7, 2009, from http://www.cdc.gov/ncbddd/single_gene/default.htm

United States Department of Health and Human Services - Office for Civil Rights. (2009). *Your rights under section 504 of the rehabilitation act.* Retrieved September 7, 2009, from http://www.hhs.gov/ocr/civilrights/resources/factsheets/504.pdf

US Department of Health and Human Services. (2010). *Personal health records and the HIPAA privacy rule.* Retrieved on February 15, 2010, from http://www.hhs.gov

US Department of Justice. (2010). *Identity theft.* Retrieved on February 20, 2010, from http://www.justice.gov/criminal/fraud/websites/idtheft.html

Vaas, L. (2001). Disability laws take flight. *eWeek, 18*(9), 50. Retrieved September 6, 2009, from Academic Search Premier Database.

Van Oranje, C., Schindler, R., Valeri, L., Vilamovska, A. M., Hatziandreu, E., & Conkin, A. (2009). *Study on the requirements and options for radio frequency identification (RFID) application in healthcare (RFID No. TR-608-EC).* Cambridge, UK: Rand Europe.

Verheijden, M., Bakx, J., Van Weel, C., & Van Staveren, W. (2005). Potentials and pitfalls for nutrition counseling in general practice. *European Journal of Clinical Nutrition, 59*, S122–S129. doi:10.1038/sj.ejcn.1602185

VeriChip. (2009). *About us.* Retrieved September 25, 2009, from http://www.verichipcorp.com/about_us.html

Vijayann, J. (2003). Offshore ops to get stronger privacy lock. [from Academic Search Premier Database.]. *Computerworld, 37*(22), 1. Retrieved September 6, 2009.

Vissers, J., & Beech, R. (2005). *Health operations management: Patient flow logistics in healthcare care.* UK: Routledge.

Waldren, S., Kibbe, D., & Mitchell, J. (2009). Will the feds really buy me an EHR? and other commonly asked questions about the HITECH act. [from ABI/INFORM Global.]. *Family Practice Management, 16*(4), 19–23. Retrieved September 29, 2009.

Walters, L. (1982). Ethical aspects of medical confidentiality. In Walters, L., & Beauchamp, T. (Eds.), *Contemporary issues in bioethics* (2nd ed., pp. 198–203).

Walton, G. (2003). *Medication administration: A wireless safety net.* Retrieved from http://www.ehealthinternational.org/pdfs/Walton.pdf

Wang, Y., Cahill, V., Gray, E., Harris, C., & Liao, L. (2006). *Bayesian network based trust management.* Paper presented at the 3rd International Conference in Autonomic and Trusted Computing (ATC), 3-6 Sept 2006, Wuhan, China.

Warren, S. D., & Brandeis, L. D. (1984). The right to privacy. *Harvard Law Review, 4*(5).

Washington Division of Developmental Disabilities. (2009). *Vision statement.* Retrieved July 12, 2009, from http://www1.dshs.wa.gov/pdf/adsa/ddd/reports/Overview2_03.pdf

Wasko, N. (2001). Internet Technology makes clinical data systems technically and economically practical: Are they politically feasible? [from SocINDEX with Full Text Database.]. *Journal of Technology in Human Services, 18*(3/4), 41–62. Retrieved September 6, 2009. doi:10.1300/J017v18n03_04

Wasserstrom, R. (1984). The legal and philosophical foundations of the right to privacy. In Mappes, T. A., & Zembatty, J. S. (Eds.), *Biomedical Ethics* (pp. 109–116). New York: McGraw-Hill.

Webster, P. (2010). Concern raised over control of cost-benefit research in United States. [from ProQuest Medical Library.]. *Canadian Medical Association Journal, 182*(2), E127–E128. Retrieved May 9, 2010. doi:10.1503/cmaj.109-3140

Wechsler, J. (2009). Pharma girds for healthcare reform. *Pharmaceutical Technology, 33*(8), 22, 24, 26-27. Retrieved May 8, 2010, from ABI/INFORM Global.

Weier, M.H. (January 19, 2008). Wal-Mart gets tough on RFID. *InformationWeek.*

Weiner, M. (2003). Using Information Technology to improve the healthcare of older adults. *Annals of Internal Medicine, 139*(5), 430–436.

Welander, P. (2007). 10 control system security threats. *Control Engineering, 54*(4), 38-44. Retrieved from http://search.ebscohost.com.library.capella.edu

Wickramasinghe, N. (2010). The Role for Knowledge Management in Modern Healthcare Delivery. *International Journal of Healthcare Delivery Reform Initiatives, 1*(2), 1–9.

Wicks, A. M., Visich, J. K., & Li, S. (2006). Radio frequency identification applications in hospital environments. *Hospital Topics, 84*(3), 3. Retrieved from http://proquest.umi.com.library.capella.edu/pqdweb?did=1086998281&Fmt=7&clientId=62763&RQT=309&VName=PQD. doi:10.3200/HTPS.84.3.3-9

Wilson, E. V., & Lankton, N. K. (2004). Interdisciplinary research and publication opportunities in Information Systems and healthcare. *Communications of the Association for Information Systems, 14*, 332–343.

Wilson, E. V., & Tulu, B. (2010). The rise of a health-IT academic focus. *Communications of the ACM, 53*(5), 147–150. doi:10.1145/1735223.1735259

Winslade, W. J. (1995). *Confidentiality.* (pp. 451-459). Encyclopedia of Bioethics. New York: Macmillan Library Reference.

Wong, R. (2007). Sensitive data in the online environment: Time for a change? *Journal of Internet Law, 10*(9), 11–17. Retrieved from http://search.ebscohost.com.library.capella.edu.

World Health Organisation. (2009). *eHealth for health care delivery.*

World Trade Organization. (2009). *Standards concerning the availability, scope and use of intellectual property rights.* Retrieved September 10, 2009 from http://www.wto.org/english/tratop_e/trips_e/t_agm3_e.htm

Xiong, L., & Liu, L. (2004). PeerTrust: Supporting Reputation-based Trust for Peer-to-Peer Electronic Communities. *IEEE Transactions on Knowledge and Data Engineering, 16*(7), 843–857. doi:10.1109/TKDE.2004.1318566

Xiong, L., & Liu, L. (2003). *A reputation-based trust model for Peer-to-Peer eCommerce communication.* Paper presented at the IEEE International Conference onE-Commerce (CEC '03), 24-27 June 2003, Newport Beach, USA.

Xu, Y., & Kwak, C. (2007). *Comparative trend analysis of characteristics of internationally educated nurses and U.S.-educated nurses in the United States.* International Council of Nurses.

Xu, Y., & Zhang, J. (2005). One size doesn't fit all: Ethics of international nurse recruitment from the conceptual framework of stakeholder interests. *Nursing Ethics, 12*(6), 571–581. doi:10.1191/0969733005ne827oa

Yamamoto, M., & Aso, Y. (2009). Placing physical restraints on older people with dementia. *Nursing Ethics, 16*(2), 192. Retrieved from http://proquest.umi.com.library.capella.edu/pqdweb?did=1651874511&Fmt=7&clientId=62763&RQT=309&VName=PQD. doi:10.1177/0969733008100079

Yasnoff, W. A., Humphreys, B. L., Overhage, J. M., & Detmer, D. E. (2004). A consensus action agenda for achieving the national health information infrastructure. [from ProQuest Medical Library.]. *Journal of the American Medical Informatics Association, 11*(4), 332–338. Retrieved May 16, 2010. doi:10.1197/jamia.M1616

Ye, J., & Wei, Q. (2004). *Legal problems concerning health discrimination in employment.* Retrieved from http://www.humanrights.cn/zt/magazine/200402004921170301.htm

Yu-Che, C., & Thurmaier, K. (2008). Financing e-government business transactions: An enterprise pricing framework for G2B services. *Public Administration Review, 68*(3), 537–548.

Zineddine, M. (2008). *Compliance of the healthcare industry with the health insurance portability and accountability act security regulations in Washington state: A quantitative study two years after mandatory compliance.* Ph.D. dissertation, Capella University.

Zorkadis, V., & Donos, P. (2004). On biometrics-based authentication and identification from a privacy-protection perspective. *Information Management & Computer Security, 12*(1), 125–137. doi:10.1108/09685220410518883

About the Contributors

Steven A. Brown is an experienced published professional with over 25 years of technical and business experience in telecommunications, data networks, strategic communications, organizational design, electronic commerce, security, and business management. Projects have included security assessments, project risk analysis, network security, cybersecurity and terrorism, homeland security, and forensic investigations. I've also worked on business planning, strategy development, government technology restriction. He holds an undergraduate degree in Electrical Engineering, a Masters of Business Administration degree, and a Doctor of Business Administration degree, concentrated in Information Systems Technology Management. He also holds several leading security certifications such as CISSP-ISSAP. He is currently responsible for curriculum development in the information assurance and security curriculum areas for the PhD and Masters programs at Capella University, and responsible for managing Capella's NSA Center of Excellence in information security initiative, and making sure Capella stays on the cutting edge of Information Security curriculum, and making the site a strategic resource for Capella students and the overall public to share information security information.

Mary Brown is an experienced professional with many years of experience in the field of information security and health informatics. She has extensive experience in the health care industry and contributes to security and health informatics education efforts including giving presentations, webinars, and workshops on a variety of related topics, Recent examples include a couple of ISC2 Think Tank webinars on security regulations and application security and a presentation at the Minnesota Government IT Symposium on the topic of the National Health Information Network. She is involved in a number of IT and information security professional organizations. She was selected as the Minnesota ISSA Security Professional of the Year for 2006 and received the Harold Able Distinguished Faculty award in 2009. Mary Brown has earned CISSP and CISA certifications and has an MS in Information Security. She is currently finishing up a PhD in IT Education with an emphasis in health informatics education. Mary teaches undergraduate courses in information assurance and security and health informatics for Capella University. She is responsible for development of the curriculum and for ensuring that the curriculum provides a complete education that covers the range of skills needed by today's information security and health informatics professionals.

* * *

Bandar Alhaqbani is an Assistant Professor of Health Informatics in the College of Public Health and Health Informatics, King Saud bin Abdulaziz University for Health Sciences, Saudi Arabia. His research interests span different topics in the area of information security, including, but not limited to, access control models, identity management, reputation systems, network security, and security of workflow management systems (WfMS). Also, he has over 8 years of experience in the Information Technology field within the healthcare domain.

Omotunde (Tunde) Adeyemo is a Senior Security Consultant at TEKsystems Inc. He has been working in Information Technology and Information Assurance and Security (IT/IAS) for about 16 years. He currently leads security efforts for systems integration and development projects (including those related to electronic health systems) at a US Fortune 50 insurance company. In his role at the client's site, Mr. Adeyemo provides consulting for security architecture designs, assessment of potential external vendors' for security maturity and criticality/risk assessment. He has helped many projects involving electronic health records with data assurance consulting. Prior to consulting, Mr. Adeyemo held IT leadership titles such as Network Manager for Young & Rubicam's Canadian offices until 2006 and later that year co-founded Fountium Technologies, an IT/IAS consulting/training company. In 1999, he worked at SecureCard Trust Company Nigeria as Head, Systems and Network Administration where he led a national electronic-purse smartcard project executed in partnership with ProtonWorld International, Belgium. He holds a BSc degree in Electronic and Electrical Engineering from Obafemi Awolowo University, Nigeria and a MSc degree in Electrical Engineering from University of Lagos. Mr. Adeyemo is currently completing his PhD degree in Information Security and Assurance at Capella University and has been researching security and privacy concerns associated with the current digitization of the US healthcare industry for his doctoral work. His other research interests include Governance, Risk and Compliance (GRC) management, IAS best-practice frameworks and strategic alignment of IAS plans and business objectives. Mr. Adeyemo is a member of ISACA, ISC2, BCI and AHIMA. He holds the CISM, CISSP and AMBCI certifications.

Dennis Backherms, a published author and contributor to academia, lives with his family in South Florida. He is currently a Systems Administrator for the Town of Palm Beach and has worked for the town since 1997. Dennis's expertise has successfully flourished from a rewarding and professional IT background spanning 15 years. He has written several technical support papers and continues to contribute to academia. Dennis was awarded a master's in Information Systems and is currently working on his Ph.D. in Information Technology. He also holds several professional business certifications from organizations such as Microsoft and Six Sigma.

Keith Bauer received his BA in philosophy and classics from Mary Washington College, a MSW from Virginia Commonwealth University, and a Ph.D. in philosophy with a concentration in healthcare ethics from the University of Tennessee, Knoxville. From 2000-2001, Dr. Bauer was a fellow at the Institute for Ethics at the American Medical Association in Chicago. From 2002-2008, he held the position of Assistant Professor of Philosophy at Marquette University. Most recently, Dr. Bauer served as Associate Professor and Director of Humanities & Social Sciences at the Jefferson College of Health Sciences in Roanoke, VA. His current research continues to explore the ethical and social implications of using information and communication technologies to deliver and manage patient care.

Elena Beratarbide (born 1969, San Sebastián, Spain) is an eHealth researcher and a senior IT Service Manager at the NHS (National Health Service) in Fife, Scotland. Her twenty-two year career with Touché&Ross (now Deloitte), KPMG and Fujitsu prior to her appointment at the NHS Fife included senior Business and IT consulting, Information Systems, Software design and development and teaching, receiving Excellence Awards on several occasions for her professional input (2002-2005 Fujitsu). She's playing a role transforming the NHS Fife IT support service in line with eHealth Governance best practices and, as a researcher, contributing with new knowledge and understanding of how eHealth Governance is happening across the healthcare organisations in Scotland and making relevant recommendations to the Scottish Executive (2009). Her research activity during the last 4 years on this area, has been conducted in collaboration with St. Andrews University, Polytechnical University of Valencia and the NHS in Scotland. Beratarbide developed her career from a multidisciplinary approach, combining her qualifications as Information Engineer, business management (processes, methods and logistics), Computer science (physical systems) and Certified Information Systems Auditor (CISA). She is best known for her contribution to the integration of new technologies within public and private organisations, producing strategic plans to help local government adapting to the information society, using technology to get government and citizens closer, but also implementing and optimising ICT and auditing systems not only within the public sector but also private organisations in a variety of industry sectors in different countries. Since 1988 when she initially published *Integrated Systems* (Venezuela), Beratarbide developed a variety of resources supporting training on both IT and business managements areas like *Information Quality Assessment: A Methodology for External Financial Auditors* (Venezuela, 1991), *Business management for young entrepreneurs* (Spain, 1995), a series of training notebooks on *Excel: a financial analysis approach* (1997), *Office automation* (2001), and *LAN/WAN networks* (2001). After this stage, Beratarbide started publishing more senior work in collaboration with other authors, such as: Vicente Delás (*IT strategies for local government*, Spain, 2001), Pablo Borges (*IT Governance implementation in the health sector: NHS case studies,* Scotland, 2009) and Tom Kelsey (*IT Governance - a key enabler of better eHealth better care,* Massachusetts, 2009-2010*).* Previous work in IT and eHealth Governance involves also her *Causal model of factors involved in the adaptation of NHS to the Information Society* (Spain, 2008) and a reviewed version after a *model localisation through a Delphi exercise* (Germany, 2010) and recently a *Multi-case analysis of the eHealth Governance factor* (Germany, 2010*).* Beratarbide is now preparing her next publication along with Tom Kelsey (St. Andrews University) on a longitudinal analysis of eHealth Governance within the NHS in Scotland and a cross-sectoral and cross-national comparison of eHealth Governance (Springer, 2011) coordinated by Middlesex University, UK. Beratarbide presented her contribution on IT and eHealth Governance in conferences like ITSMF UK, NHSScotland, AXIOS and IADIS. *"Elena helped me in implementing the business plan for IT consulting and logical security projects in all spheres of the General Administration of the Spanish State." July 12, 2009. M. Timoteo, Account Manager, Fujitsu Services Spain*

John Beswetherick received his MBA from California State University San Jose and is currently finishing up his PhD at Capella University with a Security concentration in Information Technology. John is on the Board of Directors for the Seattle United Way affiliate agency Helping Hands for the Disabled. He is also involved in the community by helping new businesses get started and compete in a recovering economy. John is a Certified Secure Software Lifecycle Professional, Senior Quality Assurance Engineer at Microsoft Corporation and will frequently write about smart home technologies, software quality assurance, software accessibility and disability issues.

Terry Dillard is the founding and current President of the North Oakland Chapter of the Information Systems Security Association (ISSA), which is located in Auburn Hills, Michigan. As a 20-year veteran of Information Technology, Management Information Systems, and Information Assurance, Mr. Dillard has serviced the information management needs of K-12 Educators, as well as small to mid-sized enterprise throughout Southeast Michigan. Prior to establishing Dillard Systems LLC, Mr. Dillard served as Director of Information Technology, and Chief Technology Officer for several privately owned firms throughout the State of Michigan. Terry continues to engage industry in many capacities as an Information Technology Consultant and Information Security practitioner. He is an Adjunct Professor at Northwood University and Baker College, where he teaches courses in Management Information Systems, and Information Assurance to undergraduate and graduate learners. Terry Dillard is a Certified Information Systems Security Professional (CISSP), and holds a Bachelor of Science degree in Business Information Systems, Master of Science degree in Information Assurance, and is currently completing the degree of Doctor of Philosophy of Business Information Technology from Capella University. Mr. Dillard is an active member of the Association of Computing and Machinery (ACM), Institute of Electrical and Electronics Engineers (IEEE), and FBI InfraGard.

Colin Fidge is a Professor of Computer Science in the Faculty of Science and Technology, Queensland University of Technology, where he teaches software engineering. His active research interests include security-critical systems, business process modelling, and large-scale industrial asset management.

Ed Goldberg teaches and mentors doctoral candidates online at Capella University, serving as adjunct faculty from 2003 until 2007 and Core Faculty since then in their School of Business and Technology PhD program. He has extensive course development experience as well. Prior to Capella, Ed served as adjunct faculty at Albertus Magnus College from 1997 to 2007, teaching a wide range of graduate, MBA, and undergraduate management and IT courses. He has also taught advanced undergraduate project management for DeVry University. He has also written IT and MIS curriculum for Capella and for the Institute for Professional Development, including courses used by Albertus Magnus College. Ed currently serves as Northeast Utilities' Business Continuity Consultant in Berlin, CT., leading all of NU's business continuity and disaster recovery planning efforts. He has served as a manager and director of the IT department at Millstone Nuclear Power Station for both NU and Dominion Resources. Ed Goldberg is a licensed Professional Engineer with more than 25 years of IT and technical management experience. His management and hands-on experience include extensive Business Continuity and Disaster Recovery planning experience in conventional and nuclear settings. He is a Certified Business Continuity Planner (CBCP), a Certified Business Continuity Auditor, served from 2005 to 2009 as president of the Connecticut chapter of ACP (Association of Contingency Planners), and was elected to the National ACP board, serving now as its Education Director. Ed earned a BS in electrical engineering and an MBA concentrated in Computer Information Systems, both from the University of New Haven. He earned an advanced Graduate Certificate in Computer Communication Networks from Rensselaer Polytechnic Institute, and a Doctorate in Management and Organizational Leadership from the University of Phoenix. In addition to his extensive work in business continuity and disaster recovery planning, his areas of interest include organizational culture. He is an expert on safety-conscious work environments and the creation and maintenance of such culture in nuclear and other industrial settings. Ed has used his varied background in machine computer control design to gain extensive experience in high-tech engineering and business management. He has first hand design experience with military computer systems, fire alarm control panels, web offset printing press accessories, and electrofinishing/plating computerized control equipment. He has a patent for a sub-ambient fluid circulation system used in the printing industry.

Matthew Waritay Guah is Associate Professor for Business Systems at the School of Business, Claflin University in South Carolina. He previously worked in the Accounting Department of Erasmus University Rotterdam. His research concentrate on IFRS, IT impact on accounting practices, management controls for healthcare reform, and financial accountability (Internet Fraud, Corporate Social Responsibility, ERP in auditing). His theoretical foundations include: institutional theory, socio-economic, risk management, and project management/escalation. Dr. Guah obtained his PhD from Warwick Business School, MSc from Manchester University and BSc from Salford (all in the UK) and served as track chair for ICIS-2009 and 2011 (healthcare IT track); VP for Accounting Information System (special-interest-group) within the Association for Information Systems (http://home.aisnet.org). He has published 3 books, 12 journals, 8 chapter contributions, and presented at more than 20 international conferences. He is editor-in-chief for the International Journal of Health Delivery Reform Initiatives. Other editorial memberships include *JCIT, SJI, JIQ, JMIS* and *IJEC*. Dr. Guah also served as visiting scholar in the Accounting Department of Hawaii University at Manoa (Honolulu, USA) and Management School of Innsbruck University (Austria). Recent speaking engagements by invitation at research seminars include Universitá Cattolica (Milan, Italy), Salford University (Manchester, UK), Westminster University (London, UK), and Warwick Business School (UK). He is external examiner for Cape Peninsula University of Technology (Cape Town, South Africa). He came into academia with a wealth of industrial experience spanning over ten years (including Merrill Lynch, HSBC, British Airways, and United Nations).

Tom Kelsey (born 1961, Aylesford, England) is a senior research fellow at the School of Computer Science of the University of St Andrews in Scotland. His primary research interests are in Bio-medical Modelling, Medical Informatics, and Computational Mathematics. Kelsey started his career in Logistics Management, involved in sourcing, deploying and evaluating Resource Planning systems for multinational corporations such as North American Philips, Acatos & Hutcheson plc and SA Uniconfis. Having a Bachelors Degree in Mathematics from Heriot-Watt University, Edinburgh, Kelsey returned to academia in 1995 to take a Masters Degree in Numerical Analysis & Programming at the University of Dundee, followed by a PhD in Computational Mathematics at the University of St Andrews, graduating in 2000. Kelsey then obtained funding for postdoctoral research at St Andrews into formalised computer algebra in conjunction with NAG Ltd., followed by a postdoctoral research position studying symmetry-breaking methods in Constraint Satisfaction Problems (an NP-hard class of problems – such as planning, scheduling and resource allocation - that often arise in industrial and commercial settings). After a year working as a Teaching Fellow, Kelsey was promoted to Senior Research Fellow and given University funds to undertake further studies into Constraint Satisfaction and Bio-medical Modelling. In 2006 Kelsey was appointed to a tenured position at the University of St Andrews, as part of a £1.3 million grant from the UK Engineering & Physical Sciences Research Council (EPSRC) covering interdisciplinary research into Computational Mathematics. Kelsey is currently a co-investigator on a further EPSRC award into modelling and abstraction themes in Constraints research, and is an active member of the prestigious Centre for Interdisciplinary Research in Computational Algebra (CIRCA) based in the schools of Mathematics and Computer Science at the University of St Andrews. In addition to his University work, Kelsey is Technical Director of the Wallace-Kelsey Research Foundation, a charitable trust that funds investigations into the fertility of survivors of childhood cancer. Kelsey is a member of the International Society for Computational Biology (ISCB), the British Machine Vision Association, and the Royal Society of Medicine. He is on the executive board of the NHS Scotland Managed Clinical Network governing paediatric oncology in Scotland. Kelsey has published extensively in high-impact journals such as Public Library of Science One, Human Reproduction, The International Journal of Radiation Biology, Oncology & Physics, and Reproductive Biomedicine Online. His work relating ovarian volume to human age at menopause, his calculation of the Effective Sterilising Dose of radiation for human females, and his publication of the first model of human ovarian reserve from conception to the menopause have led to extensive international media interest, with news reports on the BBC, NBC, Fox, CNN, etc. And news articles and features in the Times, the Scientific American, the Wall St Journal, Nature News Update, Le Monde, El Pais, etc. Kelsey is currently working with researchers from Glasgow, Edinburgh and Montevideo on studies that link the Wallace-Kelsey model of ovarian reserve to other reproductive indicators such as serum Anti-Muellerian Hormone (AMH) levels, ovarian volumes, and numbers of eggs harvested during in-vitro fertilisation cycles. Kelsey has given invited talks at major international conferences, symposia and meetings. Recent examples include talks at the Asian Symposium on Computer Mathematics in December 2009, and the ISCB Latin America meeting in March 2010. Kelsey will be a keynote speaker at the Reproductive Function and Dysfunction conference being held in September 2011 (the 15th International Development and Function of Reproductive Organs conference series). *"Tom is a leading world expert in medical and biomedical research. His results have not only increased our awareness of important aspects of human fertility, but also stimulated important research projects across the globe." July 18, 2010. W. Hamish B. WALLACE MB.BS., MD (Lond)., FRCP (Edin)., FRCPCH., FRCS - CATSCAN Clinical Lead, Royal Hospital for Sick Children, Edinburgh, UK.*

Sarah Matulis graduated summa cum laude with her BSN from Pace University Lienhard School of Nursing in 2009, and began Family Nurse Practitioner studies in 2010. Working as a graduate assistant, she enjoyed researching nursing ethics and reinforcing undergraduate students' clinical skills in the learning resource center. Sarah currently works as an emergency room staff nurse as she continues her graduate studies.

John McGaha grew up in a small town in the Midwest. Shortly after graduating from high school he enlisted in the U.S. Navy to see the world. It was only a few months after joining the Navy when John returned home to marry his high-school sweetheart, Peggy. The two are blessed with three talented, lovely daughters. Always striving to learn and take on more responsibilities, John earned a BS in computer programming and subsequently awarded a commission as Ensign. During his 22 years of active duty service, he served as a technician, supervisor, instructor, division officer, communications officer, cryptographic materials officer, security officer, top security custodian, command duty officer, surface warfare officer, and engineering officer. After completing an MS in information technology management, he entered the naval intelligence community. John's last years in the navy were spent back home in the Midwest working for NORAD and the U.S. Space Command. As an intelligence officer in the Missile Analysis Center, he directed military intelligence analysts that processed sensitive information used to monitor compliance to strategic arms treaties. Upon retirement from active duty, John has been teaching computer science and information security courses for three Midwestern institutions. He is completing doctoral course-work at Capella University with hopes of beginning his dissertation in January 2011.

Robert Stephen McIndoe is a senior consultant currently employed full time by Logica UK, the global technology company, based in London, but working internationally. He holds Masters Degrees in Fine Arts from St.Andrews University, Scotland, Business Administration from the Open University, England and in Theatre and Performance Studies from Rose Bruford College of Performing Arts in England. When he isn't earning a living as a technology consultant he earns a living in professional performance and writing. He has worked in Healthcare, Entertainment, Energy and Distribution. Robert can be contacted at mcindoer@aol.com.

H. R. Rao is a Professor of MIS at SUNY Buffalo and Adjunct Professor of CSE. His research has been funded in part by Sogang Business School's World Class University Project (R31-20002) funded by Korea Research Foundation.

Marilyn Jaffe-Ruiz is a professor of nursing at the Lienhard School of Nursing, Pace University. Her specialties are nursing education, psychiatric mental health nursing, communication, cultural diversity, and leadership. Dr. Marilyn Jaffe-Ruiz had been Pace University's Chief Academic Officer from 1994 and with the title of Provost and Executive Vice President for Academic Affairs from 1998-2003, until her return to being a professor of nursing in fall 2004. Formerly, she was Vice Provost and, prior to that, Dean of the Lienhard School of Nursing at Pace, a position she held for seven years. Dr. Jaffe-Ruiz has held faculty positions at Pace University and Columbia University. She has had extensive experience in Psychiatric/Mental Health Nursing, including as a private practitioner. Dr. Jaffe-Ruiz holds both the Ed.D. and M.Ed. from Teachers College, Columbia University, and an M.A. in Adult Psychiatric Mental Health Nursing from New York University. In addition to being a dynamic speaker and teacher, Dr. Jaffe-Ruiz has used her broad expertise to design presentations, mediate disputes, and facilitate numerous change management and strategic planning initiatives. Dr. Jaffe-Ruiz has led the University's effort in diversity that has resulted in enrichment of the learning and work environment. She has chaired the Task Force on Diversity, lectured on managing cultural diversity in the workforce and consulted on cultural diversity in healthcare. Other areas of particular interest in which she has published and lectured are healthcare and Family Systems of the Mentally Retarded and the Developmentally Disabled. She is a sibling of a person with mental retardation and has been a prime advocate for the mentally retarded/developmentally disabled and their families, principally by being on the board of directors of the New York City Chapter of the Association for the Help of Retarded Children since 1984 and the President of the chapter from 1997-1999. Dr. Jaffe-Ruiz was a member of the Board of Directors of the Visiting Nurse Service, Westchester, the Catholic Healthcare Network in New York City, Hope for A Healthier Humanity, and served as Vice-President of the Council of Deans of Nursing of Senior Colleges and Universities of the State of New York and on the Editorial Board of the Journal of the New York State Nurses Association. Dr. Jaffe-Ruiz was inducted into the Teachers College Nursing Hall of Fame by the Teachers College Nursing Educational Alumni Association and made an honorary member of the Golden Key International Honor Society at Pace University. In 2002, she received the Diversity Leadership Award at Pace University. Dr. Jaffe-Ruiz received the University's Diversity Leadership Award in 2002 and the Martin Luther King Social Justice Award in 2006.

Vasupradha Vasudevan was a student cum Research Assistant at the MIS department at SUNY Buffalo, class of 2008. She holds a Bachelors in IT, Masters in MIS and has pursued research for 6 months as a Project Associate from IIT Madras, ending June 2010.

Index

U

UK National Health Service (NHS) 213, 214, 216
Unique Patient IDs (UPI) 191
United States 43, 46, 47, 48
U.S. Department of Veterans Affairs 153
U.S. nursing shortage 200

V

VeriChip 169, 170, 178

Veterans Administration (VA) healthcare system 27, 28
Voice biometric data analysis 161

W

Wellpoint Group Ltd. 67
Wellpoints 67, 68, 70, 71
World Privacy Forum (WPF) 116

Y

Y2K problem 7, 8, 20